CRASH COURSE
Obstetrics and Gynaecology
FIRST EDITION

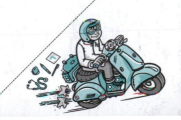

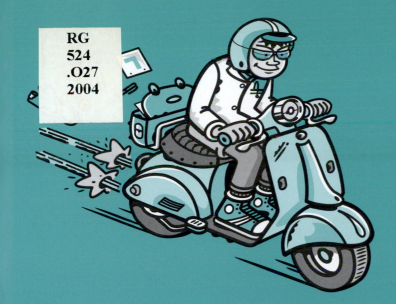

Series editor
Daniel Horton-Szar
BSC (Hons) MB BS (Hons)
GP Registrar
Northgate Medical Practice
Canterbury
Kent

Obstetrics and Gynaecology

FIRST EDITION

Nick Panay BSc MRCOG MFFP
Consultant Obstetrician & Gynaecologist, Hammersmith Hospitals NHS Trust, London

Ruma Dutta BSc MBBS MRCOG
Specialist Registrar in Obstetrics & Gynaecology, St George's Health Care NHS Trust, London

Audrey Ryan MBBS MRCOG
Specialist Registrar in Obstetrics & Gynaecology, Poole Hospital NHS Trust, Dorset

J A Mark Broadbent BSc FRCOG MFFP
Consultant Obstetrician & Gynaecologist, Barnet and Chase Farm NHS Trust, Hertfordshire

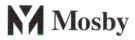 Mosby

Edinburgh • London • New York • Oxford • Philadelphia • St Louis • Sydney • Toronto 2004

MOSBY
An imprint of Elsevier Limited

Commissioning Editor	**Fiona Conn**
Project Development Manager	**Fiona Conn & The Partnership Publishing Solutions Ltd**
Project Manager	**Frances Affleck**
Designer	**Andy Chapman**
Illustration Management	**Bruce Hogarth**

First edition 2004

ISBN 0723431515

British Library Cataloguing in Publication Data
A catalogue record for this book is available from the British Library

Library of Congress Cataloging in Publication Data
A catalog record for this book is available from the Library of Congress

Note
Medical knowledge is constantly changing. Standard safety precautions must be followed, but as new research and clinical experience broaden our knowledge, changes in treatment and drug therapy may become necessary or appropriate. Readers are advised to check the most current product information provided by the manufacturer of each drug to be administered to verify the recommended dose, the method and duration of administration, and contraindications. It is the responsibility of the practitioner, relying on experience and knowledge of the patient, to determine dosages and the best treatment for each individual patient. Neither the Publisher nor the authors assumes any liability for any injury and/or damage to persons or property arising from this publication.

The Publisher

your source for books, journals and multimedia in the health sciences

www.elsevierhealth.com

The Publisher's policy is to use **paper manufactured from sustainable forests**

Printed in Spain

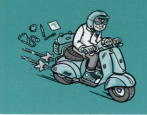

Preface

It is often difficult for medical students to develop a genuine understanding of the thought processes of practising obstetrics and gynaecology clinicians. Even the best-read student can find it difficult to relate the theory in standard reference textbooks to the day-to-day running of gynaecology clinics, emergency gynaecology units, antenatal clinics and the labour ward.

The aim of this book is to bring to life the theory of obstetrics and gynaecology in a succinct, practical way and to enable students to feel that they are learning as they would if they were closely involved with real-life case scenarios in the hospital setting. This has been made possible in two ways. First, the style of this Crash Course series is to deal initially with how patients might present to the clinician, before discussing the thought processes (through algorithms, diagrams and hints and tips) that lead to the instigation of appropriate investigations and eventual diagnosis and treatment. Second, the book is written not only by consultants but also by two specialist registrars who are currently 'at the coalface', thus helping to make the book entirely relevant from the point of view of modern, day-to-day practice.

The self-assessment section in the final part of the book allows you to test your newly acquired diagnostic skills and knowledge. Containing short answer questions, extended matching questions, patient management problem scenarios and multiple choice questions, it is entirely relevant to the way the contemporary medical student is assessed. This should provide you with the techniques and confidence that you will require to pass you examinations, so that you can put what you have learnt into practice!

Nick Panay BSc MRCOG MFFP

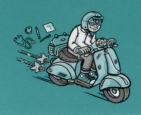

Preface

Over the last six years since the first editions were published, there have been many changes in medicine, and in the way it is taught. These second editions have been largely rewritten to take these changes into account, and keep *Crash Course* up to date for the twenty-first century. New material has been added to include recent research and all pharmacological and disease management information has been updated in line with current best practice. We've listened to feedback from hundreds of medical students who have been using *Crash Course* and have improved the structure and layout of the books accordingly: pathology and disease management material has been moved closer to the diagnostic skills chapters; there are more MCQs and now we have Extended Matching Questions as well, with explanations of each answer. We have also included 'Further Reading' sections where appropriate to highlight important papers and studies that you should be aware of, and the clarity of text and figures is better than ever.

The principles on which we developed the series remain the same, however. Clinical medicine is a huge subject, and teaching on the wards can sometimes be sporadic because of the competing demands of patient care. The last thing a student needs when finals are approaching is to waste time assembling information from different sources, or wading through pages of irrelevant detail. As before, *Crash Course* brings you all the information you need in compact, manageable volumes that integrate an approach to common patient presentations with clinical skills, pathology and management of the relevant diseases. We still tread the fine line between producing clear, concise text and providing enough detail for those aiming at distinction. The series is still written by junior doctors with recent exam experience, in partnership with senior faculty members from across the UK.

I wish you the best of luck in your future careers!

Dr Dan Horton-Szar
Series Editor

Dedications

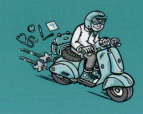

To Justine, Isabelle and Thomas for their unconditional love and incredible tolerance during the preparation of this book.   **NP**

To my dad, who would have been really proud to see my name in print, and to my mum who is. Also to Paul for his patience.   **RD**

To Rob, for reading the manuscript and for the many hours of baby-minding whilst this was being written, but also for his love, encouragement and support.   **AR**

Thanks to Mosby for their patience in putting up with the delays in preparing the text.   **MB**

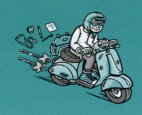

Contents

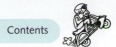

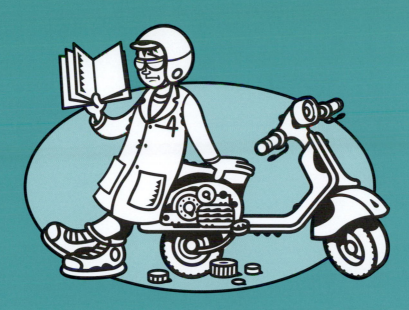

THE PATIENT PRESENTS WITH

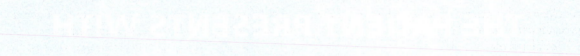

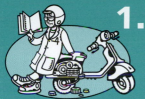

1. Abnormal Bleeding

Absent periods

The absence of periods is called amenorrhoea and can be either:

- primary, when menstruation has never occurred, or
- secondary, when menstruation has occurred but not for at least 6 months.

The causes of amenorrhoea can be broken down into the following five major categories, which are shown in greater detail in Fig. 1.1:

- Central nervous system.
- Gonadal dysfunction.
- Genital tract disorders.
- Endocrine disorders.
- Drug therapy.

A history of post-pill amenorrhoea is usually the result of pre-existing pathology that has been masked by the COCP.

History

There are so many causes of amenorrhoea that it is important to focus the history onto the relevant systems. These can be broadly grouped into five main areas:

- Gynaecological.
- Central nervous system.
- General health.
- Drugs.
- Endocrine disorders.

Gynaecological

A full gynaecological history is mandatory. By definition, menarche will not have occurred in women with primary amenorrhoea. In women with secondary amenorrhoea, the timing of menarche and pubertal development will establish whether this is normal, precocious or delayed (see Chapter 32). The duration of amenorrhoea and the presence of symptoms of pregnancy or the menopause should be noted (see Chapter 30).

Menstrual irregularity or oligomenorrhoea from the time of menarche can suggest polycystic ovary syndrome, especially if associated with obesity and hirsutism. Cyclical pain might indicate congenital or acquired outflow obstruction to menstrual fluid.

Pituitary failure can occur after massive postpartum haemorrhage (Sheehan's syndrome) and so a full obstetric history should be taken. This should include early pregnancy loss with subsequent uterine curettage, which can lead to Ashermann's syndrome. Relevant gynaecological surgery includes cervical surgery, which can cause stenosis and, more obviously, oophorectomy and hysterectomy.

Central nervous system

A past history of head injury or more recent symptoms of central nervous system (CNS) tumour such as headache and vomiting should be elicited. Visual field disturbance might indicate an expanding pituitary tumour and galactorrhoea could indicate hyperprolactinaemia.

General health

The general health of the patient should be assessed. Emotional stress, from any cause, can precipitate amenorrhoea, as can weight loss from dieting, anorexia nervosa or severe systemic illness. The reduced peripheral fat stores and body mass index (BMI) that are commonly seen in female athletes can cause amenorrhoea even though these women are fit and well.

Endocrine disorders

Thyroid disease and diabetes mellitus can present with amenorrhoea and symptoms of these disorders should be elicited. Hirsutism and virilism can be caused by congenital adrenal hyperplasia, polycystic ovary syndrome (PCOS) or an androgen-secreting tumour of the ovary or adrenal (see Chapter 32).

Drugs

Many prescribed drugs can cause amenorrhoea by producing either hyperprolactinaemia or ovarian

Causes of primary and secondary amenorrhoea	
Primary	**Secondary**
Central nervous system	*Central nervous system*
Hypothalamus:	Hypothalamus:
Kallmann's syndrome:	Kallmann's syndrome:
tumour/trauma	tumour/trauma
hypothalamic amenorrhoea:	hypothalamic amenorrhoea:
weight loss	weight loss
stress	stress
athleticism	athleticism
Pituitary:	Pituitary:
tumour necrosis (Sheehan's syndrome)	tumour necrosis (Sheehan's syndrome)
hyperprolactinaemia:	hyperprolactinaemia:
prolactin-secreting tumours	prolactin-secreting tumours
hypothyroidism	hypothyroidism
drugs	drugs
Gonads	*Gonads*
Streak gonads	Streak gonads (rarely)
Polycystic ovary syndrome:	Polycystic ovary syndrome:
hormone secreting tumour of ovary	hormone secreting tumour of ovary
androgen insensitivity	ovarian failure or removal
hermaphroditism	radiotherapy/chemotherapy
Uterus	*Uterus*
Pregnancy	Hysterectomy
Congenital absence	
Ashermann's syndrome	
Cervix	
Postsurgical stenosis	
Vagina	
Congenital absence	
Imperforate hymen	
Endocrine	*Endocrine*
Diabetes	Diabetes
Thyroid disease	Thyroid disease
Adrenal disease	Adrenal disease
Drugs	*Drugs*
Phenothiazines	Phenothiazines

Fig. 1.1 Causes of primary and secondary amenorrhoea.

failure, and a detailed drug history should be taken (see Chapter 32 for more details).

Examination

A general examination should be performed, with particular emphasis on signs of thyroid disease and diabetes mellitus. The BMI should be calculated (kg divided by m²). Anosmia (absent sense of smell) is associated with Kallmann's syndrome. The typical appearance of Turner's syndrome should be apparent; short stature, webbing of the neck, increased carrying angle at the elbow and coarctation of the aorta. The presence of galactorrhoea should be noted.

A full gynaecological examination is mandatory. Assessment of development of secondary sexual development must be made and Tanner's system can be used for this (see Fig. 1.2). Absent secondary sexual characteristics might constitute delayed puberty (see Chapter 32). Incongruous pubertal

Tanner staging of puberty					
Stage	**I**	**II**	**III**	**IV**	**V**
Breast	Pre-pubertal	Budding	Small adult breast	Areola and papilla form secondary mound	Adult breast
Pubic hair	Pre-pubertal	Sparse growth of slightly pigmented hair	Darker, coarser, begining to curl and spread over the symphysis	Hair has adult characteristics but not adult distribution	Adult

Fig. 1.2 Tanner staging of puberty

development might also suggest underlying pathology. For example, normal breast development in the presence of absent pubic or axillary hair is often found in women with androgen insensitivity. Poor breast development with normal pubic and axillary hair or hirsutism, virilism and obesity can be signs of raised circulating androgens secondary to PCOS, congenital adrenal hyperplasia (CAH), adrenal tumours or androgen-secreting ovarian tumours.

Pelvic examination should assess the patency of the vagina. If a haematocolpos is present it often causes a blue-coloured bulge at the introitus. An enlarged uterus might represent a pregnancy, and ovarian masses might be palpable.

Investigations

The following group of investigations should be performed as indicated:
- Chromosomal analysis.
- Hormone profiles.
- Imaging studies.

Chromosomal analysis

Chromosomal analysis should be performed on women with primary amenorrhoea where a chromosomal abnormality is suspected. Buccal smears or blood samples can be taken for this purpose.

Hormone profiles

The first hormone test to be performed is a urinary pregnancy test. This detects the presence of β-human chorionic gonadotrophin (hCG) and can be performed quickly in the outpatient setting.

Serum gonadotrophin levels are important. Levels of follicle stimulating hormone (FSH) and luteinizing hormone (LH) are raised with ovarian failure, and in 'hypothalamic' or hypogonadotrophic amenorrhoea the levels will be at the lower limits of normal (see

Chapter 32 for more details on hypogonadotrophic hypogonadism). In PCOS the LH:FSH ratio is usually greater than 2.5.

Serum prolactin levels should be checked to exclude hyperprolactinaemia. Thyroid stimulating hormone and free thyroxine levels should be tested if there is clinical suspicion of thyroid dysfunction or if hyperprolactinaemia is confirmed.

Serum testosterone levels might be normal or raised with PCOS, although free testosterone is usually raised. If serum testosterone levels are high then an androgen-secreting tumour of the ovary or adrenal should be suspected.

Imaging studies

An ultrasound scan of the pelvis should be performed. This will identify the typical ultrasound appearances of polycystic ovaries (enlarged ovaries with increased central stroma associated with multiple peripherally sited follicles). The presence of an intrauterine pregnancy, haematometra or haematocolpos should also be identified.

 A pelvic ultrasound scan (preferably performed vaginally) is virtually mandatory in the investigation of abnormal bleeding.

CNS tumours can be excluded by performing computed tomography (CT) or magnetic resonance imaging (MRI) scans of the head, and a lateral skull X-ray will identify pituitary fossa changes associated with an enlarging pituitary tumour.

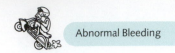
Causes of menorrhagia	
Types of cause	Specific of cause of menorrhagia
Systemic disorders	Thyroid disease
	Clotting disorders
Local causes	Fibroids
	Endometrial polyps
	Endometrial carcinoma
	Endometriosis/adenomyosis
	Pelvic inflammatory disease
	Dysfunctional uterine bleeding
Iatrogenic causes	Intrauterine contraceptive devices
	Oral anticoagulants

Fig. 1.3 Causes of menorrhagia.

Heavy periods

Heavy periods are a common gynaecological complaint. Only about half of women complaining of heavy periods actually have menorrhagia, which is defined as more than 80 mL of menstrual blood loss per period. Both local and systemic conditions can cause menorrhagia (Fig. 1.3).

History

A full gynaecological history should be taken. Particular emphasis should be made as to the pattern of menstruation: irregular menstruation implies the possibility of anovulation. Subjective assessment of menstrual flow does not correlate well with objective menstrual loss. However, the presence of clots and flooding, wearing double protection (internal and external), nocturnal soiling and interference with work or social events, all imply increased menstrual loss. Symptoms of iron deficiency anaemia might be present, including lethargy and breathlessness.

Menstrual pain, or dysmenorrhoea, is often associated with menorrhagia and it is usually experienced when the flow is heaviest. Premenstrual pain can indicate endometriosis, which is discussed further in Chapter 21. Fever, pelvic pain, dyspareunia and vaginal discharge are common symptoms of pelvic inflammatory disease (PID; see Chapter 25).

A history of PCOS increases the risk of endometrial hyperplasia and carcinoma. Symptoms of thyroid disease or clotting disorders can indicate a systemic cause of menorrhagia. Clotting disorders presenting with menorrhagia usually do so in the teenage years.

A contraceptive history is important. Recent cessation of the combined oral contraceptive pill (COCP) might indicate menstrual intolerance (the return of normal periods that appear heavier than the withdrawal bleeds associated with the COCP). Symptoms of heavy or painful periods dating from the insertion of an intrauterine contraceptive device (IUCD) would suggest that this is the cause.

Examination

General examination should be aimed at identifying signs of iron deficiency anaemia, thyroid or clotting disorders. Abdominal examination might reveal a mass arising from the pelvis.

Speculum examination could reveal vaginal discharge and cervical pathology, including cervicitis or frank malignancy. Occasionally, endometrial polyps or pedunculated fibroids will be seen prolapsing through the cervical os. Bimanual examination might reveal an enlarged uterus due to fibroids, pelvic tenderness associated with endometriosis or PID and any adnexal masses.

Investigation

Investigation is aimed at excluding the systemic and local causes of menorrhagia and includes:

- Blood tests.
- Ultrasound.
- Hysteroscopy.

A full blood count should be performed in all cases. Thyroid function and clotting studies should only be performed if clinically indicated.

A pelvic ultrasound will identify uterine enlargement caused by fibroids and adnexal masses. Endometrial polyps or submucous fibroids should be suspected if the endometrial thickness is excessive.

An endometrial biopsy should be performed, either in the outpatient clinic or at the same time as hysteroscopy. This might show endometrium inappropriate to the menstrual cycle secondary to anovulation, endometrial hyperplasia or carcinoma. A cervical smear should be performed if indicated.

Abnormal bleeding before the age of 40 does not usually require endometrial sampling.

Causes of intermenstrual and postcoital bleeding	
Affected region/system	**Specific cause**
Cervical	Ectopy
	Polyps
	Malignancy
	Cervicitis
Intra-uterine	Polyps
	Submucous fibroids
	Endometrial hyperplasia
	Endometrial malignancy
	Endometritis
Hormonal	Breakthrough bleeding

Fig. 1.4 Causes of intermenstrual and postcoital bleeding.

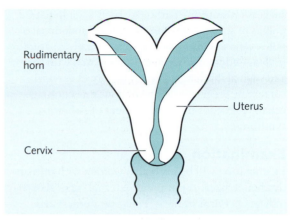

Fig. 1.5 A rudimentary uterine horn.

The most effective way of excluding intrauterine pathology is by diagnostic hysteroscopy. This can be performed in the outpatient setting with minimal analgesia and will identify endometrial polyps and submucous fibroids.

Intermenstrual and postcoital bleeding

Intermenstrual and postcoital bleeding are common symptoms that can indicate serious underlying pathology. Intermenstrual bleeding occurs between the menstrual periods and can be caused by local lesions of the cervix or intrauterine cavity (Fig. 1.4). Postcoital bleeding is precipitated by intercourse and is caused by similar conditions. Investigation should aim to exclude local causes for menorrhagia.

Painful periods

Pain associated with menstruation is called dysmenorrhoea and can be either primary or secondary. There are two definitions of primary and secondary dysmenorrhoea:
- Primary dysmenorrhoea occurs from menarche, whereas secondary dysmenorrhoea occurs in women who previously had normal periods.
- Primary dysmenorrhoea occurs from menarche but secondary dysmenorrhoea describes painful periods that are caused by, or are 'secondary' to, pathology.

Causes of secondary dysmenorrhoea	
Affected region/structure	**Cause of secondary dysmenorrhoea**
Uterine	Fibroids
	Endometrial polyps
	Ashermann's syndrome
	Infection
Cervical	Stenosis
Pelvic	Pelvic inflammatory disease
	Endometriosis

Fig. 1.6 Causes of secondary dysmenorrhoea.

Severe primary dysmenorrhoea occurs in up to 10% of women. The cause is not well understood but prostaglandins, which can cause uterine contractions and vasoconstriction, have been implicated. Rarely, primary dysmenorrhoea can be caused by a particular Mullerian abnormality whereby a rudimentary, functioning uterine horn does not connect with the vagina (Fig. 1.5).

Secondary dysmenorrhoea can be caused by conditions occurring in the uterus, cervix and the pelvis (Fig. 1.6).

History
Dysmenorrhoea is usually described as cramping pain that often radiates into the back or the upper thighs. Primary dysmenorrhoea presents in young women in their early teens and usually starts within the first year of menarche as ovulation is established. There is often a family history.

Women with secondary dysmenorrhoea will previously have had normal periods; pain develops or worsens at a later date. Menstrual irregularity can suggest intrauterine pathology such as endometrial polyps or submucous fibroids. Lower abdominal or pelvic pain and dyspareunia suggests pelvic pathology such as endometriosis, and, if associated with fever and vaginal discharge, PID. A history of cervical surgery or pregnancy associated uterine curettage usually precedes the development of Asherman's syndrome.

Examination

Examination will be normal in women with primary dysmenorrhoea. A pin-point external cervical os may indicate cervical stenosis. Pelvic tenderness and cervical excitation pain are usually present in the presence of pelvic pathology.

Investigation

A young woman presenting with primary dysmenorrhoea who has a normal pelvic examination does not usually require any further investigation. Suitable investigations for secondary dysmenorrhoea include:

- Hysteroscopy, to exclude intrauterine pathology including adhesions.
- Laparoscopy, to exclude pelvic pathology.
- Pelvic ultrasound scan, which can identify uterine fibroids; an increased endometrial thickness is suggestive of intrauterine pathology.
- Microbiological swabs to identify infection, especially *Chlamydia*.

Treatment

Primary dysmenorrhoea is nearly always associated with ovulatory cycles and abolition of ovulation using the COCP often improves dysmenorrhoea. Non-hormonal medical treatment includes simple analgesia and the non-steroidal anti-inflammatory drugs (prostaglandin synthetase inhibitors). A rudimentary horn might require surgical excision.

Submucous fibroids, endometrial polyps and uterine adhesions can be treated using operative hysteroscopy techniques. Open myomectomy might be required for larger fibroids, especially in women who wish to conserve their uterus. The treatment of PID and endometriosis is discussed in Chapters 25 and 21, respectively.

Postmenopausal bleeding

Vaginal bleeding more than 6 months after the menopause is called postmenopausal bleeding

Causes of postmenopausal bleeding	
Affected structure	**Cause of postmenopausal bleeding**
Ovary	Carcinoma of the ovary
	Oestrogen-secreting tumour
Uterine body	Myometrium:
	submucous fibroid
	Endometrium:
	atrophic changes
	polyp
	hyperplasia: simple or atypical
	carcinoma
Cervix	Atrophic changes
	Malignancy:
	squamous carcinoma
	adenocarcinoma
Vagina	Atrophic changes
Urethra	Urethral caruncle
	Haematuria
Vulva	Vulvitis
	Dystrophies
	Malignancy

Fig. 1.7 Causes of postmenopausal bleeding.

(PMB). This is a common condition and should be investigated promptly because it could indicate the presence of malignancy.

Figure 1.7 shows the causes of PMB using the anatomy of the female genital tract as a guide. There are many causes of PMB and using this method will help to remember them all. Atrophic changes to the genital tract are the most common cause but must not be assumed to be the cause until other pathology, especially malignancy, has been excluded.

Figure 1.8 provides an algorithm for the diagnosis and investigation of abnormal uterine bleeding.

History

Atrophic changes to the genital tract – the most common cause of PMB – usually present with small amounts of bleeding. Local symptoms of oestrogen deficiency include vaginal dryness, soreness and superficial dyspareunia. Pruritus vulvae can indicate the presence of non-neoplastic disorders of the vulva (traditionally known as vulval dystrophies) and the presence of a lump, whether painful or painless, can suggest a vulval neoplasm.

Profuse or continuous vaginal bleeding or the presence of a bloodstained offensive discharge is an ominous sign and can indicate cervical or endometrial malignancy. PMB is usually the only presenting symptom of other endometrial cavity pathology, such as endometrial polyps or submucous fibroids.

Fig. 1.8 Algorithm for abnormal uterine bleeding.

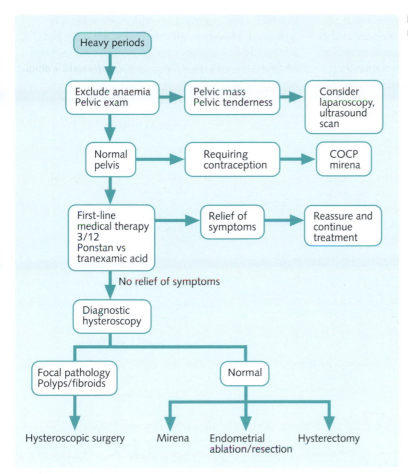

Early ovarian malignancy can be asymptomatic or present with non-specific upper abdominal symptoms such as epigastric discomfort or indigestion. Advanced ovarian malignancy can produce pelvic or abdominal pain and abdominal distension due to ascites.

Examination

A full gynaecological examination should be performed. Abdominal examination might reveal ascites or a mass arising from the pelvis. Vulval lesions should be evident on examination. The vagina and cervix should be inspected using a speculum and a bimanual examination performed. Postmenopausal ovaries should not be palpable on bimanual examination.

Investigation

The following investigations should be performed on all women with PMB:

- Ultrasound examination of the pelvis.
- Hysteroscopic examination of the uterine cavity.
- Endometrial biopsy.

Hysteroscopy will identify the presence of intrauterine pathology and can be performed without general anaesthesia in the outpatient setting. An alternative to hysteroscopy is ultrasound scanning to assess the endometrial thickness combined with endometrial sampling (discussed further in Chapter 19). Ultrasound is also used to assess the ovaries.

When indicated the following investigations should also be performed:
- Vulval biopsies.
- Cervical cytology or colposcopy.
- Cystoscopy.
- Sigmoidoscopy.
- Oestradiol levels.

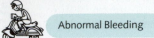
Occasionally, it is not always obvious whether the bleeding is vaginal, rectal or from the bladder, and in these cases cystoscopy and sigmoidoscopy as well as hysteroscopy should be performed. In the very elderly, bimanual examination might not be possible, in which case examination under anaesthesia is indicated. However, elderly frail women are not always ideal candidates for general anaesthesia and less invasive investigations, such as ultrasound, might have to be relied upon.

2. Pelvic Pain and Dyspareunia

Differential diagnosis

Pelvic pain, as for any type of pain, can be either:
- Acute, or
- chronic.

Chronic pelvic pain is often associated with 'dyspareunia', the term used to describe painful sexual intercourse. This is classified as superficial or deep, depending on whether it is experienced superficially at the area of the vulva and introitus or deep within the pelvis.

Figures 2.1 and 2.2 show the differential diagnoses that should be considered when the patient presents with these symptoms.

History to focus on the differential diagnosis of pelvic pain and dyspareunia

Because the differential diagnosis is so diverse, a thorough history is important.

Presenting complaint

A detailed history of the pain is essential to distinguish between pain of acute onset and chronic pain. The following characteristics should be elicited:
- Whether the pain is continuous or intermittent.
- The duration of the pain.
- The nature of the pain – whether it is sharp or dull.
- The position of the pain – is it unilateral or bilateral?
- The relation of the pain to the menstrual cycle.
- Its relation to bowel habit.
- Radiation of the pain to the back or the legs.
- Associated symptoms, such as nausea and vomiting, vaginal discharge, vulval irritation.

For example, the pain related to torsion of an ovarian cyst is typically of acute onset, worse on one side of the pelvis than the other, associated with nausea and vomiting, and radiating to the upper thighs. It is important to make this diagnosis promptly because an operation to relieve the torsion might save the ovary from irreversible ischaemia.

Mittelschmerz is an acute pain associated with ovulation. To make this diagnosis, it is therefore essential to know the timing of the pain in relation to the patient's menstrual cycle. Endometriosis is also related to menses, typically starting up to 2 weeks before the period and usually being relieved when the bleeding starts (also known as secondary dysmenorrhoea). Deep dyspareunia is commonly associated with this condition.

PID may or may not be associated with vaginal discharge. The pain is typically felt across the whole of the lower abdomen and there might be a history of fever.

In relation to bowel habit, appendicitis can be associated with nausea and vomiting, whereas diverticulitis is more likely to be associated with constipation and affect the older population.

Past gynaecological history

The date of the patient's last menstrual period (LMP) is important to exclude current pregnancy and the possibility of a miscarriage or ectopic pregnancy. The date and result of the last cervical smear test should also be checked, as well as a history of irregular or postcoital bleeding, which might be associated with malignancy.

The LMP could also be relevant if the patient has symptoms suggesting perimenopausal changes.

Recent gynaecological procedures that involve instrumentation of the uterus could put the patient at risk of developing PID (e.g. insertion of an IUCD, termination of pregnancy or hysteroscopy).

Previous PID or gynaecological surgery could have resulted in adhesion formation. This is more likely to result in a picture of chronic pain, and can be difficult to treat. Pelvic floor repair can alter the vagina in such a way as to cause deep dyspareunia. Recent childbirth is a common cause of superficial dyspareunia, particularly if suturing of vaginal lacerations or episiotomy was necessary.

Congenital malformations of the genital tract are rare and are likely to present before the patient is sexually active and experiencing dyspareunia. There might be a history of previous operations to restore normal anatomy.

Differential diagnosis of pelvic pain	
Acute	**Chronic**
Pelvic inflammatory disease (see Chapter 25) sexually transmitted infection Tubo-ovarian abscess post-termination of pregnancy post-insertion of IUCD post-hysteroscopy	Adenomyosis (see Chapter 21) Endometriosis
	Adhesions secondary to: gynaecological operation pelvic inflammatory disease appendicitis
Early pregnancy complications (see Chapter 29) miscarriage ectopic pregnancy	
Gynaecological malignancy (see Chapter 23)	
Ovarian cyst (see Chapter 22) rupture haemorrhage torsion	Gastrointestinal pathology diverticulitis irritable bowel syndrome
Fibroid necrosis (see Chapter 20)	
Ovulation pain (Mittelschmerz)	
Abscesses Bartholin's cyst labial	
Urinary tract infection Renal calculi	
Appendicitis	

Fig. 2.1 Differential diagnosis of pelvic pain.

Differential diagnosis of dyspareunia	
Superficial	**Deep**
Congenital vaginal atresia vaginal septum	Congenital incomplete vaginal atresia vaginal septum
Infection vulvovaginitis (see Chapter 3)	Infection PID (see Chapter 25)
Postsurgery relating to childbirth pelvic floor repair	Postsurgery relating to childbirth pelvic floor repair
Vulval disease Bartholin's cyst vulval dystrophies carcinoma of vulva	Pelvic disease endometriosis fibroids ovarian cyst / tumours
Psychosexual vaginismus	Psychosexual vaginismus
Atrophic changes postmenopausal	

Fig. 2.2 Differential diagnosis of dyspareunia.

Past medical/surgical history

A history of appendicectomy excludes one of the common differential diagnoses of pelvic pain.

Drug history

A postmenopausal patient who has not been using hormone replacement therapy might have superficial dyspareunia secondary to atrophic changes.

Sexual history

Current use of contraception must be checked, both to exclude pregnancy and to determine the risk of PID. A recent change of partner, particularly if no barrier contraception has been used, increases the risk.

With regards to dyspareunia, there might be a history of difficulty with intercourse, suggesting vaginismus. This might be a difficult subject for the patient and care should be taken to broach it in a sympathetic manner.

Social history

A useful guide to the severity of symptoms in patients presenting with chronic pelvic pain is how it affects their normal life, for example, going to school or taking time off work.

A history of sexual abuse has been shown to be relevant to presentation with chronic pain. Again, a sensitive approach is essential in questioning.

Examination of patients with pelvic pain and dyspareunia

- General examination.
- Abdominal palpation.
- Vulval/vaginal/cervical inspection.
- Bimanual pelvic examination.

General examination

Pyrexia and tachycardia are associated with PID. Rupture of an ovarian cyst can cause intraperitoneal bleeding and, subsequently, hypotension with tachycardia. A ruptured ectopic pregnancy would also present with these signs. It should be noted that hypotension is a late sign and its absence does not exclude these diagnoses.

Gynaecological malignancy is more likely to present with symptoms other than pelvic pain, more commonly in the older age group. However, signs such as cachexia and anaemia should be excluded.

Abdominal palpation

The site of the pain should be elicited, as should the presence of guarding or rebound tenderness, which suggest peritonism. An abdominal mass arising from the pelvis, such as an enlarged fibroid uterus, might be present. This could give symptoms of deep dyspareunia or of acute pelvic pain, if there is fibroid necrosis.

Vulval/vaginal/cervical inspection

Figure 2.3 shows the diagnoses responsible for both pelvic pain and superficial dyspareunia that might affect the vulva and vagina. A speculum examination should be performed to look for discharge.

Bimanual pelvic examination
Tenderness

Generalized tenderness, including uterine, is more common with PID. This condition is also associated with cervical excitation. The tenderness may be unilateral with an ovarian cyst or an ectopic pregnancy. A common site for endometriosis is the pouch of Douglas, and tender nodules can be palpated in the posterior fornix.

A pregnancy test to exclude an ectopic pregnancy is mandatory in a patient of reproductive age who presents with acute abdominal pain. This is essential even if the symptoms suggest a gastrointestinal cause rather than a gynaecological one, because the presentation of ectopic pregnancy can be atypical.

Mass

The following conditions may present with a pelvic mass:
- Tubo-ovarian abscess.
- Ovarian cyst.
- Endometriotic cyst.
- Fibroid.
- Ectopic pregnancy.

The uterus is enlarged in pregnancy and the cervical os might be open if the patient is miscarrying. A

Vulval/vaginal inspection	
Symptom	**Cause(s)**
Postmenopausal changes (see Chapter 30)	Vulval and vaginal skin appears thin and atrophic. This can cause superficial dyspareunia
Vulval dystrophies (see Chapter 24)	There might be patches of inflammation, leukoplakia and ulceration, which cause superficial dyspareunia
Episiotomy/lacerations (see Chapter 41)	Injury secondary to childbirth commonly causes superficial dyspareunia
Abscesses	A Bartholin's abscess is an abscess of the gland situated towards the posterior fourchette; labial abscesses are commonly situated on the labia majora. Both types cause acute pain and need incision and drainage

Fig. 2.3 Vulval/vaginal inspection.

fixed, tender, retroverted uterus could be a result of endometriosis or PID. The uterus typically feels tender and bulky with adenomyosis.

Investigations of patients who have pelvic pain and dyspareunia

A summary list of the investigations used in patients who present with pelvic pain and dyspareunia is shown in Fig. 2.4. Figure 2.5 is an algorithm for the diagnosis, investigation and treatment of pelvic pain; Fig. 2.6 provides the same information for dyspareunia.

Blood tests

A full blood count (to check haemoglobin) and group-and-save sample are necessary if there is an early pregnancy complication with bleeding from the vagina or intraperitoneal bleeding.

A white blood cell count and a C-reactive protein (CRP) level will aid diagnosis of infection, along with the clinical signs.

A serum hCG or urine pregnancy test is done to exclude early pregnancy complications. This is mandatory in any patient of reproductive age who presents with acute pelvic pain, to exclude a potentially fatal ectopic pregnancy.

Infection screen

A midstream urine (MSU) sample should be sent to exclude a urinary tract infection. Swabs should be sent to check for PID, as listed in Fig. 2.4, most importantly including an endocervical swab to confirm *Chlamydia* infection.

Investigation of patients who have pelvic pain and dyspareunia	
Investigation	**Procedure**
Blood tests	FBC G&S CRP hCG
Infection screen	Midstream urine sample Vulval/high vaginal swabs Endocervical/urethral swabs
Radiological investigations	Pelvic ultrasound scan Abdominal X-ray
Biopsy for vulval disease	
Laparoscopy to check for: endometriosis ovarian cyst ectopic pregnancy adhesions PID	

Fig. 2.4 Investigation of patients who have pelvic pain and dyspareunia.

Even with a chronic pain history as opposed to an acute one, it is still appropriate to take swabs for sexually transmitted infections.

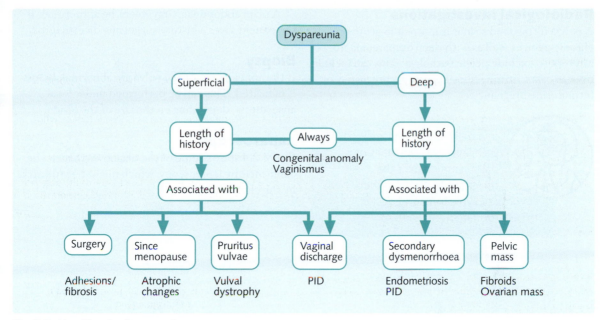

Fig. 2.5 Algorithm for dyspareunia.

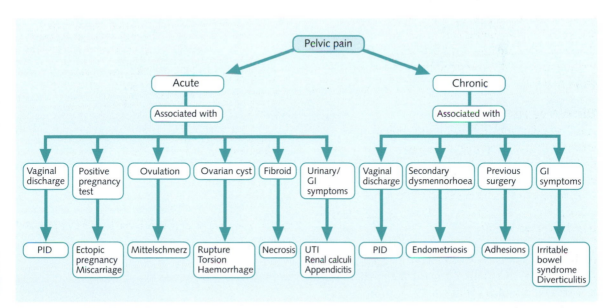

Fig. 2.6 Algorithm for pelvic pain.

Radiological investigations

A pelvic ultrasound scan is important in acute or chronic pain, as well as with deep dyspareunia, to attempt to exclude pelvic pathology. This can include ovarian cysts, uterine fibroids, ectopic pregnancy or intrauterine pregnancy.

In a patient with chronic pain, assessing activities of daily living enables the physician to establish the severity of symptoms and decide on appropriate management.

A plain abdominal X-ray might be appropriate if the patient gives a history suggesting diverticulitis.

Biopsy

If the appearances of the vulva are abnormal, biopsy is indicated. This can be performed under local anaesthesia, depending on the size of the lesion.

Laparoscopy

Figure 2.4 shows some of the diagnoses that can be confirmed by laparoscopy, which might be indicated by the clinical picture.

3. Vaginal Discharge

Differential diagnosis

Vaginal discharge can be either:

- Physiological, or
- pathological.

Physiological discharge varies with the changing oestrogen levels associated with the menstrual cycle and pregnancy. The diagnosis is usually one of exclusion, that is, pathological causes need to be excluded. Then the patient can be reassured that her symptoms are normal. Possible causes of physiological vaginal discharge are:

- Vestibular gland secretions.
- Vaginal transudate.
- Cervical mucus.
- Residual menstrual fluid.

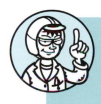 Don't forget that vaginal discharge might simply be physiological, related to the menstrual cycle or to pregnancy.

The differential diagnoses of pathological vaginal discharge are shown in Fig. 3.1. The most common group is the infections.

History to focus on the differential diagnosis of vaginal discharge

The patient should be asked about the nature of the discharge. This includes:

- Timing of onset.
- Colour.
- Odour.
- Presence of any blood.
- Irritation.

For example, candidal infection is associated with a thick, itchy, white discharge, whereas with bacterial vaginosis there is typically a grey, fishy-smelling discharge. An allergic reaction is usually associated with itching. Urinary symptoms, such as dysuria and frequency, might be present with a sexually transmitted infection.

Lower abdominal pain, backache and dyspareunia are suggestive of PID (see Chapter 25), more commonly in a younger woman. In relation to malignancy, the patient age group is usually older than the infective group (see Chapter 23). General symptoms such as weight loss and anorexia should be excluded.

Past gynaecological history

The date of the menopause and the last cervical smear test are relevant, particularly if malignancy is suspected.

A ring pessary might previously have been sited to relieve genital prolapse (see Chapter 27). This should be changed every 6 months. Previous history of hysterectomy could be linked with development of a uretero- or vesicovaginal fistula. This results in constant vaginal loss that is actually urine. A history of obstructed labour, more common in developing countries, also puts the patient at risk of a vesicovaginal fistula.

Past medical history

A history of diabetes mellitus predisposes the patient to candidal infection.

 Generalized symptoms can be indicative of different pathologies, depending on the age of the patient. Lower abdominal pain, backache and dyspareunia suggest infection in a younger woman but malignancy in older age groups.

Sexual history

The patient's current method of contraception is important with regards to the risk of a sexually transmitted infection, as is a recent new partner.

Drug history

Recent antibiotic therapy can precipitate candidal infection.

Differential diagnosis of pathological vaginal discharge	
Diagnosis	**Cause of discharge**
Infective	Sexually transmitted infection *Chlamydia trachomatis* *Trichomonas vaginalis* *Neisseria gonorrhoea* Infection not sexually transmitted *Candida albicans* Bacterial vaginosis
Inflammatory	Allergy to soap/contraceptives etc Atrophic changes Postoperative granulation tissue
Malignancy	Vulval carcinoma Cervical carcinoma Uterine carcinoma
Foreign body	Retained tampon/condom Ring pessaries
Fistula	From bowel, bladder and ureter to vagina

Fig. 3.1 Differential diagnosis of pathological vaginal discharge.

Investigations for vaginal discharge	
Investigation	**Cause of discharge**
Microbiological swabs	Vulval/high vaginal swab (HVS) *Candida albicans* *Trichomonas vaginalis* Endocervical/urethral swab *Chlamydia trachomatis* *Neiserria gonorrhoea*
Midstream urine specimen	Infection
Cervical cytology	Cervical disease
Endometrial sampling/ hysteroscopy	Uterine disease
Pelvic ultrasound scan	Pelvic mass
Laparoscopy	Pelvic inflammatory disease Pelvic malignancy

Fig. 3.2 Investigations for vaginal discharge.

Examination of patients with vaginal discharge

- General examination.
- Abdominal palpation.
- Speculum examination.
- Bimanual palpation.

General examination should be aimed at identifying signs of systemic infection (tachycardia, pyrexia, local lymphadenopathy) or malignancy (cachexia, generalized lymphadenopathy).

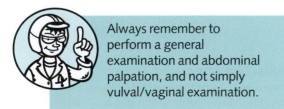

Always remember to perform a general examination and abdominal palpation, and not simply vulval/vaginal examination.

Abdominal palpation should exclude any localized tenderness, which may be present if the patient is developing PID, or an abdominal mass if malignancy is suspected.

The vulva and vagina should be inspected carefully and a speculum examination should be performed to check the cervix and to confirm or exclude:
- Vaginal discharge.
- Inflammation.
- Ulceration.
- Foreign bodies.
- Local tumours.

Bimanual pelvic examination will reveal pelvic tumours. It might also elicit tenderness and cervical excitation, suggesting PID.

Investigation of patients with vaginal discharge

- Microbiological swabs vulval/high vaginal/endocervical/urethral.
- MSU specimen.
- Cervical cytology/biopsy.
- Endometrial sampling/hysteroscopy.
- Pelvic ultrasound scan.
- Laparoscopy.

Figure 3.2 shows the relevant investigations for vaginal discharge. Figure 3.3 is an algorithm for the diagnosis and investigation of vaginal discharge.

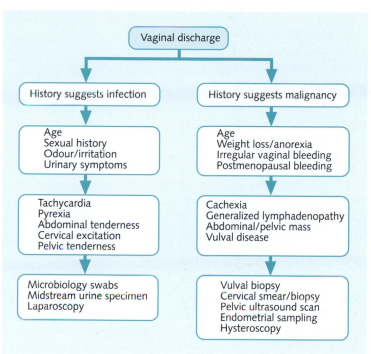

Fig. 3.3 Algorithm for vaginal discharge.

4. Vulval Symptoms

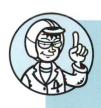

Itching or irritation of the vulval region is called pruritus vulvae. This debilitating and socially embarrassing symptom is common and can be caused by a whole host of conditions. These are grouped into four broad categories (Fig. 4.1):
• Infection.
• Vulval dystrophy.
• Neoplastic.
• Dermatological.

> Symptoms complained of in the vulval area might be due to a generalized skin problem or to systemic illness.

History

The age of the patient is important because younger women are generally more likely to have an infectious aetiology, and vulval dystrophies (more correctly termed non-neoplastic epithelial disorders of the vulva) and neoplasms are more likely in older women. Acute onset of symptoms occurs frequently with infection whereas other causes of pruritus vulvae can have a more chronic and insidious onset. Embarrassment often delays presentation. A history of postmenopausal bleeding is important.

Exacerbating and relieving factors can give clues as to the aetiology. Symptoms of yeast and herpetic infection might worsen premenstrually. A recent change in soap or washing powder, or overzealous hygiene can suggest a contact dermatitis. Self-treatment with emollients and antifungals is common and should be noted, as should the response.

Cervical intraepithelial neoplasia (CIN) and vulval intraepithelial neoplasia (VIN) are thought to share a common aetiology, so a history of CIN should be noted. Abnormal vaginal discharge can suggest infection and, if suspected, a detailed sexual history should be taken. The discharge of infection with

Trichomonas vaginalis and bacterial vaginosis has a typically 'fishy' odour.

Dermatological conditions such as psoriasis and eczema can affect the vulva and a history of these conditions elsewhere on the body might be relevant. Symptoms suggestive of diabetes mellitus, renal and liver failure should be noted.

Examination

General examination of the patient includes assessment of skin surfaces prone to dermatological conditions: face, hands, wrists, elbows, trunk and knees. Signs of chronic renal failure and liver disease should be looked for.

Examination of the vulva, urethral meatus and perianal region in a good light is essential. The vagina and cervix should be inspected carefully with the aid of a speculum. Colposcopic examination of the vulva might be useful if no apparent lesion can be seen with the naked eye and to perform directed biopsies. Inguinal lymphadenopathy can occur secondary to infection or malignancy.

> Even if no lesion is seen it might still be prudent to perform colposcopic examination of the area and take biopsies.

Infection
Generalized vulvitis, vaginal discharge and ulcers suggest an infective cause, although ulceration should alert the examiner to the possibility of malignancy. Genital warts might be seen on the vulva, perianally, in the vagina or on the cervix.

Vulval dystrophies
Labial fusion, adhesions, stenosis of the introitus, leucoplakia (literally meaning 'white plaque') and atrophic changes are frequent signs of lichen

Differential diagnosis of pruritus vulvae

Type of cause	Description
Infection	Fungal
	Candida
	Tinea
	Parasitic
	Trichomonas vaginalis
	Enterobius (pinworm)
	Pediculosis pubis
	Bacterial
	Bacterial vaginosis /vaginitis
	Viral
	Herpes simplex virus
	Human papilloma virus
Vulval dystrophy	Lichen sclerosis
	Hypertrlphic vulval dystrophy
Neoplastic	Vulval intraepithelial neoplasia (VIN)
	Squamous carcinoma
	Paget's disease of the vulva
Dermatological	Psoriasis
	Eczema
	Contact dermatitis

Fig. 4.1 Differential diagnosis of pruritus vulvae.

sclerosis, the most common of the vulval dystrophies. The lesions of hyperplastic dystrophy can be localized or extensive, and typically show thickening of the affected skin with variable colour change. Thickened plaques of leucoplakia might be present.

Neoplasia

VIN lesions are variable and can be papular (similar to genital warts) or macular with irregular borders.

Pigmentation (brown or black) is common and leucoplakia and ulceration can occur. Invasive squamous carcinoma of the vulva usually appears as an exophytic tumour, often with surface ulceration. Paget's disease of the vulva can be unifocal or multifocal and the lesions are typically clearly defined, scaly, erythematous plaques with varying degrees of ulceration and leucoplakia.

If no physical cause is found for vulval symptoms there might be a psychosomatic problem.

Dermatological

Psoriasis might appear as the typical scaly plaques but it can also be smooth, erythematous and fissured.

Investigating pruritus vulvae

Where systemic disease is suspected, relevant testing should include liver function, renal function and glucose tolerance. Urinalysis might reveal the presence of haematuria, proteinurea and glycosuria.

The relevant bacteriological swabs should be performed to exclude yeast infection (Fig. 4.2) and sexually active women should be screened for sexually transmitted diseases. Pinworms might be identified by naked-eye visualization of the adult female worms in the perianal region or by microscopic identification of the ova.

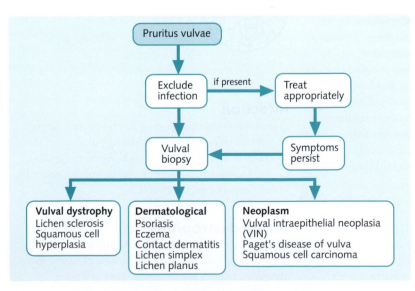
Fig. 4.2 Algorithm for pruritus vulvae.

Although certain conditions of the vulva have a typical appearance, many are difficult to distinguish with the naked eye. The mainstay of diagnosis of vulval dystrophies, dermatoses and neoplasms is histological. Punch biopsies of the vulva can be performed under local anaesthetic in the outpatient setting, with or without the aid of a colposcope. Discrete lesions can be excised in their entirety, as excision biopsies under general anaesthesia. Hysteroscopy or dilatation and curettage (D&C) is indicated to exclude endometrial pathology when postmenopausal bleeding has occurred.

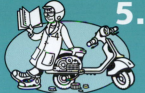

5. Urinary Incontinence

Urinary incontinence is an objectively demonstrable involuntary loss of urine that is a social or hygienic problem. The two most common causes of urinary incontinence are genuine stress incontinence (GSI) and detrusor overactivity (DO), which account for approximately 90% of incontinent women. These, and other causes, are shown in Fig. 5.1 in order of frequency of occurrence.

History

A detailed history is mandatory because of the presence of multiple symptoms that are not always apparent on cursory questioning. The two symptoms stress incontinence and urge incontinence are commonly used synonymously with the conditions GSI and DO, respectively (see Fig. 5.2 for definitions of common urogynaecological terms). This is inaccurate and can lead to inappropriate treatment because many incontinent women will admit to both symptoms, although in only 5% of women will GSI and DO coexist.

A patient who gives a history of stress incontinence might still have detrusor instability.

Genuine stress incontinence

The most common symptom of GSI is stress incontinence, usually small amounts of urinary leakage. However, one-third of women with GSI will also admit to urge incontinence and up to a half will experience urgency of micturition. Frequency of micturition and nocturia are also common symptoms.

GSI is associated with the following factors and these must be highlighted in the history:

- Increasing age.
- Increasing parity.
- Genital prolapse.
- Postmenopausal status.
- Previous pelvic floor surgery.

Detrusor overactivity

The vast majority of women with DO will complain of urgency, urge incontinence, frequency and nocturia. However, up to one-quarter might complain of stress incontinence because raised intra-abdominal pressure can stimulate an unstable bladder to contract and produce the symptom of stress incontinence.

The following factors should be highlighted in the history:

- Age.
- History of nocturnal enuresis.
- Neurological history.
- Previous incontinence surgery.
- Drug history.

Sensory urgency

Sensory urgency differs from detrusor overactivity (motor urgency) in that the urgency occurs in the absence of detrusor activity. The presenting symptoms are the same as for detrusor overactivity although incontinence is not such a common feature.

Voiding disorders

Voiding disorders can result in chronic retention leading to overflow incontinence. As well as urgency and frequency, the classic symptoms of 'prostatism' might be present: hesitancy, straining to void, poor flow and incomplete emptying. Large residual volumes of urine due to incomplete emptying predispose to urinary tract infection, which aggravates the symptoms of incontinence, urgency and frequency. Stress incontinence might be a presenting symptom.

Fistulae

Fistulae are very rare in the UK but should always be suspected when incontinence is continuous during the day and at night.

Examination

Chronic dampness can cause excoriation of the vulva. The best way to demonstrate stress incontinence is to ask the patient to cough while standing with a moderately full bladder. Stress incontinence is not always demonstrable, especially with the patient in the supine position. Examination of the vaginal walls, using a Sims' speculum, will identify scarring from previous surgery and the presence of uterovaginal prolapse; especially important is a cysto-urethrocele. Bimanual examination should identify a pelvic mass.

As neurological disease can present with urinary symptoms, including incontinence, a neurological examination should be performed.

A neurological examination should always be carried out to exclude this cause for the incontinence problems.

Investigations

As suggested above, the bladder is an 'unreliable witness' and judicious investigation is important if inappropriate treatment is to be avoided. It is essential to exclude a urinary tract infection (UTI), a common cause of sensory urgency, because the UTI might be the cause of the presenting symptoms and infection could be exacerbated by further invasive investigations (Fig. 5.3).

No patient should undergo incontinence surgery prior to having urodynamic studies. A wrongly diagnosed and treated patient could end up with a worse problem than she started with.

Female urinary incontinence

1. Genuine stress incontinence (GSI)
2. Detrusor overactivity (DO)
3. Mixed GSI and DO
4. Sensory urgency
5. Chronic voiding problems (chronic retention)
6. Fistula

Fig. 5.1 The causes of female urinary incontinence in order of frequency of occurrence.

Fig. 5.2 Definitions of commonly used urogynaecological terms.

Commonly used urogynaecological terms

Term	Definition
Cystometry	The measurement of bladder pressure and volume
Detrusor overactivity	An overactive bladder is one that is shown objectively to contract spontaneously or on provocation during the filling phase while the patient is attempting to inhibit micturition
Frequency of micturition	Voiding more than seven times per day
Genuine stress incontinence	The involuntary loss of urine when the intravesical pressure exceeds the maximum urethral pressure in the absence of detrusor activity
Nocturia	Voiding more than twice per night
Nocturnal enuresis	The involuntary passage of urine at night
Stress incontinence	Involuntary loss of urine associated with raised intra-abdominal pressure
Urge incontinence	Urinary leakage associated with a strong and sudden desire to void
Urgency of micturition	A strong and sudden desire to void
Urinary incontinence	Involuntary loss of urine that is a social or hygienic problem and is objectively demonstrable
Uroflowmetry	The measurement of urine flow rate
Videocystourethrography	Combines radiological with pressure and flow studies

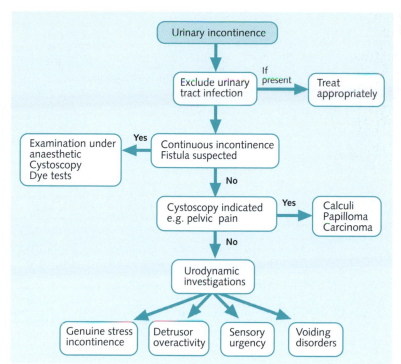

Fig. 5.3 Algorithm for urinary incontinence.

Urodynamics

It could be argued that all incontinent women should have urodynamics performed (see Chapter 26). This is especially so in women about to undergo incontinence surgery.

Uroflowmetry will identify low peak urine flow rates, which suggests a voiding disorder. Cystometry is probably the single most useful urodynamic investigation and will confirm or exclude DO. Cystometry will not diagnose GSI but will suggest this diagnosis by exclusion of other disorders such as DO.

Videocystourethrography (VCU) combines radiological with pressure and flow studies and gives the most information about bladder function. VCU can positively identify GSI as well as DO and other disorders. It is a very useful test to perform prior to incontinence surgery, although not all units provide this service.

Cystoscopy

Although cystoscopy allows inspection of the anatomy of the bladder and bladder neck, it does not give information regarding their function. Anatomical assessment of the bladder neck is important in the presence of voiding disorders; polyps, calculi and malignancies will be obvious, as will trabeculation. True bladder capacity can be measured under general anaesthesia.

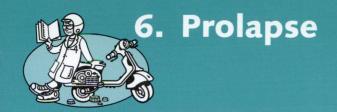

6. Prolapse

Differential diagnosis

A prolapse is the protusion of an organ or a structure beyond its normal anatomical site. In the female genital tract, the type of prolapse depends on the organ involved and its position in relation to the anterior or posterior vaginal wall (Fig. 6.1; see also Fig. 27.1, p. 142).

Cystocoele/cystourethrocoele

A cystocoele is a prolapse of the upper anterior wall of the vagina, which is attached to the bladder by fascia. This type of prolapse can extend to include the lower anterior vaginal wall as the urethra is displaced down ; this is known as a cystourethrocoele.

Rectocoele

A rectocoele is a weakness in the levator ani muscles that causes a bulge in the mid-posterior vaginal wall, which includes the rectum.

Enterocoele

An enterocoele is a true hernia of the pouch of Douglas. It is a prolapse of the upper third of the posterior vaginal wall and contains loops of small bowel.

Uterine descent

The uterus lies outside the vagina and might be associated with a cystocoele and/or a rectocoele; third-degree uterine descent is also known as a procidentia.

History to focus on the differential diagnosis of prolapse

Most commonly, the patient presents with a history of local discomfort or a feeling of 'something coming down', as the prolapsed organ pushes into the vagina and bulges towards the introitus. It might interfere with sexual function or be exacerbated by increasing intra-abdominal pressure, such as with coughing or straining to pass stools. Other symptoms depend on the organ/organs involved.

The two most common presenting symptoms are feeling 'something coming down' and backache. Don't forget that there might be other causes of backache, especially in elderly patients.

Urinary symptoms

These occur with a cystocoele or a cystourethrocoele. There might be urinary frequency or incomplete emptying of the bladder, which predisposes to urinary infection; there might even be overflow incontinence. Stress incontinence might be present if there is descent of the urethrovesical junction (bladder neck).

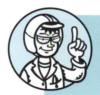

The urinary system and the bowel are involved. Related symptoms must therefore be excluded in the history.

Bowel symptoms

A rectocoele may cause incomplete bowel emptying. This can be relieved if the patient pushes back the prolapse digitally.

Uterine descent

Uterine descent often gives symptoms of backache, although other causes of backache must be excluded, especially in older patients. A procidentia causes discomfort as it rubs on the patient's clothing and this might cause a bloody, sometimes purulent, discharge.

Figure 6.2 shows factors that should be elicited in the history that may predispose the patient to prolapse in general.

Differential diagnosis of prolapse

- Cystocoele
- Cystourethrocoele
- Rectocoele
- Enterocoele
- Uterine descent

Fig. 6.1 Differential diagnosis of prolapse.

Prolapse

Type of factor	Specific factor
Congenital	Spina bifida
	Connective tissue disorder
Acquired	Obstetric factors:
	prolonged labour
	precipitate labour
	instrumental delivery
	fetal macrosomia
	increasing parity
Chronically raised intra-abdominal pressure	Chronic cough
	Constipation
Iatrogenic	Hysterectomy
	Colposuspension
Postmenopausal atrophy	

Fig. 6.2 Factors that might predispose the patient to prolapse.

Examination for prolapse

- Abdominal palpation.
- Sims' speculum examination.
- Bimanual pelvic examination.

Following abdominal palpation to exclude a mass, the patient should be examined in the left lateral position using a Sims' speculum. With the posterior vaginal wall retracted, any anterior wall prolapse will be demonstrated if the patient is asked to bear down. Conversely, if the anterior vaginal wall is retracted, then an enterocoele or rectocoele will be seen.

Examination for prolapse is with the patient in the left lateral postion and using a Sims' speculum. Abdominal palpation and bimanual examination must always be performed.

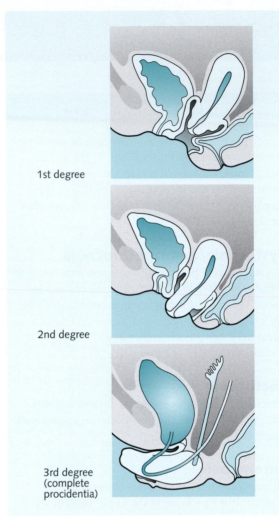

1st degree

2nd degree

3rd degree (complete procidentia)

Fig. 6.3 Classification of uterine descent.

Uterine descent is assessed by examining the position of the cervix in the vagina, again with the Sims' speculum (Fig. 6.3):
- First degree: any descent of the cervix within the vagina.
- Second degree: descent of the cervix to the introitus.
- Third degree: descent of the cervix outside the introitus (procidentia).

If the patient has a full bladder, stress incontinence can be demonstrated by asking the patient to cough. A bimanual pelvic examination is mandatory to exclude a pelvic mass as the cause of the prolapse.

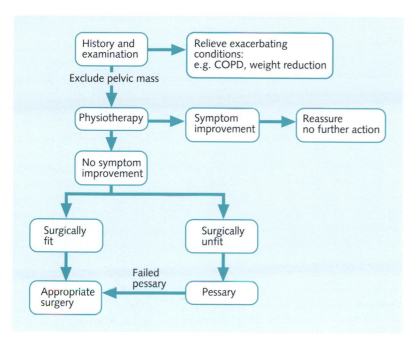

Fig. 6.4 Algorithm for prolapse.

Investigation of prolapse

There are few relevant investigations for prolapse because it is basically a clinical diagnosis dependent on examination findings (Fig. 6.4). In relation to patients with urinary symptoms, the following tests might be appropriate:

- Mid-stream urine specimen.
- Urodynamics.

31

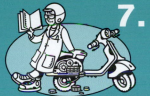
The history, examination and investigations must be aimed at distinguishing an ectopic pregnancy from a miscarriage (Fig. 7.1), while remembering that any woman who has pain or bleeding in pregnancy will be anxious. Any uncertainty about the diagnosis, and the reasons for it, should be explained to the patient carefully. Explain the plan for investigating the cause further. Note that the definitions in Fig. 7.2 refer to miscarriage. Traditionally, miscarriage was termed 'abortion' in gynaecology but as this is taken to mean 'termination' in common parlance, 'miscarriage' is the term preferred for spontaneous abortion.

History for bleeding/pain in early pregnancy

Last menstrual period

The first day of the last menstrual period (LMP) will allow you to calculate the gestation, which is important when scanning – the absence of a fetal pole in the uterus can be explained by the fact that the pregnancy is still very early, although if the woman was further on in the pregnancy this would raise the suspicion of an ectopic pregnancy. It is important to establish whether the woman is sure of the date and whether her cycle is regular; if not, the estimate may be wrong. If she conceived while taking the pill then the last period cannot be relied upon to predict the gestation because it was a hormonally induced withdrawal bleed.

Presenting complaint
Bleeding

Some women might not realise that there is a problem with their pregnancy until they have a scan (see Fig. 7.2). Miscarriage does not always start with heavy bleeding, and the loss seen with ectopic pregnancy is variable, so the amount of bleeding cannot be used to predict the problem unless the woman has seen products of conception mixed with the bleeding, in which case she is having an inevitable miscarriage. Products may be described as 'pieces of tissue'. Heavy blood flow will form clots that can be described as being 'like liver' – it is worth asking the woman the size of the clots in relation to coins ('Were they 5p-sized or 50p-sized?'). You can often quantify the blood flow by asking how many pads she has needed to change in a day.

The woman might connect the onset of bleeding to an event such as intercourse or exercise. It is possible for the cervix, which is more friable in pregnancy, to bleed postcoitally but actual miscarriage is not provoked by intercourse. The woman might feel guilty and blame herself, and it is important to reassure her.

Pain

Miscarriage typically causes cramping, central, low abdominal pain. The patient might describe it as 'like period pains' or 'like contractions'. It might have started suddenly or could have been preceded by days or weeks of spotting.

The pain of a tubal ectopic pregnancy will be worse on one side than the other, and centred around the iliac fossa. There might have been dyspareunia on that side over the previous few days and, as a result of blood irritating the bowel, the woman might have had some diarrhoea. If an ectopic pregnancy ruptures it causes pain all over the abdomen and referred shoulder-tip pain because of blood irritating the inferior surface of the diaphragm.

Past obstetric history

A history of miscarriage or ectopic pregnancy increases the risk of these problems happening again (see Chapter 29).

Past medical history

This should focus on any conditions that predispose to ectopic pregnancy (see Fig. 7.3 and Chapter 29). Also remember that a woman who has a non-viable or an ectopic pregnancy might need an operation so attention should be paid to conditions that may affect fitness for anaesthetic.

Examining women with pain and/or bleeding in early pregnancy

Observations

The woman might be experiencing significant pain if the uterus is expelling clots or products, or if an ectopic pregnancy has ruptured. Check her pulse and blood pressure.

Miscarriage is unlikely to cause shock due to hypovolaemia but, rarely, cervical shock is seen, in which there is a vagal response to the dilatation caused by products of conception distending the cervical canal. In this case pulse and blood pressure would both be low.

Haemorrhage from a ruptured ectopic pregnancy can be massive; the pulse will be weak and tachycardic and blood pressure will be low. The patient will look pale, sweaty and unwell and might collapse.

Differential diagnosis for bleeding in early pregnancy

- Threatened miscarriage, ongoing pregnancy (see Chapter 29)
- Non-viable pregnancy (complete, incomplete or delayed miscarriage; see Chapter 29)
- Molar pregnancy (see Chapter 29)
- Ectopic pregnancy (see Chapter 29)
- Local cause, e.g. cervical ectropion or carcinoma (see Chapter 23)

Fig. 7.1 Differential diagnosis for bleeding in early pregnancy.

Conditions predisposing to ectopic pregnancy

Factor	Reason
Pelvic inflammatory disease	Tubal damage and pelvic scarring
Tubal surgery, e.g. previous ectopic or sterilization	Tubal damage
Peritonitis or pelvic surgery in past, e.g. appendicitis	Pelvic scarring
Endometriosis	Tubal damage and pelvic scarring
IUCD in situ	Abnormal implantation
IVF pregnancy	Abnormal implantation

Fig. 7.3 Conditions predisposing to ectopic pregnancy.

Types of miscarriage

Type of miscarriage	Description
Threatened	Bleeding occurring before 24 weeks, where the cervix is closed on examination
Inevitable	Bleeding occurring before 24 weeks, where the cervix is open on examination
Missed/delayed/silent	Scan shows a non-viable fetus or an empty intrauterine gestation sac. The cervix is closed on examination. Patient might not have had any bleeding
Complete	Scan shows that there are no products of conception left in the uterus in a case where the patient has had bleeding. The cervix will be closed on examination
Incomplete	Scan shows that there are products of conception left inside the uterus in a case where the patient has bleeding. The cervix will be open on examination

Fig. 7.2 Types of miscarriage.

Most ectopic pregnancies do not present with an acute abdomen but the diagnosis of ectopic pregnancy should be considered in any woman who collapses and is shocked.

Abdominal examination

With miscarriage, the abdomen will be soft. If more than 12 weeks, or if the uterus is fibroid, it might be palpable above the symphysis pubis. With ectopic pregnancy the uterus will not be palpable abdominally. Before it ruptures there will be tenderness on the affected side, and there might be some guarding and rebound. Once ruptured, the entire abdomen will be tense and tender with guarding and rebound.

Cusco's speculum examination

The cervix should be visualized and swabs taken from the endocervix and vagina. An ectropion or, rarely, a cervical carcinoma, might be visible. It might be possible to see if the os is open or closed but this is best determined by palpation.

An ectropion is not pathological – it is simply an extension of endocervical columnar epithelium, which bleeds easily, onto the ectocervix and is common in pregnancy due to the influence of oestrogen. Bleeding from an ectropion is usually light but can be heavier if provoked by intercourse or in the presence of infection, so cervical swabs should be taken. No treatment is necessary unless infection is proven.

Vaginal examination

Is the os open or closed? This finding is vital to help the diagnosis until a scan is available. In early pregnancy, if the woman has had a labour in the past, the external os will be open ('multip's os') but the internal os should be closed, so this question refers to the internal os. If it is open there will be no

resistance, and the cervix will admit a finger. An open os indicates an inevitable miscarriage; a closed os might be seen with miscarriage (see Fig. 7.2) or with ectopic pregnancy. The uterine size in weeks should be estimated. The adnexae should be examined – an ectopic pregnancy will cause fullness and tenderness on the affected side. Cervical excitation is present with an ectopic pregnancy.

Cervical excitation is sudden severe pain that occurs when the cervix is moved at the time of vaginal examination. This is different from the discomfort that many women feel at the time of examination.

Investigation of bleeding and/or pain in early pregnancy

Figure 7.4 provides an algorithm for the diagnosis and investigation of bleeding and/or pain in early pregnancy.

Blood tests

- Full blood count: the woman is unlikely to be anaemic due to the bleeding of miscarriage but there might be pre-existing anaemia, which will be important from an anaesthetic point of view. An ectopic, if ruptured, may result in severe anaemia. Electrophoresis, if appropriate, must also be requested.
- Blood group: women who are Rhesus negative will require anti-D after an operation for ectopic pregnancy, after an evacuation of the retained products of conception (ERPC) at any gestation or after an episode of bleeding after 12 weeks.
- The serum β-hCG level cannot be used to diagnose an ectopic pregnancy but two samples taken 48 h apart will not show the doubling in level expected in an intrauterine pregnancy.

Ultrasound scan

Transvaginal scans give the best view in early pregnancy (Fig. 7.5). The uterus is examined, looking for a gestation sac and fetal pole, and then for a fetal heartbeat. If the uterus is empty, raising the

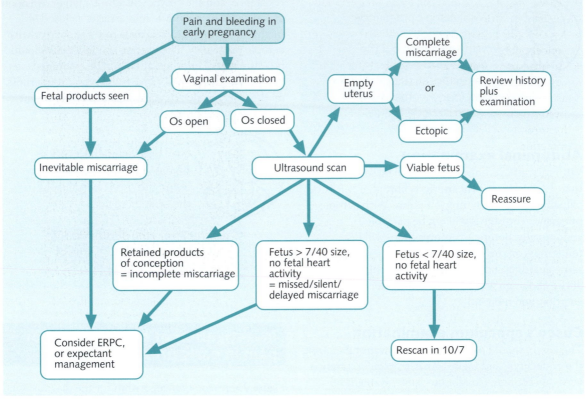

Fig. 7.4 Algorithm for bleeding and/or pain in early pregnancy.

possibility of ectopic pregnancy, the adnexae are scanned, looking for a mass. Sometimes a live ectopic is seen, where the ectopic gestation sac contains a fetus with a heartbeat. Free fluid, due to bleeding from the ectopic pregnancy, might be seen in the pouch of Douglas. In miscarriage, retained products of conception may be seen.

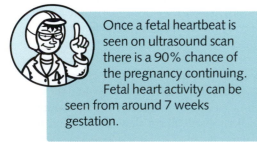

Once a fetal heartbeat is seen on ultrasound scan there is a 90% chance of the pregnancy continuing. Fetal heart activity can be seen from around 7 weeks gestation.

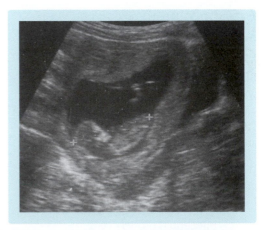

Fig. 7.5 Transvaginal scan showing intrauterine pregnancy, 7-week-sized fetus. Reproduced with kind permission from *Obstetric Ultrasound* (2nd edn), published by Churchill Livingstone.

Recurrent miscarriage

A woman who has had three or more consecutive 1st trimester miscarriages should have the same history and examination as above, remembering to consider the causes listed in Chapter 29. Extra investigations should also be ordered:

- Karyotyping of both partners and of products of conception.
- An ultrasound scan (USS) to assess the uterine cavity and the ovaries. This has been shown to be as useful and more acceptable to patients as hysterosalpingography. It is also, unlike the hysterosalpingogram (HSG), without the risk of infection.
- A high vaginal swab (HVS) to screen for bacterial vaginosis.
- Antiphospholipid antibodies assay on two occasions at least 6 weeks apart. The test is performed twice to avoid the false negatives that occur due to fluctuations in antibody levels, and the false positives caused by a temporary rise in levels at times of viral illness. If the two results are different, take the test again. The diagnosis is made after two positive tests.
- Cervical weakness is best diagnosed by careful history taking, where there will be a story of painless cervical dilatation or spontaneous rupture of membranes in the second trimester. Transvaginal scan of the cervical canal can aid diagnosis, showing an open internal os and short canal.

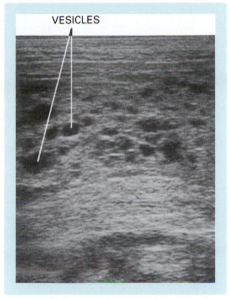

Fig. 7.6 Molar pregnancy. Reproduced with kind permission from *Obstetric Ultrasound* (2nd edn), published by Churchill Livingstone.

Trophoblastic disease

Presentation can occur in several ways:
- Bleeding in early pregnancy, investigated by USS, which reveals a molar pregnancy with a characteristic 'bunches of grapes' appearance (Fig. 7.6). A partial mole pregnancy might not appear abnormal on scan.
- USS for dating in early pregnancy, which might have been routine or was perhaps ordered because the uterus was larger than expected by dates of LMP.
- Exaggerated symptoms of pregnancy due to the high levels of β-hCG (e.g. hyperemesis gravidarum).
- Products of conception following miscarriage and ERPC are reported by the histopathologist as showing partial or complete mole.
- Persistently raised hCG following ectopic pregnancy, miscarriage or term delivery.

8. Subfertility

Ninety percent of couples will conceive within 2 years; those that don't should be seen and investigated as a couple – although they are referred to a gynaecology clinic, the problem might not lie with the woman (Fig. 8.1).

Infertility affects 1 in 7 couples in the UK:
- 22% = male factor alone
- 21% = female and male factors
- 57% = female factor alone

First, consider what is necessary for conception. An XX woman and an XY male must have penetrative intercourse resulting in male ejaculation. Conception occurs in the 4 days around ovulation – sperm can survive for 3 days and an egg can be fertilized for 1 day after it is released. The sperm must pass through the cervical mucus, the uterine cavity and into the fallopian tube. The egg must have been picked up at the fimbrial end of the tube and transported down to meet the sperm so that fertilization can take place, and the fertilized embryo must be able to implant in the uterus.

Taking the history

It is helpful to bear the above sequence in mind when taking the history and examining the subfertile couple to diagnose the cause of the problem (Fig. 8.2).

History of the couple

This should include the length of time that they have been trying to conceive and whether they are having regular intercourse. Night shifts or a partner who works away or abroad could be reducing their chances of conception. The issue of sexual dysfunction should be broached, as female vaginismus or male impotence might be the problem.

History from the woman
Past obstetric history

It should be established whether this is primary or secondary infertility, that is, whether the woman has had a pregnancy before and, if so, whether this was with a different partner. Details of previous pregnancies must be recorded, paying particular attention to a history of ectopic pregnancy, which could point to a tubal reason for infertility.

Past gynaecological history

A menstrual history will identify heavy periods, which might be due to fibroids, and painful periods, which might suggest endometriosis. Endometriosis can cause tubal problems, either by scarring the tubes or by interfering with the ciliary action of the tubal lining. Asherman's syndrome – the presence of intrauterine adhesions that form after curettage or termination of pregnancy – causes severe dysmenorrhoea. If the cycle length is between 21 and 35 days and is regular, ovulation is more likely.

A history of chlamydial infection, IUCD use, tubal surgery or ectopic pregnancy can all raise the suspicion of PID, which can cause tubal damage. Dyspareunia is an important symptom, suggesting PID or endometriosis.

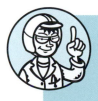

One episode of PID gives a 10% chance of tubal blockage; three episodes of PID give a 50% chance of tubal blockage.

Women who have had treatment at colposcopy following an abnormal smear have a small risk of cervical stenosis.

Past medical history

Chronic medical conditions (e.g. renal disease, hypothyroidism and hyperthyroidism) and eating disorders – especially anorexia nervosa – decrease the number of ovulatory cycles, reducing the chance of conception.

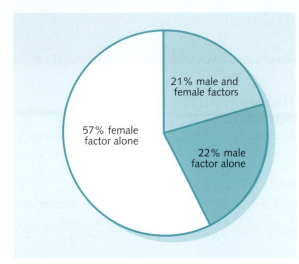

Fig. 8.1 Pie chart for infertility.

Causes of female infertility	
Type of problem	**Cause of infertility**
Ovulatory problem	Chronic systemic illness
	Eating disorders
	Abnormal pituitary/hypothalamic
	• endocrine profile polycystic
	• ovarian syndrome
	• hyperprolactinaemia
	• hypo-/hyperthyroidism
	Cannabis use
	NSAIDs
Tubal problem	Previous tubal surgery
	Previous ectopic pregnancy
	Endometriosis
Uterine problem	Submucosal fibroid
	Uterine septum
	Ashermann's syndrome
Coital problem	Intercourse not occurring often enough
	Impotence
	Vaginismus

Fig. 8.2 Causes of female infertility.

Drug history

All drugs being taken, prescription or otherwise, must be detailed. Any drugs that are not recommended for use in pregnancy can be reviewed at this visit and alternatives suggested if appropriate. All women trying to conceive should be taking folic acid supplements.

The regular use of non-steroidal anti-inflammatory drugs, or of cannabis, is known to decrease the number of ovulatory cycles.

Social history

Smoking is known to decrease fertility, although the mechanism is unclear.

History from the man
Past surgical history

Ask about surgery, including that which was performed as a baby or small child. Repair of inguinal hernia might have led to obstruction of the vas deferens in its inguinal portion; undescended testes are known to predispose to poorer semen quality (regardless of timing of orchidopexy) and testicular torsion is associated with reduced fertility. Bladder neck surgery, including transurethral resection of the prostate (TURP) can result in retrograde ejaculation.

Past medical history

Epididymo-orchitis, most commonly caused by sexually transmitted infections such as chlamydia (sometimes put under the category of non-specific urethritis, NSU) can result in epidiymal obstruction. This is also common in cystic fibrosis sufferers. Postpubertal mumps orchitis can cause significant testicular atrophy resulting in very poor quality sperm, and chronic medical conditions (e.g. renal disease) impair spermatogenesis. Diabetes can lead to retrograde ejaculation.

Drug history

Anabolic steroids, cannabis, cocaine, sulfasalazine (taken for inflammatory bowel disease), colchicine (used to treat gout), nitrofurantoin and tetracyclines (antibiotics) have all been shown to decrease sperm numbers and/or function. α-Blockers (used for treatment of benign prostatic hypertrophy) and some antidepressants are known to interfere with ejaculation; β-blockers cause impotence.

Social history

Smoking can impair the quality of the sperm but alcohol (if the intake is moderate) does not affect fertility.

Regarding occupation, it is possible that if the testes are kept at a high temperature (e.g. the job entails driving all day), the sperm count might be lower. Heavy metals, solvents and agricultural chemicals are all associated with oligospermia.

Examination

Examination of the woman
General
The BMI is calculated from height and weight (kg divided by m²). Those at the extremes, that is, women who are obese (BMI > 30) or underweight (BMI < 19), are less likely to be ovulating. Hirsutism and acanthosis nigricans can indicate PCOS and other syndromes linked to infertility have other typical facies (e.g. hyper/hypothyroidism, Cushing's syndrome, Turner's syndrome). The presence or absence of secondary sexual characteristics should be noted.

Abdominal examination
Scars from previous surgery might be seen on inspection (e.g. laparoscopy for endometriosis/PID). On palpation, the presence of a mass could point to a large fibroid uterus or ovarian cyst, and tenderness could be due to pelvic adhesions from endometriosis or PID.

Vaginal examination
The practice of female genital mutilation is widespread in some parts of the world and can make penetrative sex impossible. Occasionally, an intact hymen is discovered. Vaginal discharge can be physiological or due to PID – if there is doubt, send swabs. The uterus is palpated; a non-mobile uterus could be due to adhesions from endometriosis or PID; an enlarged uterus is likely to be due to fibroids. The ovaries are often difficult to palpate but might be bulky if polycystic.

Examination of the man
Obesity is known to decrease testosterone, so BMI should be calculated. The presence of secondary sexual characteristics is noted – inadequate virilization could be due to abnormal karyotype. Scars from inguinal hernia repair might point to an obstructive problem. Finally, underwear! Tight underwear raises the scrotal temperature and can impair sperm function.

Testicular presence and size is measured against an orchidometer, and the presence of the vas deferens on both sides is checked by palpation.

Investigation of subfertility

Basic investigations for all couples
Blood tests
Check the following in the woman:
- Progesterone: the level rises after ovulation. The test should be performed a week before the next period is due, e.g. day 21 of a 28-day cycle, or day 28 of a 35-day cycle. If > 32 nmol/L, ovulation has occurred.
- Rubella immunity: this is not an investigation of infertility but must be checked in any woman who is intending to conceive so that she can be vaccinated if not immune to prevent infection in pregnancy.

Ultrasound
This can be transvaginal or transabdominal, and is performed to look for:
- Presence of uterus and ovaries.
- Congenital abnormalities of the uterus.
- Bulky ovaries with multiple peripheral follicles in PCOS.
- Hydrosalpinx if PID appears in the history.

Microbiology
Chlamydia screening for the woman and the man in the form of urethral swabs, serum or urine (or endocervical swab for the woman) is performed. Infection is asymptomatic in up to 70% of women so there might be no clues in the history, but diagnosis is important. Although treatment will not improve fertility, failure to treat prior to HSG or laparoscopy and dye (see below) can lead to an exacerbation of infection when these investigations are carried out, which may worsen infertility.

Test of tubal patency
These tests are performed in the first half of the cycle to ensure that the patient is not already pregnant.

Hysterosalpingogram (HSG) is performed without anaesthetic (Fig. 8.3). The cervix is cannulated, radio-opaque dye is introduced into the uterus and an X-ray is taken to look for passage of the dye. Blockage inside or outside the tubes can prevent the dye flowing; however, tubal spasm in response to the dye can also prevent flow.

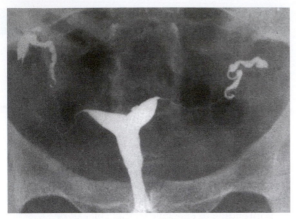

Fig. 8.3 Hysterosalpingogram. Reproduced with kind permission from *Self Assessment Picture Test Obstetrics and Gynaecology* (1st edn), published by Mosby Wolfe.

Normal parameters of semen analysis	
Volume	1.5–5 mls
Count	>20 million/ml
Progression	>50%
Normal forms	>30%

Fig. 8.4 Normal parameters of semen analysis.

Laparoscopy and dye is performed under general anaesthetic. It enables visualization of the pelvis, looking for endometriosis or scar tissue secondary to PID, the ovaries and the tubes. Blue dye is introduced through the cervix by a second operator and its progress through and out of the tubes can be seen with the laparoscope. Lack of 'fill and spill' of dye indicates tubal occlusion.

The choice of investigation should be dictated by the history and examination. If there is no suspicion of tubal blockage or other intra-abdominal pathology, a HSG is preferable because it avoids the anaesthetic risk; in all other cases laparoscopy should be performed.

Hysterosalpingo contrast sonography (HyCoSy) is an ultrasound investigation in which the cervix is cannulated and the passage of fluid through the uterus and tubes is monitored using Doppler. This is a recently developed alternative to HSG; the results are comparable and it is said to be less uncomfortable for the patient. At present it is not widely used in the UK.

Semen analysis
The man is asked to provide a specimen after 3 days abstinence from ejaculation and after a period of good health – a systemic illness within the previous 72 days could have affected the quality of sperm produced. The sample should be processed within 1 hour of production. The sperm are counted and evaluated for motility, progression and morphology, and the volume of the specimen is recorded (Fig. 8.4 gives the normal parameters). The presence of more than 10^6 white blood cells suggests epididymo-orchitis. Ideally, at least two samples should be processed. These must be produced at least 12 weeks apart to sample different populations of sperm.

Further investigations
These might be prompted by specific points in the history or examination, and include:
- Thyroid function, prolactin, LH/FSH if the woman has an irregular cycle.
- Prolactin: if either partner has galactorrhoea.
- Karyotyping: if secondary sexual characteristics are absent.
- Testosterone: if the man appears hypoandrogenic (non-hirsute, small soft testes) or if the woman is overly hirsute.
- Postcoital test: if unsure whether proper sexual intercourse is taking place, or if the man refuses to provide a semen specimen for analysis (e.g. on religious grounds), a sample can be taken from the vagina, suspended in saline and examined for the presence of sperm. This test was once more widely done to look for evidence of cervical hostility, but has now been shown to be a poor predictor.
- Antisperm antibodies: should only be performed in tertiary centres. Both women and men might have antibodies to sperm. In men they occur on the sperm surface, in the seminal plasma and in the blood serum, whereas in women they are found in blood and in cervical mucus. They affect sperm motility and function but their presence is not a significant predictor of infertility – they are

found in 5–10% of infertile men but also in 2% of fertile men.

- Hysteroscopy: should only be performed if the ultrasound suggests abnormality (e.g. intrauterine adhesions, endometrial polyps or fibroids). Polyps and submucosal fibroids are associated with infertility but the exact causal relationship is unclear.

9. The Menopause

Presentation and differential diagnosis

The strict definition of the menopause is 'cessation of menstruation', but this is not always helpful as a basis for management because amenorrhoea is often preceded by many years of oestrogen-dependent symptoms. From a biological viewpoint it is unlikely that the ovaries are suddenly switched off; their function is more likely to decline gradually, with the cessation of periods as an endpoint that is reflected by the occurrence of irregular periods, decreased fertility, increasing premenstrual syndrome and climacteric depression before the amenorrhoea of the menopause. This can result in difficulties in differential diagnosis, depending on which of the following menopausal symptoms predominate.

Menstruation is a poor sign of menopausal status.

Bleeding disturbances

For example oligomenorrhoea and secondary amenorrhoea. See Chapters 1 and 19 for the differential diagnosis.

Vasomotor symptoms

For example, hot flushes, night sweats, palpitations, headaches and dizziness. The differential diagnosis is outlined in Fig. 9.1.

If a woman has symptoms and is suspected of being menopausal but still has a regular cycle she should be treated empirically with HRT.

Differential diagnosis of vasomotor symptoms during menopause

- Cardiovascular problems, e.g. arrhythmias, coronary heart disease, valvular lesions, cardiomyopathies
- Central nervous system problems, e.g. transient ischaemic attacks, small cerebrovascular accidents, tumours
- Other endocrinopathies, e.g. hypo-/hyperthyroidism, hyperprolactinaemia, Cushing's syndrome
- Haematological problems, e.g. myeloma
- Infective causes, e.g. tuberculosis
- Other, e.g. malignancy

Fig. 9.1 Differential diagnosis of vasomotor symptoms during the menopause.

These symptoms affect 75% of women during a natural menopause but are more common and severe in women experiencing an acute menopause after bilateral oophorectomy or radiotherapy.

One of the greatest difficulties in diagnosing the menopause is that vasomotor symptoms can occur for up to 5 years before menstruation ceases. It is vital that the diagnosis is considered and treatment started empirically if women are not to be left to suffer unnecessarily.

Night sweats can be due to conditions other than the menopause, such as tuberculosis or lymphoma.

Psychological symptoms

For example, mood swings, worsening premenstrual syndrome, decreased libido, poor concentration. The differential diagnosis is given in Fig. 9.2.

The origin of psychological symptoms is complex and likely to involve both biological and psychosocial factors. Epidemiological studies have confirmed an increase of psychological symptoms in women in the perimenopausal years. The orthodox psychiatric view is that the effect of depression is entirely

Differential diagnosis of psychological symptoms during menopause
• Psychiatric disorders, e.g. endogenous depression, anxiety, neurosis, bipolar disorders • Lesions of the central nervous system • Other endocrinopathies, especially hypothyroidism • Severe premenstrual syndrome • Other, e.g. malignancy

Fig. 9.2 Differential diagnosis of psychological symptoms during the menopause.

Differential diagnosis of intermediate menopause symptoms
Dermatological conditions, e.g. eczema, psoriasis Connective tissue disorders, e.g. scleroderma, systemic lupus erythematosus Other endocrinopathies, e.g. hypothyroidism The 'natural ageing process' Mechanical trauma, e.g. joint sprain Rheumatological conditions, e.g. rheumatoid arthritis

Fig. 9.3 Differential diagnosis of intermediate menopause symptoms.

environmental, related to domestic stress, loss of youth and fertility, the 'empty nest' syndrome and death of parents.

Depression is common in the perimenopause because of fluctuating hormone levels, but other pathology such as hypothyroidism should be excluded.

There is no doubt that these psychosocial aspects are important factors in depression but that hormonal changes also play a part is suggested by the finding that the predominance of depression in women occurs only between puberty and the menopause, and is most common at times of greatest hormonal change, such as premenstrually, postnatally and during climacteric depression. Conversely, during the last trimester of pregnancy, when hormone levels are stable, depression rarely occurs.

Again, these symptoms can occur years before menstruation ceases and menopause must be considered as a diagnosis in women who present with depression in their 30s, 40s and 50s (and occasionally younger) and especially after surgical oophorectomy without adequate HRT.

Intermediate menopause symptoms

- Vulvovaginal: dyspareunia, vaginal bleeding.
- Urinary: dysuria, frequency, haematuria, incontinence.

- Skin: bruising, infection, poor healing.
- Joints: pain.

The differential diagnosis is shown in Fig. 9.3 (see also Chapters 2, 4 and 5).

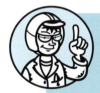

Urinary and vaginal symptoms are often the first presenting symptoms of the menopause.

Oestrogen deficiency results in the rapid loss of collagen, which contributes to the generalized atrophy that occurs after the menopause. In the genital tract this is manifested by dyspareuria and vaginal bleeding from fragile atrophic skin, and in the lower urinary tract by dysuria, urgency and frequency, commonly termed the urethral syndrome. More generalized changes are seen in older women as increased bruising and thin translucent skin, which is vulnerable to trauma and infection. A similar loss of collagen from ligaments can cause many of the generalized aches and pains that are so common in postmenopausal women.

Long-term symptoms of the menopause

Osteoporosis-related minimal injury fracture

Factors that might have contributed to an early presentation osteoporosis related fracture include:
- Smoking.
- Low BMI.
- Long episodes of amenorrhoea.

- Early age of menopause.
- Family history of osteoporosis.
- Systemic disease, e.g. renal disease.
- Drug usage, e.g. steroids, chemotherapy.

Osteoporosis, or osteopenia, is a disorder of the bone matrix resulting in a reduction of bone strength to the extent that there is a significant increased risk of fracture.

Osteoporosis itself is generally symptomless unless a fracture has occurred. Very rarely, the first presentation of the menopause will be when a woman suffers an osteoporosis-related fracture. This could have occurred because one of the contributory factors shown above prevented that woman achieving her genetically pre-programmed peak bone mass.

There has been some enthusiasm for the implementation of a national osteoporosis screening programme to measure bone density because prediction of osteoporosis from clinical risk factors and the intensity of short-term symptoms is unreliable. However, this is premature because no studies have yet demonstrated that bone densitometry is suitable for mass screening.

Figure 9.5 provides an algorithm for the investigation and management of the menopause.

Differential diagnosis of osteoporosis-related fracture during menopause

- Fracture due to 'appropriate' trauma
- Pathological fracture (due to malignancy), e.g. myeloma
- Bone disease, e.g. Paget's, osteomalacia
- Genetic/congenital disorders

Fig. 9.4 Differential diagnosis of osteoporosis-related fracture during the menopause.

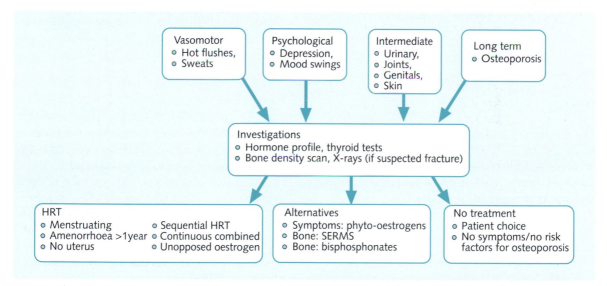

Fig. 9.5 Algorithm for the management of menopause (see Chapter 30 for details on investigation and treatment).

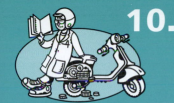

10. Bleeding in the Second and Third Trimesters of Pregnancy

Differential diagnosis of bleeding

Antepartum haemorrhage (APH) is defined as vaginal bleeding after 24 weeks gestation, that is, it is a separate entity from bleeding in early pregnancy associated with miscarriage (see Chapter 7). Figure 10.1 gives an overview of the differential diagnoses. Approximately 50% of cases of APH are caused by either a placenta praevia or a placental abruption; in the remaining 50% the bleeding is unexplained.

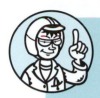 With any bleeding in pregnancy, the patient must be assessed and the amount of bleeding should be measured as accurately as possible; resuscitation of the patient must be initiated if necessary.

It is important to note that perinatal mortality following even minor episodes of bleeding is double that of a normal pregnancy. Also, a patient who presents with an APH has an associated risk of a postpartum haemorrhage.

History to focus on the differential diagnosis of bleeding

Figure 10.2 gives an algorithm for diagnosis of antepartum haemorrhage. Important points to elicit are:
- The amount of bleeding.
- Whether the blood is fresh or old.
- Any association with mucoid discharge.

There might be an obvious trigger event such as recent sexual intercourse (causing bleeding from a cervical lesion) or a road traffic accident (causing a placental abruption). The result of the patient's last smear test is relevant to exclude a cervical cause for the bleeding. The patient should be asked about the presence of fetal movements.

The presence or absence of constant abdominal pain is particularly important because it will help in the clinical differentiation between a placenta praevia and an abruption (see Chapter 37). Remember that a placental abruption does not have to be associated with visible bleeding – a concealed abruption (see Chapter 37).

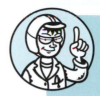 The presence of abdominal pain typically distinguishes placental abruption from placenta praevia

The pain might be caused by uterine contractions. In the case of an abruption, the uterine myometrium becomes infiltrated by blood, which can initiate contractions or simply make the uterus irritable.

Examination of patients who have bleeding in the second and third trimesters

The aim is to assess maternal and fetal well-being.

Maternal well-being
- Pulse and blood pressure.
- Maternal pallor.
- Abdominal palpation to elicit uterine tenderness and/or uterine contractions.
- Speculum examination – *only if placenta praevia has been excluded* – to exclude cervical abnormalities.
- Digital examination – *only if placenta praevia has been excluded* – and the patient appears to be in labour, to assess cervical change.

Fetal well-being
- Abdominal palpation to assess the lie and presentation of the fetus, as well as engagement of

49

the presenting part; it might be difficult to palpate fetal parts in the case of an abruption.

- Auscultation of the fetal heart to determine fetal viability.

Differential diagnosis of antepartum haemorrhage	
Source of haemorrhage	**Type of haemorrhage**
Uterine source (see Chapter 37)	Placenta praevia
	Placental abruption
	Vasa praevia
	Circumvallate placenta
Lower genital tract source (see Chapter 23)	Cervical ectropion
	Cervical polyp
	Cervical carcinoma
	Cervicitis
	Vaginitis
	Vulval varicosities
Unknown origin	

Note: Bloody mucoid vaginal loss might be the 'show' associated with the onset of labour

Fig.10.1 Differential diagnosis of antepartum haemorrhage.

Investigation of patients who have bleeding in the second and third trimesters

Blood tests

Initial investigations include taking blood for a haemoglobin level and to group and save serum. Blood might need to be cross-matched if the bleeding is heavy, especially with a major placenta praevia. If a patient is Rhesus negative, she should be given anti-D immunoglobulin to prevent haemolytic disease of the newborn in a future pregnancy.

Even with a minor degree of antepartum bleeding, the patient should be given anti-D immunoglobulin if she is Rhesus negative, after 12 weeks gestation.

Fig.10.2 Algorithm for antepartum haemorrhage.

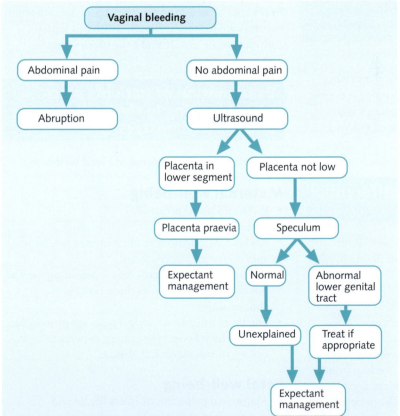

Fetal monitoring

A cardiotocograph (CTG) should be done to confirm fetal well-being. It will also assist in monitoring uterine activity, either established contractions or an irritable uterus.

Ultrasound scan

Part of the routine 20-week anomaly scan is to check the placental site. An ultrasound scan should be arranged if it has not already been done. This can be performed by the transvaginal route to check the position of the leading placental edge in relation to the internal cervical os, particularly if the placenta is posterior. It is important to differentiate between major and minor placenta praevia (see Chapter 37).

The scan might also reveal a retroplacental haematoma suggesting placental abruption, but this diagnosis is normally made on clinical grounds – a small haematoma might be missed, especially if the placenta is posterior.

Management of patients who have bleeding in the second and third trimesters

Management of the pregnancy depends on the amount of bleeding, the condition of the mother and the fetus and the likely cause of the bleeding. If a cervical cause is suspected, the patient might need to be referred for further investigations, such as colpscopy (see Chapter 23).

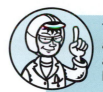

The patient who has had an antepartum haemorrhage is at risk of a postpartum haemorrhage.

Placenta praevia

Conservative management is appropriate if the bleeding is only mild to moderate in the second trimester, especially in a preterm pregnancy. If delivery is anticipated in such a case then intramuscular steroids should be administered to improve fetal lung maturity (see Chapter 38).

Inpatient care is advised for women with major placenta praevia in the third trimester because of the unpredictability of the timing of labour and the potential for heavy vaginal bleeding. If the placenta is within 2 cm of the internal cervical os, caesarean section is necessary and should be performed by a senior obstetrician.

Placental abruption

Again, with mild to moderate bleeding, expectant management is appropriate. However, depending on the clinical scenario, including the amount of bleeding and the status of the fetus, immediate delivery might be necessary in the interests of the mother and the fetus.

11. Large- or Small-For-Dates

Differential diagnosis

The growth of a pregnancy is estimated by measuring the symphysis–fundal height (see Chapter 46). This takes into account the size of the fetus, the liquor volume and the maternal structures, including the uterus. Before deciding whether it is abnormal or not, the dates of the last menstrual period and the previous scan reports should be checked to confirm the gestation of the pregnancy, and also whether it is a singleton.

The differential diagnoses of the large-for-dates (LFD) or small-for-dates (SFD) abdomen can be considered in two categories:
1. Fetal/placental.
2. Maternal.

A fetus found to be SFD can be categorized according to its growth pattern:
- small for gestational age (SGA): the fetus is small for the expected size at a certain gestation but continues to grow at a normal rate
- intrauterine growth restriction (IUGR): the fetus is small or normal-sized for the expected size at a certain gestation but the growth rate slows down as the pregnancy advances.

History to focus on the differential diagnosis of a LFD or SFD abdomen

Past obstetric history
With respect to the LFD abdomen, a patient who had gestational diabetes in a previous pregnancy is at risk of developing the same condition again (see Chapter 36). This disorder puts the pregnancy at risk of fetal macrosomia and polyhydramnios (increased liquor volume).

A previous history of a baby that was SGA or IUGR, whether in relation to pre-eclampsia or not, increases the risk of a future pregnancy being affected.

Past gynaecological history
The patient might have been diagnosed with uterine fibroids or with an ovarian cyst, either prior to pregnancy or in early pregnancy. Both conditions can cause the symphysis–fundal height to palpate as LFD.

Past medical history
Diabetes mellitus increases the chance of fetal macrosomia and polyhydramnios. The abdomen will palpate LFD, as in gestational diabetes. Fetal infection with Toxoplasmosis CMV, Rubella or Herpes, may produce polyhydramnious so the mother should be asked about recent flu-like illness or rash.

Current maternal disease increases the risk of IUGR and therefore a SFD abdomen (see Chapter 36):
- Renal disease including renal transplantation.
- Hypertension.
- Congenital heart disease.
- Severe anaemia.
- Sickle-cell disease.
- Systemic lupus erythematosus.
- Cystic fibrosis.

Family history
In relation to a LFD uterus, it is important to ask about a family history of diabetes mellitus. This will put the patient at increased risk of developing gestational diabetes in her current pregnancy.

There is also evidence that a family history of pre-eclampsia is relevant, and this disorder can be associated with IUGR (see Chapter 35).

Social history
The ethnic group of the patient can be relevant in a SFD patient. The growth charts used in most units were derived from Caucasian populations, in whom the average birthweight is greater than, for example, an Asian population. Hence some units have developed customized growth charts for each particular patient group.

Smoking in pregnancy is a major cause of a fetus being SGA, so that the abdomen palpates as SFD. It affects growth in the third trimester. Alcohol and illegal drug use are also causes of being SGA and so all these factors must be checked in the antenatal history.

 If the symphysis–fundal height is larger or smaller than expected for the gestation, the first check is that the dates of the last menstrual period and the first dating scan agree.

Examination of the patient with a LFD or SFD uterus

Chapter 46 discusses examination of the pregnant patient and the uterus. This should include checking blood pressure, and urinalysis for proteinuria or glycosuria. The following should be noted on abdominal palpation in relation to LFD or SFD:

- Symphysis–fundal height.
- Number of fetuses.
- Fetal lie.
- Liquor volume.
- Presence of uterine fibroids.
- Presence of adnexal masses.

Investigation of the patient with a LFD or SFD uterus

Figures 11.1 and 11.2 provide algorithms for the investigation of the LFD and SFD uterus.

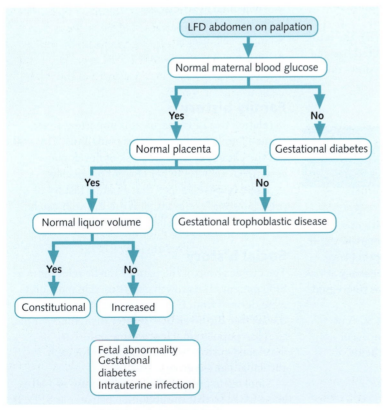

Fig. 11.1 Algorithm for a large-for-dates abdomen.

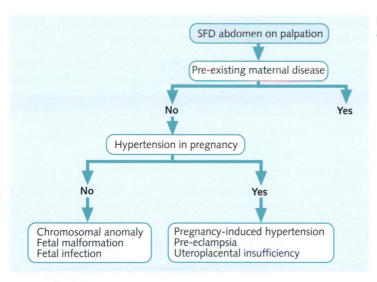

Fig. 11.2 Algorithm for a small-for-dates abdomen.

If there is no evidence of uteroplacental insufficiency, the other causes of the fetus being small-for-dates should be excluded. Ultrasound scan should examine for fetal abnormalities and check for signs of in utero infection. Prior screening for chromosomal abnormalities should be reviewed.

LFD or SFD. In the case of SFD, then serial measurements, at least 2 weeks apart, should be taken to distinguish between SGA and IUGR.

There are two types of IUGR. Typically, asymmetrical IUGR is associated with uteroplacental insufficiency, whereas symmetrical IUGR is more commonly seen with other conditions. With uteroplacental insufficiency, the fetus preferentially diverts blood to the vital organs. There is less blood to the kidneys, and therefore reduced production of liquor (oligohydramnios), as well as less storage of glycogen in the fetal liver. This results in a discrepancy between the growth of the fetal head and the abdomen.

Blood tests

In the case of a LFD patient, a glucose tolerance test should be arranged to establish whether gestational diabetes has developed (see Chapter 36). If polyhydramnious is found in the absence of diabetes, fetal infection may be the cause so maternal antibodies (IgM and IgG) to Toxoplasma, Rubella, CMV and Herpes should be investigated.

A patient who is SFD and is also hypertensive should be investigated for pre-eclampsia (see Chapter 35). The blood investigations include platelet count, liver function tests and uric acid level.

The fetal causes of oligohydramnios are related to its ability to produce urine and thus liquor.
The fetal causes of polyhydramnios are secondary to its inability to swallow liquor.

Ultrasound
Fetal ultrasound

Plotting ultrasound measurements of biparietal diameter, head circumference, abdominal circumference and femur length on a growth chart is the main method of monitoring fetal growth, either

Placenta/ liquor ultrasound

Trophoblastic disease is usually excluded at the 12-week dating scan by checking the structure of the placenta (see Chapter 29). Otherwise, this condition can present later in pregnancy with a uterus that palpates LFD.

A scan can also be used to measure the liquor volume. The amniotic fluid index (AFI) is the sum of the fluid pockets in four quadrants of the abdomen.

Maternal ultrasound

Ultrasound scan is useful to diagnose uterine fibroids or the presence of ovarian cysts.

Doppler studies

In conjunction with growth scans and measurement of the liquor volume, Doppler waveforms of the blood flow in the uteroplacental and fetoplacental circulations can be used to assess the SGA or IUGR fetus. Increased placental vascular resistance, for example in pre-eclampsia, changes the pattern of the flow in the umbilical artery. There is normally flow towards the placenta during fetal diastole. However, as the placental resistance increases, diastolic flow becomes absent and then reversed. Other vessels can also be examined within the fetus, including the middle cerebral artery and the ductus venosus, to look for patterns of flow redistribution if the placental blood flow is insufficient.

Cardiotocography

The CTG can be used to assess the IUGR fetus. When not in labour, the tracing might be abnormal when the uteroplacental insufficiency is severe. The presence of the following should be excluded:

- Reduced variability.
- Bradycardia.
- Tachycardia.
- Decelerations.

The SGA fetus can only be distinguished from the IUGR fetus by serial growth scans. Further investigation includes Doppler studies and cardiotocography.

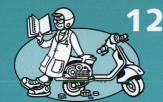

12. Abdominal Pain in the Second and Third Trimesters of Pregnancy

Differential diagnosis of abdominal pain in pregnancy

The important differential diagnosis when assessing abdominal pain in pregnancy is whether the cause is obstetric or non-obstetric. Figure 12.1 shows the systems that might be involved.

Don't forget the non-obstetric causes of abdominal pain. Some of them are more common than the obstetric causes, such as a urinary tract infection.

History to focus on the differential diagnosis of abdominal pain in pregnancy

With diverse differential diagnoses, the history is very important to identify the cause of the pain. Figure 12.2 gives a summary of the points elicited from the history and examination that help to make the diagnosis.

Current obstetric history
This should include the current gestation and the parity. The antenatal history might be relevant. For example, if the patient has a history of pregnancy-induced hypertension (see Chapter 35) then she is at risk of pre-eclampsia and placental abruption (see Chapter 10). She might have already been admitted earlier in the pregnancy with suspected preterm labour (see Chapter 38). A urinary tract infection might have been treated earlier in this pregnancy.

Presenting symptoms
As with any history of pain, its characteristics are important:

Differential diagnosis of abdominal pain in 2nd and 3rd trimesters	
System involved	**Pathology**
Obstetric	Labour preterm/term
	Placental abruption
	Symphysis pubis dysfunction
	Ligament pain
	Pre-eclampsia/HELLP syndrome
	Acute fatty liver of pregnancy
Gynaecological	Ovarian cyst rupture/torsion/haemorrhage
	Uterine fibroid degeneration
Gastrointestinal	Constipation
	Appendicitis
	Gallstones/cholecystitis
	Pancreatitis
	Peptic ulcer
Genitourinary	Cystitis
	Pyelonephritis
	Renal stones/renal colic

Fig. 12.1 Differential diagnosis of abdominal pain in the second and third trimesters of pregnancy.

- Nature: continuous or intermittent.
- Quality: stabbing or burning or tightening.
- Duration.
- Site: generalized or specific.
- Radiation: to the pelvis or to the back.
- Exacerbating factors.

It is important to ask about other symptoms, particularly gastrointestinal and genitourinary, such as dysuria, frequency of bowel habit or nausea.

Past obstetric history
There might be a history of pre-eclampsia or preterm labour in a previous pregnancy, which puts the patient at increased risk in her current pregnancy.

Past gynaecological/medical/surgical history
Ultrasound scans earlier in the current pregnancy might have alerted the medical staff to the presence of an ovarian cyst or uterine fibroids. There might be a history of peptic ulcer disease or gallstones. The

Making a diagnosis from the history and examination	
Differential diagnosis	**Clinical features**
Labour (see Chapter 40)	Intermittent pain, usually regular in frequency, associated with tightenings of the abdominal wall. The presenting part of the fetus is usually engaged. Vaginal examination shows cervical change
Placental abruption (see Chapter 37)	Mild or severe pain, more commonly associated with vaginal bleeding. The uterus is usually tender on palpation and can be irritable or tense. There might be symptoms and signs of pre-eclampsia
Symphysis pubis dysfunction	Pain is usually low and central in the abdomen just above the symphysis pubis, which is tender on palpation. Symptoms are worse with movement
Ligament pain	Commonly described as sharp pain, which is bilateral and often associated with movement
Pre-eclampsia/HELLP syndrome (see Chapter 35)	Epigastric or right upper quadrant pain, associated with nausea and vomiting, headache and visual disturbances. On examination, there is hypertension and proteinuria
Acute fatty liver of pregnancy	Epigastric or right upper quadrant pain, associated with nausea, vomiting, anorexia and malaise
Ovarian cyst (see Chapter 22)	Unilateral pain, which is intermittent and might be associated with vomiting
Uterine fibroid (see Chapter 20)	Pain is localized and constant. Fibroid is noted on palpation and is tender
Constipation	Usually suggested by the history, can cause lower abdominal discomfort and bloating
Appendicitis	Pain associated with nausea and vomiting. Tenderness with guarding and rebound might be localized to the right iliac fossa
Gallstones / cholecystitis	Right upper quadrant or epigastric pain, which might radiate to the back or to the shoulder tip. Tenderness in the right hypochondrium and pyrexia with cholecystitis
Pancreatitis	Epigastric pain radiating to the back, associated with nausea and vomiting. Occurs most commonly in the third trimester
Peptic ulcer	Epigastric pain associated with food. There might be heartburn, nausea and even haematemesis
Cystitis	Usually suggested by history, with pain and tenderness in the low abdomen or suprapubically
Renal stones / renal colic / pyelonephritis	Loin pain that might radiate to the abdomen and groin, possibly associated with vomiting and rigors. Pyrexia is present with pyelonephritis

Fig. 12.2 Making a diagnosis from the history and examination.

patient might have had a previous appendicectomy or a cholecystectomy.

Examination of the patient who has abdominal pain in pregnancy

General examination

As with any clinical examination, the general condition of the pregnant patient should be assessed, including:

- Temperature.
- Pulse.
- Blood pressure.
- Respiratory rate.
- Cardiovascular system.
- Respiratory system.

Abdominal palpation

The abdomen should be inspected for any previous operation scars. In the presence of a gravid uterus, abdominal palpation to establish the cause of the symptoms might not be straightforward. Compared with examining a non-pregnant patient, the site of the tenderness might not be typical. Examining a non-pregnant patient who has an ovarian cyst torsion is likely to elicit tenderness and guarding in the iliac fossa. Depending on the gestation, this might not be so specific in a pregnant patient because the gravid uterus might be interfering with the usual anatomical markings. Tenderness at McBurney's point, which is typical of appendicitis (see *Crash Course in Surgery*) might also be difficult to elicit in a patient who is late in the second or in the third trimester of pregnancy.

When examining an obstetric patient, remember that she might feel faint if she lies flat on her back for too long, secondary to pressure on the large vessels reducing venous return to the heart and causing supine hypotension. She should be examined with left lateral tilt.

The uterus should be palpated to determine:

- Lie, presentation, engagement depending on gestation (see Chapter 46).
- Presence of uterine contractions.
- Generalized or specific uterine tenderness.
- Presence of uterine fibroids.

Vaginal examination

A speculum examination is appropriate if there is vaginal bleeding, to exclude cervical causes (see Chapter 37). A vaginal examination may be indicated if the history and abdominal palpation suggest that the patient is in labour, in order to determine if there is cervical change (see Chapter 46).

Investigation of the patient who has abdominal pain

Figure 12.3 gives a summary of the investigations that should be considered and Fig. 12.4 provides an algorithm for the investigation of abdominal pain.

Summary of abdominal pain investigations

- Full blood count
- Clotting studies
- Group and save (G&S) sample
- Urea/electrolytes
- Liver function tests (LFTs)
- Glucose
- Urinalysis/midstream urine (MSU)/24-h urine collection for protein
- Cardiotocograph (CTG)
- Ultrasound scan of the uterus, ovaries, kidneys, liver and gall bladder

Fig.12.3 Summary of investigations to be considered in a patient with abdominal pain.

Blood tests
Full blood count/clotting studies

The full blood count can show a reduced haemoglobin if the patient has been bleeding, for example in the case of a placental abruption. The platelet count might be low in association with pre-eclampsia or HELLP (hypertension, elevated liver enzymes, low platelets) syndrome, possibly associated with abnormal clotting studies. A group and save sample of serum is appropriate if there is bleeding, in case cross-matched blood is required for transfusion. With the non-obstetric causes of pain, the white blood cell count will be raised if there is infection, for example, with pyelonephritis or cholecystitis.

Urea/electrolytes/glucose/liver function tests

These tests might be abnormal in pre-eclampsia or HELLP syndrome, with raised urea and creatinine suggesting haemoconcentration, and with raised liver transaminases. Serum uric acid is high in pre-eclampsia and in acute fatty liver, whereas in the latter, there is also hypoglycaemia.

Urinalysis/midstream urine sample

In pre-eclampsia, there is proteinuria on dipstick urinalysis and a 24-h urine collection to quantify the amount of protein might be indicated to determine the severity of the disease. Proteinuria can also be present with a urinary tract infection and might be associated with microscopic haematuria, particularly in the presence of renal stones.

Cardiotocograph

The fetal heart should be auscultated before 24 weeks gestation with a pinard or a sonicaid. A cardiotocograph is performed after this gestation (see Chapter 16) and will help determine fetal well-being, particularly in the case of placental abruption. The recording will also detect uterine activity including the presence and frequency of uterine contractions.

Ultrasound scan (uterus/ovaries/kidneys/liver/gallbladder)

An obstetric scan might show a retroplacental haematoma in the case of severe placental abruption. If preterm delivery is necessary, for example in acute fatty liver, fetal well-being and growth should be assessed, and the fetal weight estimated.

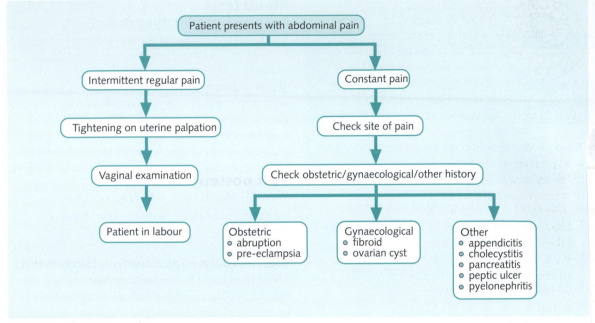

Fig. 12.4 Algorithm for abdominal pain.

For the other systems, ultrasound examination can assist diagnosis and management. An ovarian cyst might be seen if haemorrhage, rupture or torsion of the cyst is suspected. Renal stones or gallstones can be visualized.

Management of the patient with abdominal pain

This depends on the cause of the pain and the gestation of the pregnancy. With regards to the obstetric causes, caesarean section or induction of labour might need to be considered. In severe pre-eclampsia, for example, the benefits of delivery to the mother's health can outweigh the risks to the fetus of preterm birth. Placental abruption might be severe enough to compromise the fetus, and then delivery should be expedited.

However, most conditions can be managed conservatively with treatment such as analgesia, for example with renal stones, or antibiotics for pyelonephritis. Multidisciplinary management with other specialties might be appropriate, for example with gastroenterology in a patient suspected of having gallstones or a peptic ulcer. Occasionally, an operation is necessary for an acute appendicitis or for ovarian torsion.

Remember to liaise with other specialists in the management of conditions such as renal stones or cholecystitis. In the case of preterm labour, discuss management with the paediatricians.

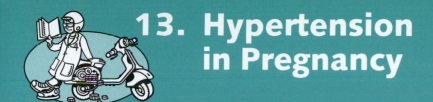
Differential diagnosis of hypertension in pregnancy

Blood pressure problems in pregnancy can be divided into two groups:

1. Pre-existing hypertension, where the blood pressure was high prior to pregnancy and therefore presents either as a woman who is known to have hypertension or because a reading taken in the first trimester is high.
2. Pre-eclampsia, a multisystem disorder, one of whose manifestations is high blood pressure, but where renal, liver and clotting functions are also affected.

History and examination are aimed at differentiating these problems, remembering that the two may coexist, as essential hypertension predisposes to pre-eclampsia.

History

Presenting complaint

The absence of symptoms does not exclude the diagnosis of pre-eclampsia.

The woman is often asymptomatic of her high blood pressure, which is picked up as part of the routine antenatal check, but she might be experiencing symptoms of pre-eclampsia (Fig. 13.1). You must ask specifically about:

- Headache.
- Visual disturbance (in the form of flashing lights, not the 'black dots' associated with postural hypotension).
- Right upper quadrant or epigastric pain (due to oedema of the liver capsule).
- Facial swelling.

Past gynaecological history

A history of high blood pressure when taking the oral contraceptive pill indicates a susceptibility to high blood pressure in pregnancy.

Past obstetric history

If the blood pressure was high in previous pregnancies because of essential hypertension it is very unlikely to be normal in this pregnancy. Pre-eclampsia, however, does not always recur with every pregnancy; it is most common in primigravida or in the first pregnancy with a new partner.

Past medical history

Conditions that predispose to hypertension include diabetes, renal and cardiac disease.

Family history

Pre-eclampsia does 'run in families', with the strongest association being if the patient's sister was affected in her pregnancy.

Drug history

Some women with hypertension prior to pregnancy might already be on medication. This might need to be changed to avoid drugs contraindicated in pregnancy (see Chapter 40).

Examination of women with hypertension in pregnancy

The points to note are shown in Fig. 13.1.

General examination

- Severe pre-eclampsia can cause an altered level of consciousness.
- Look for facial oedema – if you are not sure if her face is swollen, ask her partner or family member if she looks different.
- Check the blood pressure.

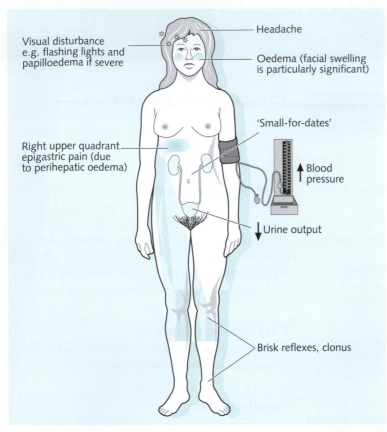

Fig. 13.1 Signs and symptoms of pre-eclampsia.

Visual disturbance e.g. flashing lights and papilloedema if severe

Headache

Oedema (facial swelling is particularly significant)

Right upper quadrant epigastric pain (due to perihepatic oedema)

'Small-for-dates'

↑ Blood pressure

↓ Urine output

Brisk reflexes, clonus

Blood pressure should be measured with the patient sitting or lying propped on pillows, with the arm the same level as the heart, using the disappearance rather than the muffling of sound as the cut-off for the diastolic. The correct size of cuff must be used; if a small cuff is used for a large woman the blood pressure will be artificially (and worryingly) high.

- Check the reflexes and examine for clonus.
- Perform fundoscopy to look for papilloedema in pre-eclampsia. Retinopathy might be seen in severe, chronic cases of essential hypertension.

Abdominal palpation
- Feel for liver tenderness.
- Palpate the uterus to see if the growth seems appropriate for the gestational age.

Investigation of women with hypertension in pregnancy

Figure 13.2 provides an algorithm for the investigation of hypertension in pregnancy.

Urinalysis

If told that you are to see a pregnant woman with raised blood pressure, one of your first questions must be 'What does the urinalysis show?'. The presence of proteinuria raises the suspicion of pre-eclampsia.

The urine should be dipped. The presence of protein might be due to pre-eclampsia but could also be the result of contamination with blood, liquor (if the membranes have ruptured) or vaginal discharge, or

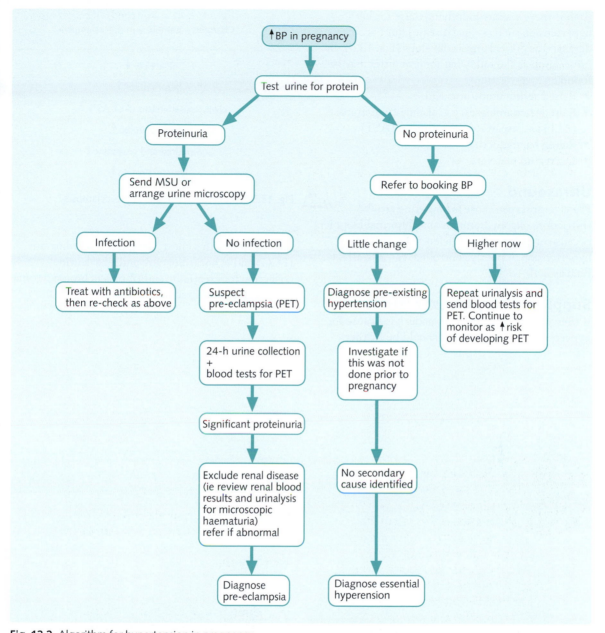

Fig. 13.2 Algorithm for hypertension in pregnancy.

be caused by a UTI. It is important that the sample is a 'clean catch'.

Check the other findings on dipping – lots of leucocytes and protein might indicate UTI, especially if nitrites and/or blood are also present. Even if a UTI is suspected, do not dismiss the proteinuria because the consequences of missing pre-eclampsia could be grave. Send an MSU for microscopy and culture but continue checking for pre-eclampsia.

To quantify proteinuria, a 24-h collection should be performed. The result is suggestive of pre-eclampsia if the 24-h urine protein is more than 0.3 g.

Blood tests

Urate, renal function tests, liver function tests, a full blood count and a clotting screen are sent. The results would be expected to be normal for pregnancy in women with essential hypertension (unless there was an underlying cause for her hypertension such as renal disease) but become deranged as pre-eclampsia develops (Fig. 13.3). In pre-eclampsia the following abnormalities may be found on investigation:

- Raised serum urate/uric acid.
- Raised transaminases, e.g. alanine transaminase (ALT) and aspartate transaminase (AST).
- Raised haematocrit.
- Decreased platelets.

Ultrasound

Pre-eclampsia can cause intrauterine growth restriction, oligohydramnios and abnormal Dopplers because of placental insufficiency. Essential hypertension, if poorly controlled, can also affect fetal growth.

Supplementary investigations

If there is any suspicion of an underlying cause for hypertension in pregnancy it should be further investigated with a chest X-ray, electrocardiogram (ECG) and echocardiogram, and a 24-h urine collection for creatinine and (if phaeochromocytoma is suspected) for catecholamines.

Changed parameters in pre-eclampsia
Platelets ↓
Serum urate ↑
Liver transaminases (ALT, AST) ↑
Serum bilirubin ↑
Serum urea and creatinine ↑
Urinary protein ↑

Fig. 13.3 Changed parameters in pre-eclampsia.

14. Stillbirth

The term 'stillbirth' is used to describe the intrauterine death of a fetus after 24 weeks gestation, which is diagnosed before or during labour, or at delivery. The woman might present with symptoms of the event that caused the baby to die, or simply attend because she has not felt fetal movements. Figure 14.1 summarizes the common causes of stillbirth.

 The national stillbirth rate in the UK is 5.3 per 1000 deliveries.

If fetal death is suspected antenatally an ultrasound scan is performed to look for absence of fetal heart activity. It is recommended that the finding of intrauterine death is confirmed by a second sonographer. The rate of stillbirth varies with maternal age (Fig. 14.2) being lowest when the mother is aged between 25 and 29.

History

Finding out when the mother last felt fetal movements can help to work out how recently fetal death occurred, but this will not help with the diagnosis of the underlying cause unless it can be linked to a particular occurrence.

History of the pregnancy
The following points might be helpful:
- Rhesus group: if the woman is Rhesus negative then Rhesus disease is a possibility.
- Down syndrome screening: if the woman is high risk, a chromosomal abnormality might be present.
- Ultrasound for anomaly/growth: any structural abnormalities or a history of IUGR increase the risk of stillbirth.
- Recurrent antepartum haemorrhage: repeated small abruptions can compromise fetal well-being and cause IUGR.

Ask about any leaking of fluid or bleeding in the recent history. Ruptured membranes allow infection to ascend and infect the membranes and placenta (chorioamnionitis) and therefore the fetus. Bleeding might be due to abruption. Abruption and chorioamnionitis would both cause uterine pain. Bleeding from placenta praevia is painless; the mother might have had a scan earlier in pregnancy that diagnosed a low-lying placenta.

Signs of maternal illness (fever, feeling unwell, flu-like symptoms, gastrointestinal upset) are also suggestive of fetal infection. Listeria, toxoplasma and parvovirus can cause only very mild illness in the mother but death in the fetus.

Rhesus disease and twin-to-twin transfusion syndrome cause sudden polyhydramnios, so the mother might describe feeling suddenly larger.

 If one twin dies in a dichorionic twin pregnancy, the chance of the other twin dying is < 5%, so if the pregnancy is preterm the mother can be managed expectantly. There is a risk that she could develop coagulopathy so her platelets need to be monitored regularly. If one of a pair of monochorionic twins dies compromise of the other twin is far more likely, so delivery is advisable.

Obstetric cholestasis causes a characteristic pattern of itching affecting particularly the palms of the hands and the soles of the feet (see Chapter 36).

Past obstetric history
If the woman has had a previous stillbirth it is important to find out if an underlying cause was discovered. Rhesus disease gets more severe with successive pregnancies, so a first child might be unaffected or suffer only mild jaundice. Gestational diabetes in a previous pregnancy is likely to recur.

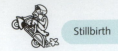

Causes of stillbirth	
Type of condition	Cause of stillbirth
Maternal condition	Diabetes (pre-existing and gestational)
	Pre-eclampsia
	Sepsis
	Obstetric cholestasis
	Acute fatty liver
	Thrombophilias, e.g. protein C and protein S resistance, factor V Leiden mutation, antithrombin III deficiency
Fetal condition	Infection: *Toxoplasma*, *Listeria*, *Syphilis*, parvovirus
	Chromosomal abnormality
	Structural abnormality
	Rhesus disease leading to severe anaemia
	Twin-to-twin transfusion syndrome (affects monochorionic twins only)
	IUGR
	Alloimmune thrombocytopaenia
Placental condition	Postmaturity
	Abruption
	Placenta praevia: significant bleed
	Cord prolapse

Fig. 14.1 Causes of stillbirth.

Rates of stillbirth in relation to maternal age	
Maternal age	Rate of stillbirth per 1000 deliveries
<25	5
25–29	4
30–34	4.3
35–39	5
40–44	6.5
45 and over	7

Fig. 14.2 Rates of stillbirth in relation to maternal age.

Past medical history

Maternal medical conditions such as diabetes and renal disease increase the risk of stillbirth. A personal or family history of thrombosis might point to an underlying thrombophilia.

Examination

General examination

The mother's pulse, blood pressure and temperature are taken. Maternal infection can cause a tachycardia and pyrexia. A significant bleed due to abruption or bleeding placenta praevia can cause hypovolaemic shock. The itching of cholestasis might be evident from scratch marks on the skin – there is no rash in obstetric cholestasis.

Examination of the uterus

Assess the following:

- Uterine size: small-for-dates suggests IUGR or that the fetus died some time ago; large-for-dates might be due to polyhydramnios (diabetes, Rhesus disease, twin-to-twin transfusion syndrome).
- Uterine consistency: abruption causes the uterus to feel tense, tender and hard, and it might be irritable (i.e. palpation provokes contractions). With chorioamnionitis the uterus will be soft and tender and might be irritable.
- Fetal presentation: breech presentation is associated with fetal abnormality.

Investigations

Urinalysis

The urine is dipped, looking particularly for protein as a sign of pre-eclampsia. If significant proteinuria is found a 24-h collection is commenced, and an MSU is sent to exclude infection.

Blood tests

The tests below are sent to investigate the cause of fetal death. At the time of diagnosis a full blood count and a sample for group and save should be sent due to the risk of disseminated intravascular coagulation (DIC) following stillbirth:

- HbA1c (glycosylated haemoglobin): if raised this suggests maternal diabetes.
- Coombs' test to look for evidence of Rhesus disease.
- Infection screen: blood cultures and antibody levels for toxoplasma, parvovirus, listeria, and syphilis.
- Kleihauer test: looks for evidence of fetomaternal haemorrhage, as can occur with abruption.
- Thrombophilia screen.

Ultrasound scan

Once the diagnosis of fetal death has been made, a scan will not add much information unless the parents do not wish post-mortem of the baby, in which case the scan is an opportunity to look for evidence of internal structural anomalies.

Pathology

Parents are encouraged to allow post-mortem examination of their baby so that all possible information is collected. They should be reassured that this will not prevent them from arranging a funeral or cremation for the baby. Post-mortem includes examination of the placenta and a fetal karyotype. If the parents do not consent to the full post-mortem they should be offered a more limited examination comprising X-rays and external examination of the baby, or solely examination of the placenta.

Management of stillbirth

In most cases, labour is induced using prostaglandins and oxytocin. Occasionally a caesarean section is performed because the mother is unwell and delivery needs to be expedited, or because induction of labour would pose a significant risk, for example if the mother had had several caesarean sections in the past.

Some women will opt to continue the pregnancy. More than 90% will spontaneously labour within 3 weeks. By 4 weeks after fetal death (which might have occurred some time before diagnosis) there is a 1 in 4 risk of developing coagulopathy, so these women should have their platelets monitored regularly.

After death the fetal body releases procoagulant factors into the mother's circulation leading to intravascular coagulation, with consumption of clotting factors and platelets, and deposition of fibrin, resulting in DIC, which can cause catastrophic haemorrhage.

After delivery the parents should be encouraged to hold their baby. Footprints, handprints and photographs can be taken and the parents might choose to have some form of blessing or religious ceremony at this stage. The mother can be given cabergoline to suppress lactation.

Follow-up

Psychological and social support is extremely important. Prior to the woman leaving hospital the GP and community midwife should be informed, and any antenatal clinic appointments cancelled. The mother should be seen for at least 10 days by the midwife for postnatal checks. Information about parent support groups (e.g. SANDS, the Stillbirth and Neonatal Death Society) should be given.

A follow-up appointment should be made with the consultant, who often chooses to see the parents in the gynaecology rather than antenatal clinic. All the results will be reviewed and any questions can be answered, even if only to explain that the stillbirth was unexplained.

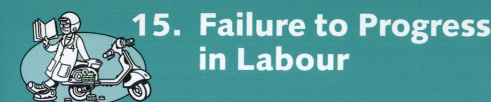

Labour and delivery require the interaction of three components – the passages, the passenger and power – as part of a dynamic process:

- Passages: the shape and size of the hard bony pelvis and soft tissues.
- Passenger: the size and presentation of the fetus.
- Power: this is both involuntary (strength and frequency of uterine contractions) and voluntary (diaphragm and abdominal muscles).

 Labour is a dynamic process that depends on many factors.

Any of these factors can be involved in the failure of labour to progress normally. Once the diagnosis of labour has been made (see Chapter 40), a primiparous patient is expected to progress at approximately 1 cm/h and a multiparous patient at approximately 2 cm/h.

A partogram (Fig. 40.1) gives a graphic representation of this progress and hence failure to progress normally can easily be detected (Fig. 15.1). Examination and investigation of the causes of the resultant prolonged labour should be considered in terms of the three factors mentioned above. Figure 15.2 shows the differential diagnoses that should be excluded.

History to focus on the differential diagnosis

Passages
Bony passages
Figure 40.16 (p. 235) gives some of the causes of abnormalities of the bony passages that can cause failure to progress in labour.

Soft passages
The patient might have previously been diagnosed – either prior to pregnancy or on antenatal ultrasound scans – with fibroids. A cervical fibroid can interfere with cervical dilatation.

A history of cervical surgery will cause scarring, which can then prevent cervical dilatation. This is particularly relevant with a knife cone procedure, but seems to be less common with the LLETZ (large loop excision of the transformation zone) procedure that is more frequently performed nowadays (see Chapter 23).

Female circumcision (also known as female genital mutilation) usually makes the vaginal introitus smaller and thus can affect progression to normal vaginal delivery in the second stage of labour.

Passenger
It is often useful, in a multiparous patient, to check the weights of previous deliveries as an assessment of ability to deliver the current infant.

A history of diabetes, either long-standing or gestational, puts the fetus at risk of macrosomia, which means that the fetal size might be out of proportion to the size of the maternal pelvis (cephalopelvic disproportion or CPD; see Chapter 40), resulting in failure to progress in labour.

Antenatal diagnosis of a fetal abnormality can inhibit normal progress. For example, a congenital goitre causes extension of the neck so that the normal process of flexion cannot occur. In anencephaly, a form of spina bifida in which the fetal skull fails to develop, the head is less able to engage and therefore labour might not progress normally.

 About one-fifth of vertex presentations in early labour are occipitoposterior.

Power
There need to be three or four uterine contractions every 10 min, each lasting approximately 60 s, to maintain adequate progress in labour. This can be assessed by asking the patient or checking the cardiotocograph.

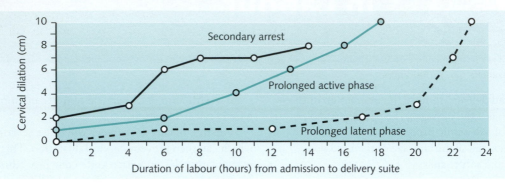

Fig. 15.1 Abnormal patterns of cervical dilatation in labour.

Causes of failure to progress in labour	
Bony passages	Abnormal shaped pelvis
	Cephalopelvic disproportion
Soft passages	Uterine/cervical fibroids
	Cervical stenosis
	Circumcision
Passenger	Fetal size
	Fetal abnormality
	Fetal malposition
	Fetal malpresentation
Power	Lack of coordinated regular strong uterine contractions

Fig. 15.2 Differential diagnosis of the causes of failure to progress in labour.

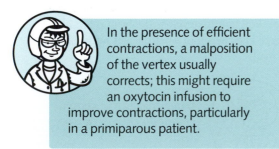

In the presence of efficient contractions, a malposition of the vertex usually corrects; this might require an oxytocin infusion to improve contractions, particularly in a primiparous patient.

Examination

Examination of the patient should always include checking the colour of the liquor to exclude meconium. This is relevant when considering fetal well-being in a patient who is making slow progress.

It should be assessed in conjunction with the fetal monitoring (see Chapter 16).

Passages and passenger

Short stature puts the patient at risk of CPD and so, traditionally, maternal height is checked at the booking visit (see Chapter 45). Chapter 46 discusses in detail the examination of the maternal abdomen and the vagina to assess the size and position of the fetus. Figure 15.3 lists the factors that should be checked.

Labour can be slow if the fetus is not in a longitudinal lie. Similarly, a malpresentation (see Chapter 39) or a malposition (see Chapter 40) causes failure to progress. The uterus should always be palpated to check engagement, that is, how much of the fetal head is palpable above the pelvic brim.

When the cervix is fully effaced at the onset of labour, it is thin. However, if progress is slow, it becomes thicker on palpation as it gets oedematous. A cervical fibroid should be excluded.

Figure 15.4 demonstrates how the station of the presenting part is assessed. Caput and moulding (see Chapter 40) increase as the progress of the labour slows. Moulding is graded according to whether the overlapping of the skull bones is reducible or not.

Power

Abdominal palpation assesses the following features of the contractions:
- Frequency.
- Strength.
- Length.

Examination of the patient who is making slow progress in labour	
Type of examination	**Procedure**
Abdominal examination	Uterine size by measuring symphysis–fundal height (SFH)
	Fetal lie
	Fetal presentation
	Fetal position
	Engagement
Vaginal examination	Cervical dilatation
	Cervical thickness or effacement
	Station
	Position of the presenting part
	Presence of caput or moulding
	Pelvic outlet (less commonly performed nowadays)

Fig. 15.3 Examination of the patient who is making slow progress in labour.

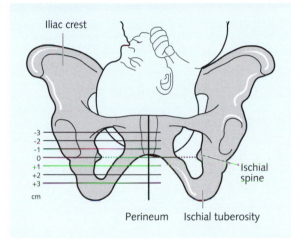

Fig. 15.4 Station of the head.

Investigation

Assessment of the passage and the passenger is made clinically as described above (Fig. 15.5). The cardiotocograph can be used to assess frequency of uterine contractions, in conjunction with uterine palpation. It also assesses the risk of fetal hypoxia (see Chapter 16).

Management

This depends on the cause. Artificial rupture of the membranes (ARM) is thought to release local prostaglandins and can increase the rate of labour progression. The strength and frequency of the

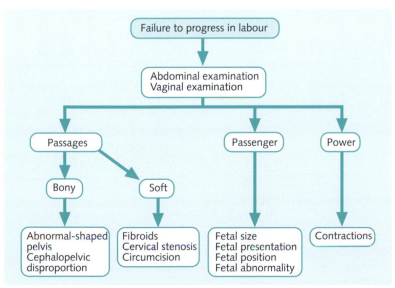

Fig. 15.5 Algorithm for failure to progress in labour.

uterine contractions can also be improved. Regular strong contractions will help to correct a fetal malposition by rotating the head against the pelvic floor muscles, as well as improving descent.

However, caution must be exercised in a multiparous patient. Generally, labour proceeds more rapidly in a second pregnancy. Therefore, if progress is slow, fetal size and the risk of CPD must be considered so that excessive contractions do not put the patient at risk of uterine rupture.

The presence of good contractions over several hours but without significant progression in terms of cervical dilatation and descent of the presenting part should alert the physician to consider delivery by caesarean section.

Failure to progress in the second stage of labour should be assessed in the manner already described and instrumental delivery considered (see Chapter 41). If the head is almost crowning then an episiotomy might be all that is necessary.

Oxytocin infusions can correct prolonged labour but particular care must be taken to exclude cephalopelvic disproportion if there is secondary arrest in a multiparous patient.

16. Abnormal Cardiotocograph in Labour

The cardiotocograph, or CTG, is a form of electronic fetal heart rate (FHR) monitoring used to evaluate fetal well-being before and during labour. It has been used increasingly in the UK since the 1970s, with the aim of detecting fetal hypoxia before it causes perinatal mortality or cerebral palsy.

However, the expected reduction in hypoxia-induced intrapartum perinatal mortality has not occurred and the role of CTG monitoring has been questioned. Recently, the need to educate staff about CTG interpretation and audit standards has been highlighted.

When presenting a CTG, note the:
- Patient's name.
- Date.
- Baseline FHR.
- Baseline variability.
- Presence of accelerations.
- Absence of decelerations if the trace is normal.

Features of the CTG

There are four features of the CTG, which should all be assessed individually and then taken together with the clinical picture to determine the appropriate management of the patient. For example, the progress of the labour or the presence of meconium-stained liquor might be important considerations. Figure 16.1 shows a normal CTG tracing.

- Baseline fetal heart rate (FHR): this is the mean level of FHR over a period of 5 to 10min. It is expressed as beats per minute (bpm) and is determined by the fetal sympathetic and the parasympathetic nervous systems. The normal range is 110–160bpm. In the preterm fetus, the baseline tends to be at the higher end of the normal range.
- Baseline variability: minor fluctuations occur in the baseline FHR at 3 to 5 cycles per minute. It is measured by estimating the difference in bpm between the highest peak and the lowest trough of change in a 1-min segment of the trace. Normal baseline variability is ≥ 5bpm.
- Accelerations: these are increases in the FHR of 15bpm or more, lasting 15s or more. These are a feature of a normal CTG.
- Decelerations: these are falls in the FHR below the baseline of more than 15bpm, lasting 15s or more. Different patterns of decelerations can be seen, depending on their timing with the uterine contractions:
  - Early decelerations: the FHR slows at the same time as the onset of the contraction and returns to the baseline at the end of the contraction.
  - Late decelerations: the FHR begins to fall during the contraction, with its trough more than 20s after the peak of the contraction and returning to baseline after the contraction.
  - Variable decelerations: the timing of the slowing of the FHR in relation to the uterine contraction varies and can occur in isolation. There is typically rapid onset and recovery. However, other features might make this type of deceleration more suspicious, such as loss of the normal baseline variability.
  - Sinusoidal pattern: there is regular oscillation of the baseline, with absent variability. The pattern lasts at least 10min and has an amplitude of 5–15bpm above and below the baseline.

Figure 16.2 shows an abnormal CTG tracing. The CTG can be categorized into :
- Normal: all four features are reassuring.
- Suspicious: one feature is non-reassuring, the others are reassuring.
- Pathological: two or more features are non-reassuring, or more than one is abnormal.

Figure 16.3 shows how the features of the CTG are categorized.

Physiology

The principle of monitoring during labour is to detect fetal hypoxia and therefore prevent acidaemia and cell damage.

Acute fetal hypoxia

This can occur secondary to:

- Uterine hyperstimulation.
- Placental abruption.
- Umbilical cord compression.

These conditions can result in a decrease in the fetal heart rate, with decelerations or bradycardia. This is produced by chemoreceptor-mediated vagal stimulation and then by myocardial ischaemia.

Chronic fetal hypoxia

If there has been chronic uteroplacental insufficiency during the pregnancy, for example secondary to pre-eclampsia, then the fetus might be at increased risk of hypoxia during labour. Reduced intervillous perfusion during uterine contractions or maternal hypotension can exacerbate underlying reduced placental perfusion. This might result in an increase in the fetal cardiac output with an increase in the baseline heart rate and could be followed by reduced heart rate variability due to brainstem hypoxia. Continuing hypoxia eventually produces myocardial damage and heart rate decelerations.

Monitoring uterine contractions

As well as monitoring the FHR, the CTG also monitors the frequency of the uterine contractions. This can be important, for example, if the patient is having intravenous oxytocin to stimulate the contractions. It is essential that frequency of contractions and the return to resting tone between contractions is noted.

The actual strength and the length of each contraction should be checked by palpation of the uterus, because the size of the peaks shown on the tracing might be related to positioning of the monitor on the maternal abdomen or thickness of the maternal abdominal wall.

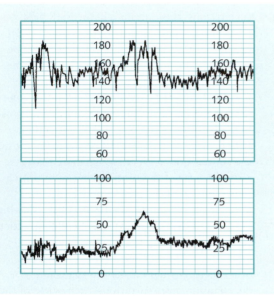

Fig. 16.1 Fetal heart acceleration during a uterine contraction with normal baseline variability.

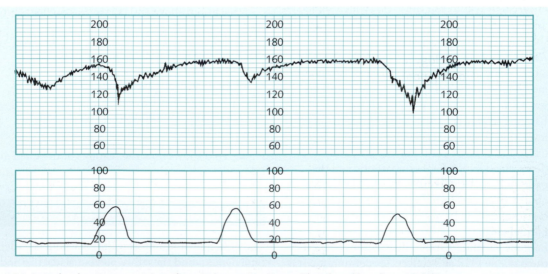

Fig. 16.2 Late decelerations occurring after uterine contractions with reduced baseline variability.

Features of the fetal heart rate				
Feature	Baseline (bpm)	Variability (bpm)	Decelerations	Accelerations
Reassuring	110–160	≥5	None present	Present
Non-reassuring	100–109 161–180	<5 for ≥40min	Early decelerations Variable decelerations/single deceleration 3 min	None present
Abnormal	<100 >180 Sinusoidal pattern	<5 for ≥90min ≥ 10min	Late decelerations Single deceleration >3 min	None present

Fig. 16.3 Categorization of the features of the fetal heart rate.

Monitoring in an uncomplicated pregnancy

Intermittent auscultation of the fetal heart rate might be appropriate for a healthy woman in labour who has had an uncomplicated pregnancy. This involves documenting the heart rate for a minimum of 60s at least:

- Every 15min in the first stage of labour.
- Every 5min in the second stage of labour.

Continuous monitoring might be recommended if any abnormal features develop or any risk factors develop, such as meconium-stained liquor.

Who should have continuous CTG monitoring?

Figure 16.4 shows the maternal and fetal indications for recommending continuous monitoring.

The maternal and fetal indications for advising continuous CTG monitoring relate to the underlying physiology related to changes in the FHR during normal and abnormal labour. Don't forget that intermittent monitoring might be appropriate in some patients.

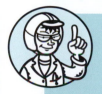

For FBS the following are required:
- Appropriate equipment.
- Cervix ≥ 2 cm dilated.
- Mother in left lateral position.

Indication for monitoring	
Maternal	Previous caesarean section Pre-eclampsia Diabetes Antepartum haemorrhage Other maternal medical disease
Fetal	Intrauterine growth restriction Prematurity Oligohydramnios Abnormal Doppler artery studies Multiple pregnancy Breech presentation
Intrapartum	Meconium-stained liquor Vaginal bleeding in labour Use of oxytocin for augmentation Epidural analgesia Maternal pyrexia Post-term pregnancy Prolonged rupture of membranes >24h Induced labour

Fig. 16.4 Indications for recommending continuous cardiotocograph monitoring.

History of the patient who presents with an abnormal CTG in labour

The need to act on an abnormal CTG in labour can be influenced by maternal, fetal and intrapartum factors. Figure 16.4 gives the indications for continuous CTG monitoring but this list also shows the relevant points in the patient's antenatal history that might make the attending physician more concerned if the CTG is suspicious.

Particularly important are the intrapartum factors. In the presence of meconium-stained liquor, for example, the CTG should be acted upon promptly. If the cervix is not yet dilated, fetal blood sampling might not be possible (see below). If progress in labour is slow (see Chapter 15), then operative delivery might be necessary.

Examination of the patient who presents with an abnormal CTG in labour

Baseline maternal observations
Temperature
A raised temperature might explain fetal tachycardia.

Pulse
This might be raised in conjunction with maternal pyrexia. In the presence of fetal bradycardia, maternal pulse should be checked to ensure that the monitoring is recording FHR and not the mother.

Blood pressure
Epidural anaesthesia can be associated with maternal hypotension as it is administered. This results in reduced flow to the uterus and can cause fetal bradycardia. Therefore, blood pressure should be regularly checked when the medication is given.

Abdominal palpation
- Size.
- Engagement of presenting part.
- Scar tenderness in a patient with a previous caesarean section.
- Uterine tone.

The size of the maternal abdomen should be assessed to check if it is large or small for dates (see Chapter 11). The engagement of the presenting part is important to assess progress in labour (see Chapters 15 and 40). In a patient who has previously had a caesarean section, the presence of scar tenderness should be elicited; scar rupture is commonly associated with an abnormal CTG and vaginal bleeding. Another cause of vaginal bleeding with an abnormal CTG is placental abruption (see Chapter 37). If this is suspected, the uterus will typically feel hard and tender.

The uterine contractions should be palpated, especially if the patient's labour is being stimulated by intravenous oxytocic agents. It is important to check that the uterus is not hyperstimulated, as this can cause an abnormal CTG. There should be resting tone between contractions.

Vaginal examination
As well as assessing the dilatation of the cervix to determine the progress in labour and the ability to perform a fetal blood sample, the presence of the fetal cord must be excluded. A cord prolapse, as it is known, is associated with a fetal bradycardia, and this is an emergency situation requiring immediate delivery by caesarean section.

Investigating the abnormal CTG

Using the criteria described above, if the CTG is suspicious, the patient can be managed conservatively (Fig. 16.5).

If the CTG is pathological, fetal blood sampling (FBS) should be performed if there are the appropriate facilities. The procedure is performed with the mother in the left lateral postion and the cervix should be dilated at least 2 cm. A sample of blood from the fetal scalp gives the fetal pH (i.e. a measure of acidosis). It might indicate that delivery is necessary (pH ≤ 7.20), or that the test should be repeated within 30 min (pH 7.21–7.24).

If FBS is not possible, delivery should be expedited. Contraindications to FBS are given in Fig. 16.6.

Fig. 16.5 Algorithm for cardiotocograph monitoring.

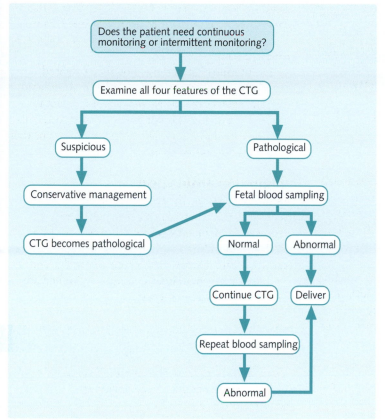

Contraindications to fetal blood sampling

- Maternal infection (HIV/hepatitis B/herpes simplex)
- Fetal bleeding disorder (haemophilia/thrombocytopaenia)
- Prematurity (< 34 weeks)

Fig. 16.6 Contraindications to fetal blood sampling.

17. Bleeding after Delivery

Postpartum haemorrhage

The presenting complaint in postpartum haemorrhage (PPH) is bleeding from the genital tract of more than 500 mL after delivery of the infant. It is classified as either primary or secondary:

- Primary PPH: bleeding more than 500 mL within 24 h of delivery.
- Secondary PPH: bleeding more than 500 mL that starts 24 h after delivery and occurs within 6 weeks.

Figure 17.1 gives the differential diagnoses that should be considered. About 90% of cases of PPH are caused by uterine atony; about 7% are due to genital tract trauma.

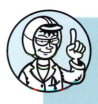

When the patient presents with primary PPH, always check that the placenta and membranes are complete to exclude retained products of conception.

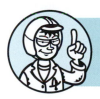

Don't forget to check the genital tract for signs of trauma once the placenta has been delivered.

History to focus on the differential diagnosis

Primary PPH
Uterine atony
Certain factors in the patient's history can increase the risk of a primary PPH secondary to uterine atony:

- Multiple pregnancy.
- Grand multiparity.
- Polyhydramnios.
- Fibroid uterus.
- Prolonged labour.

- Previous postpartum haemorrhage.
- Antepartum haemorrhage.

In a multiple pregnancy, the placental site is larger than with a singleton. There is also overdistension of the uterus (see Chapter 34). This is also seen in polyhydramnios (see Chapter 11).

Mode of delivery
The mode of delivery may increase risk of PPH. Genital tract trauma can occur with a normal vaginal delivery, either from an episiotomy (see Chapter 41) or from a vaginal or cervical tear. Bleeding is more common with an instrumental delivery especially forceps, in particular Keilland's forceps (see Chapter 41).

Average blood loss at caesarean section is 500 mL. This might be increased if there is a placenta praevia (see Chapter 37) or if delivery of the presenting part is difficult after a prolonged labour; it becomes impacted in the pelvis and delivery causes the uterus to tear.

Rarely, PPH is secondary to uterine inversion that occurs after delivery of the placenta (see Chapter 42). As well as bleeding, the patient complains of abdominal pain, which can be severe, associated with a feeling of prolapse. Rupture of the uterus is also uncommon except in association with labour in a patient who has previously had a caesarean section.

Other causes
Coagulation disorders can be acute or chronic. The chronic conditions such as inherited vascular disorders are usually known about antenatally. DIC can present acutely, secondary to placental abruption or severe pre-eclampsia for example.

Secondary PPH
In the presence of retained products of conception, either placenta or membranes, the common presenting complaint is prolonged heavy vaginal bleeding or persistent offensive discharge. If this becomes infected the patient might present with fever and lower abdominal pain.

A molar pregnancy also presents with persistent vaginal bleeding (see Chapter 29). The rarer choriocarcinoma might metastasize to the lungs, liver

Differential diagnoses of postpartum haemorrhage	
Type of PPH	**Differential diagnosis**
Primary	Uterine atony
	Genital tract trauma (cervix/vagina/perineum)
	Retained placenta/placenta accreta
	Coagulation disorders
	Uterine inversion
	Uterine rupture
Secondary	Retained products
	Endometritis
	Persistent molar pregnancy/choriocarcinoma

Fig. 17.1 Differential diagnoses of postpartum haemorrhage (see Chapter 42).

Primary postpartum haemorrhage
• Amount of blood loss
• Pulse
• Blood pressure
• Urine output
• Uterine contraction
• Fundal height
• Placenta and membranes complete
• Genital tract trauma

Fig. 17.2 Examination of the patient who presents with primary postpartum haemorrhage.

or brain. Presenting symptoms include haemoptysis and dyspnoea or neurological symptoms.

Examination

Primary PPH

The blood loss must be estimated as accurately as possible to manage the patient appropriately. Examination must include the ABC (airways, breathing, circulation) of basic resuscitation (see Chapter 18), as well as pallor, pulse and blood pressure. Abdominal palpation should assess whether the uterus is contracted or not. The fundal height should be at or below the umbilicus. If it is above, there might be retained products of conception or the uterus could be filling with clots.

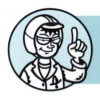 Always remember ABC and basic examination when the patient presents with PPH.

Uterine inversion should be considered if the fundus is indented or cannot be palpated. Vaginal examination will assess the degree of inversion, either up to the cervical os or complete inversion of the uterus and vagina.

If the uterus is well contracted and the placenta is out, then the bleeding might be from trauma to the genital tract. The patient should be examined in sufficient light, with adequate analgesia (either regional or general) to exclude lacerations to the cervix, vagina and perineum.

If the placenta and membranes have been delivered, they must be carefully examined to see that the cotyledons appear complete and that there is no suggestion of a succenturiate lobe. The examination is summarized in Fig. 17.2.

Secondary PPH

Basic observations should include pulse, blood pressure and temperature. There might be a tachycardia and pyrexia with endometritis. The height of the uterine fundus should be checked because the uterus will usually remain poorly contracted if there are retained products of conception. Tenderness should be excluded to rule out endometritis.

Speculum examination excludes vaginal discharge if there is suspicion of infection. Bimanual palpation examines the size of the uterus, because it might be bulky with retained products or with a molar pregnancy. Tenderness is present with endometritis. If the cervical os is open, there might be retained products of conception.

Investigations

Primary PPH

Having established intravenous access, blood should be sent for haemoglobin, platelets, clotting screen including fibrin degradation products, and serum save. Depending on the estimated blood loss, cross-matching blood might be necessary. Urea and electrolytes should be tested if the urine output is poor.

Figure 17.3 provides an algorithm for the management of primary PPH.

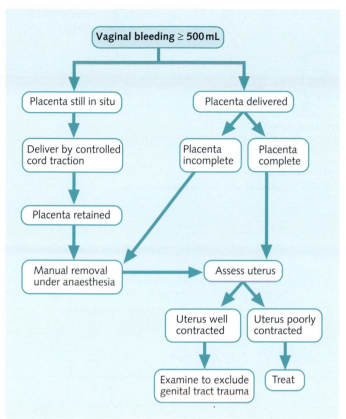

Fig. 17.3 Algorithm for the management of primary postpartum haemorrhage.

Secondary PPH

A full blood count should be taken to estimate haemoglobin and to give an indication of infection if the white blood cell count is raised. Again, cross-matching blood for transfusion might be necessary, depending on the clinical situation and the haemoglobin result. A high vaginal swab should be taken to exclude endometritis.

An ultrasound scan that is done to check that the uterus is empty will exclude retained products, including molar tissue. Care should be taken to interpret the findings in conjunction with the clinical picture because blood clot might have a similar scan appearance.

The diagnosis of a molar pregnancy is confirmed with a persistently raised serum β-hCG level. Evacuation of the uterus will yield tissue for histological analysis to confirm the diagnosis and exclude choriocarcinoma. However, if the latter is diagnosed, liver function tests and a chest X-ray should be performed to check for metastases.

Figure 17.4 provides an algorithm for the management of secondary PPH.

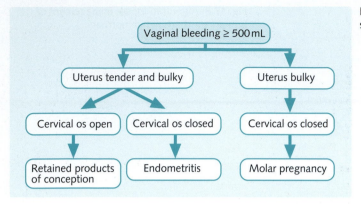

Fig. 17.4 Algorithm for the management of secondary postpartum haemorrhage.

18. Maternal Collapse

Collapse of a patient on the maternity ward or delivery suite might have an obstetric or a non-obstetric cause. The danger, when faced with a collapsed pregnant woman, is to prioritize delivery because of fears for the fetus. However, it is important to remember that maternal resuscitation is the single most effective means of improving fetal health; delivery, if necessary, should be contemplated only when the mother is stable.

The principles of first-line management are the same in all situations; check:
- airway
- breathing
- circulation

and call for help. If antenatal, establish fetal monitoring once the mother's initial resuscitation has commenced.

Haemorrhage

Antenatal bleeding sufficient to cause collapse will usually be due to placental bleeding, either placental abruption or placenta praevia. Figure 18.1 summarizes the different presentations (see also Chapter 10). Uterine rupture can also cause collapse with bleeding. Postnatal bleeding (post-partum haemorrhage) causes are shown in Fig. 18.2 and is covered in Chapter 17.

Placental abruption and placenta praevia

Major obstetric haemorrhage can be extremely rapid and is potentially fatal, so coordinated management between midwives, doctors, anaesthetists and the blood bank is vital. Abruption severe enough to cause collapse or fetal distress is likely to be associated with blood loss of at least 1500mL and a 30% incidence of coagulopathy.

Both abruption and bleeding placenta praevia increase the risk of PPH.

It can be difficult to control bleeding from the placental site during caesarean section for placenta praevia. Oxytocin infusion is used but further measures might be required, including ergometrine, the prostaglandin analogue Carboprost (Hemabate), bimanual compression, internal iliac ligation and, in extremis, hysterectomy. Recently, arterial embolization by radiologists has provided another alternative.

Uterine rupture

Uterine rupture is uncommon. Occasionally, trauma might be the cause (e.g. road traffic accident), but more commonly the woman is multiparous and in labour. Those most at risk are women with a scar on the uterus, usually a previous caesarean section; using a syntocinon infusion in this situation increases the risk still further. Symptoms and signs include:
- Scar pain and tenderness.
- Constant pain, inbetween contractions.
- PV bleeding.
- CTG abnormalities.
- Bloodstained liquor.
- Haematuria.

Resuscitation and laparotomy are needed.

Uterine atony

When the uterus fails to contract following delivery of the placenta, the blood vessels that supplied the placenta's huge circulation are not shut off by compression, so uterine bleeding continues. Risk factors include:
- Precipitate labour.
- Induced labour.
- Augmented labour (syntocinon infusion).
- Caesarean section following prolonged/augmented labour.
- Magnesium sulfate treatment.
- Multiple pregnancy.
- Chorioamnionitis.

Placental praevia versus placental abruption	
Placental abruption	**Placenta praevia**
Painful	Painless
Uterus tense, hard and tender to palpate	Uterus soft, non-tender to palpate
Amount of blood seen might not represent true loss because bleeding might be concealed	Blood loss seen reflects total loss

Fig. 18.1 Placenta praevia versus placental abruption.

Causes of postpartum haemorrhage
• Tone: uterine atony
• Tissue: retained products of conception
• Trauma: genital tract lacerations
• Thrombin: clotting abnormalities

Fig. 18.2 Causes of postpartum haemorrhage.

If medical treatment (syntocinon, ergometrine, Hemabate) fails, consider packing the uterus, radiological arterial embolization, or surgery – internal iliac artery ligation, B Lynch suture or hysterectomy.

Amniotic fluid embolism

This poorly understood condition results in transient pulmonary hypertension, profound hypoxia, left ventricular failure and secondary coagulopathy. Fetal and maternal mortality is high. The use of syntocinon and rapid labour are known to be risk factors, but amniotic fluid embolism (AFE) can also occur in non-augmented labours.

The diagnosis might only be discovered post-mortem but could also be made on the basis of the characteristic trio of:
• Cyanosis.
• Collapse.
• Clotting derangement (DIC).
Management consists of ventilatory support and correction of the coagulopathy.

Acute myocardial infarction

Antenatal myocardial infarction (MI) carries a mortality of up to 45%. The resuscitation algorithm is the same as that for non-pregnant adults but the woman must be tilted onto her left side to reduce the compression of the vena cava by the pregnant abdomen (Fig. 18.3). If it is felt that the fetus is compromising the resuscitation, delivery should be achieved. A senior cardiologist should be involved at an early stage.

Eclampsia

Chapter 42 outlines the presentation and management of eclampsia. In summary, the management begins with controlling the fit. A magnesium sulfate infusion is started as prophylaxis against further fits. The blood pressure must be reduced to mean arterial pressure (MAP) levels of less than 125 mmHg. Delivery of the fetus should be considered at this point.

Diabetic emergency

Management of diabetic coma is described in *Crash Course on General Medicine*. In the acute setting it is more likely to be due to hypoglycaemia, especially as the delicate balance of tight control in pregnancy and after delivery can be very difficult. Hyperosmolar non-ketotic coma might be seen in a diabetic woman who has been unwell at home for some time.

Hypoglycaemia

 'Hypos' are more common in pregnancy because fasting blood glucose levels are lower.

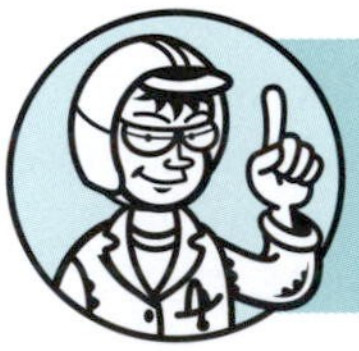

Infuse 50 mL 50% dextrose intravenously over a short space of time, followed by a saline flush. Check the blood sugar again 15 min later. Once the woman is conscious, a 20 g glucose drink is given, followed by a longer-acting carbohydrate snack or meal. The blood sugar should be rechecked 1 h later.

Hyperglycaemia

Rehydration, an insulin infusion to reduce serum glucose levels and hourly assessment of serum

A

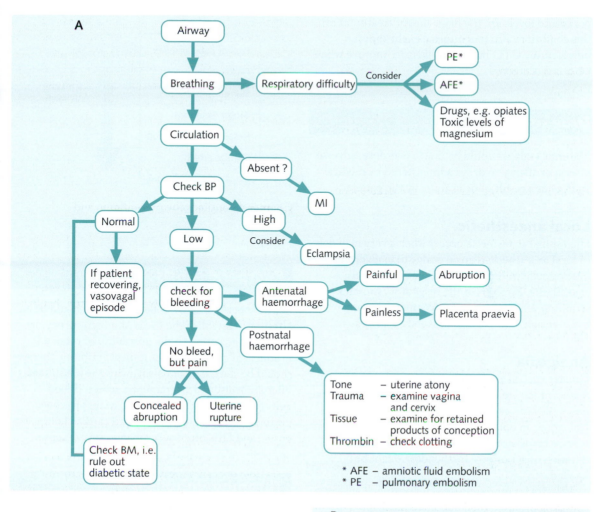

Airway → Breathing → Respiratory difficulty → Consider → PE*, AFE*, Drugs, e.g. opiates / Toxic levels of magnesium

Circulation → Absent? → MI

Check BP → Normal / Low / High → Consider → Eclampsia → MI

Normal → If patient recovering, vasovagal episode

Low → check for bleeding → Antenatal haemorrhage → Painful → Abruption / Painless → Placenta praevia

check for bleeding → No bleed, but pain → Concealed abruption / Uterine rupture

check for bleeding → Postnatal haemorrhage

Normal → Check BM, i.e. rule out diabetic state

Tone   – uterine atony
Trauma   – examine vagina and cervix
Tissue   – examine for retained products of conception
Thrombin – check clotting

* AFE – amniotic fluid embolism
* PE – pulmonary embolism

B

Wedge under the patient's right side rolls her into the left lateral position, relieving pressure on the inferior vena cava

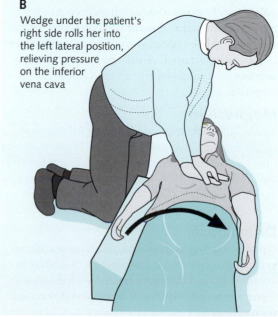

Fig. 18.3 Resuscitation. A. Algorithm. B. Position for cardiopulmonary resuscitation.

potassium levels are the main aims of treatment of this condition. Fetal monitoring might show an unreassuring CTG but this is likely to improve when ketosis is corrected.

Drug toxicity

Maternal collapse could be due to overdose, adverse effects or allergy to drugs administered by medical staff, or as a result of drug abuse by the patient.

Local anaesthetic
High spinal anaesthesia occurs when a very high dose of local anaesthetic is given or due to inadvertent intravascular injection at the time of epidural anaesthesia. Paralysis of the respiratory muscles requiring ventilation results. Warning signs are hypotension, nausea, dizziness and dyspnoea.

Analgesia
Opiates such as pethidine, morphine and diamorphine are used for pain relief in labour. In high doses they can cause respiratory depression. Naloxone, an opiate antagonist, will immediately reverse respiratory depression but has a short duration of action so a further dose might be needed.

Voltarol is commonly used for postnatal analgesia. Any drug in this family of non-steroidal anti-inflammatory drugs (NSAIDs) can precipitate bronchoconstriction in asthmatics. A severe asthma attack should be treated with IV hydrocortisone and nebulized salbutamol; ventilatory support might be necessary.

Magnesium
Magnesium sulfate is used following eclampsia as prophylaxis against further seizures. Hypermagnesia can result in coma. The signs of magnesium toxicity are shown in Fig. 18.4. Calcium gluconate injection is used to treat toxicity.

Drug abuse
Opiates, Ecstasy and cocaine can all cause collapse and coma. Convulsions can result from Ecstasy or cocaine use, and should be treated with diazepam. Opiate-induced respiratory depression is reversed with naloxone.

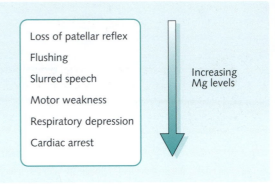

Fig. 18.4 Signs of magnesium toxicity.

Puerperal sepsis

Septic shock can cause collapse. There should be an attempt to establish the focus of infection, paying particular attention to the possibility of retained products of conception. Empirical antibiotic therapy should be started after liaising with the consultant microbiologist and after a septic screen (blood cultures, MSU, chest X-ray, and swabs) has been performed. Renal, respiratory and cardiac failure can ensue, and DIC often accompanies severe sepsis.

Thromboembolism

Pregnancy is a prothrombotic state, and thromboembolism is one of the most common causes of maternal mortality (see Chapters 36 and 43).

Pulmonary embolism
Smaller pulmonary emboli (PEs) will cause breathlessness and pleuritic pain but larger emboli can present with collapse. On examination the following may be found:
- Tachypnoea.
- Tachycardia.
- Raised jugular venous pressure (JVP).
- Loud second heart sound.

The investigation of PE is detailed in Chapter 36, with first-line investigations being arterial blood gases (to look for a low P_{O_2} and P_{CO_2}), chest X-ray (to exclude infection) and ECG, followed by a ventilation perfusion isotope (VQ) scan or spiral CT to identify the clot. Anticoagulation with heparin is the norm, but a PE large enough to cause collapse may merit treatment with streptokinase.

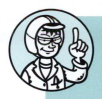

In pregnancy, arterial blood gases and ECG might be normal in the presence of a small PE, so if there is any doubt, a scan (VQ or spiral CT) must be arranged.

Cerebral vein thrombosis

This condition is uncommon but is associated with a high mortality; it usually occurs in the puerperium. There might be focal neurological signs but signs can be more 'general', with convulsions, headache, photophobia and vomiting being typical. There might be a fever and raised white cell count.

The diagnosis is made on CT or MRI. Convulsions should be treated, the patient kept well hydrated and heparin therapy considered.

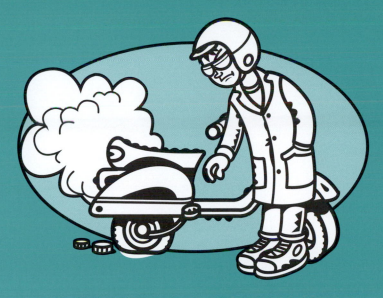

DISEASES AND DISORDERS

19. Abnormal Uterine Bleeding

Abnormal uterine bleeding is an extremely common problem experienced by most women at some time in their life. The causes can be physiological or pathological and, as long as serious pathology is excluded, might not require treatment. For normal menstruation to occur, the following are necessary:

- Hypothalamic function.
- Pituitary function.
- Ovarian function.
- Endometrial function.
- Patent cervix and vagina.

Abnormal uterine bleeding can be caused by malfunction or disease at any of these levels.

Amenorrhoea

This is the term used to describe absence of menstruation. Lack of menstruation after the age of 16 years is called primary amenorrhoea and is relatively uncommon. Secondary amenorrhoea is extremely common and implies menstruation has occurred in the past but has been absent for 6 months or more. The most common causes of secondary amenorrhoea are physiological, most frequently pregnancy and the menopause.

The causes of amenorrhoea can be broken down into the following five major categories:

- Central nervous system.
- Gonadal dysfunction.
- Genital tract disorders.
- Endocrine disorders.
- Drug therapy.

Investigation policy

Amenorrhoea can be physiological, that is, due to the premenarche, pregnancy, lactation or the menopause. When investigating primary amenorrhoea, the premenarchal state should be diagnosed only if pathology has been excluded.

Primary amenorrhoea

Primary amenorrhoea should be investigated from the age of 16 years or before if pubertal development has not started by the age of 14 years. Investigation should be determined by assessment of pubertal development (Fig. 19.1).

When no pubertal development has occurred by the age of 14 years then investigation should be as for delayed puberty (see Chapters 1 and 32).

Where pubertal development is normal, genital tract anomalies, such as an absent uterus or vagina, should be excluded by examination or ultrasound scanning. If normal then investigation should be as for secondary amenorrhoea (see below).

Incongruous pubertal development can be caused by chromosomal abnormality or increased circulating androgens. For instance, women with testicular feminization often have normal or even excellent breast development in the absence of axillary and pubic hair. Poor breast development in the presence of normal or excessive axillary or pubic hair is compatible with increased circulating androgens commonly associated with PCOS, and less commonly with CAH or androgen-secreting tumours of the ovary or adrenal.

A woman presenting with primary amenorrhoea should always have her karyotype checked.

Secondary amenorrhoea

The most common cause of secondary amenorrhoea in women of childbearing age is pregnancy, and this should be excluded before further investigation is commenced.

Having excluded physiological causes of secondary amenorrhoea, further investigation includes measurements of serum gonadotrophins, androgens and prolactin. Other useful investigations include a pelvic ultrasound scan, which will identify the typical appearance of polycystic ovaries and the presence of a haematometra, a lateral skull X-ray or CT or MRI of the head to identify a pituitary tumour and exclusion of thyroid disease and diabetes mellitus (Fig. 19.2). Women under 30 years of age who have

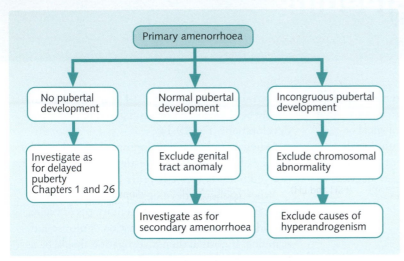

Fig. 19.1 Algorithm for primary amenorrhoea.

ovarian failure should have their chromosomes analysed.

Complications of amenorrhoea

Although amenorrhoea itself does not cause any complications, some of the underlying conditions do carry certain risks:

- Women who carry a Y chromosome have a 25% chance of developing gonadal malignancy, usually a gonadoblastoma or dysgerminoma.
- Hypo-oestrogenic states characteristic of hypothalamic amenorrhoea and premature ovarian failure are associated with an increased risk of osteoporosis and ischaemic heart disease.
- Endometrial hyperplasia and endometrial carcinoma occur more frequently in women with PCOS because of the unopposed oestrogen effect on the endometrium associated with chronic anovulation.
- Haematocolpos is associated with an increased risk of endometriosis due to retrograde menstruation.
- Amenorrhoeic women are usually subfertile.

Treatment of amenorrhoea

Certain conditions can cause primary and secondary amenorrhoea, depending on the age at which the condition presents. Their treatment is discussed under secondary amenorrhoea.

Treatment of primary amenorrhoea
Gonadal dysgenesis
Apart from the management of the psychosexual aspects of gonadal dysgenesis, these women require

HRT to protect against cardiovascular disease and osteoporosis. This will also stimulate secondary sexual development in those who have not yet been exposed to oestrogens (e.g. Turner's syndrome). Those women who carry a Y chromosome should have both gonads removed, because of the risk of malignancy, followed by long-term HRT.

Genital tract anomaly
Women with a congenitally absent vagina should be offered vaginal reconstruction to enable sexual activity. If the uterus is present, this will allow drainage of a haematometra. A haematocolpos should be drained by excision of the persistent vaginal membrane.

Treatment of secondary amenorrhoea
In young women who have no pathology, the condition is often self-limiting and might not require treatment.

Hypothalamic amenorrhoea
Where weight loss is implicated, a return of BMI to the normal range (25–30) usually results in spontaneous menstruation, as does the removal of stressful situations or treatment of systemic illness.

Polycystic ovary syndrome (PCOS)
The mainstay of treatment for PCOS is weight loss. As the BMI approaches the normal range spontaneous ovulation and menstruation often

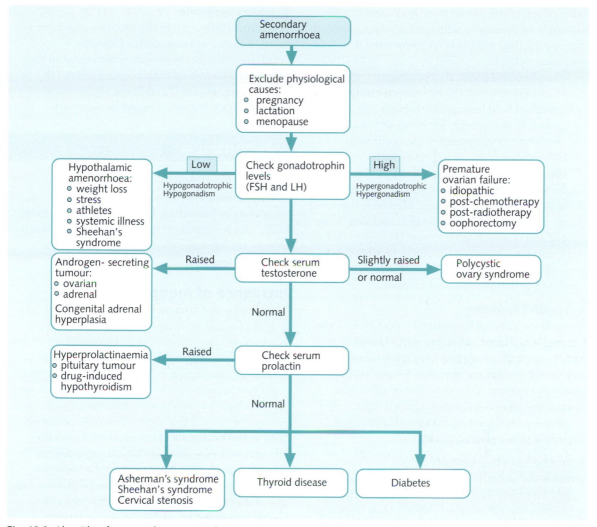

Fig. 19.2 Algorithm for secondary amenorrhoea.

occurs. Endometrial hyperplasia should be treated with progestogens. Long-term protection of the endometrium can be provided using cyclical progestogens or the COCP. Dianette (Schering) is ideal for those with hirsutism because the anti-androgenic and progestogenic effect of cyproterone acetate will reduce symptoms of hyperandrogenism and protect the endometrium from hyperplasia. A new combined pill (Yasmin; Schering) contains a progestogen (drospirenone), which has both a weak anti-androgenic and antimineralocorticoid activity.

Metformin is now being used in trials for treatment of PCOS as it is thought to be driven by insulin resistance.

Hyperprolactinaemia

The treatment of hyperprolactinaemia includes the following:

- Dopamine agonists for microadenoma.
- Dopamine agonists or surgery for macroadenoma.
- Cessation of drugs, where possible, in drug-induced hyperprolactinaemia.
- Correction of hypothyroidism.

Treatment is advisable for pituitary microadenoma to reduce the risk of osteoporosis. Dopamine agonists such as bromocriptine and cabergoline should be used to reduce the serum prolactin levels. Side-effects include nausea, dizziness, hypotension, drowsiness and headaches, and are less common with cabergoline, which can be given once weekly. Cessation of therapy usually results in recurrence of hyperprolactinaemia but is recommended if pregnancy occurs.

Transphenoidal removal of pituitary macroadenoma carries a risk of diabetes insipidus, cerebrospinal fluid leakage, panhypopituitarism and recurrence of the tumour. Shrinkage of the tumour and resolution of symptoms might occur with medical treatment, as for microadenoma.

Where hyperprolactinaemia is drug induced (Fig. 19.3), cessation of the drug results in a fall of serum prolactin levels to normal levels. However, this is not always advisable, depending on the condition being treated and where drug treatment is likely to be long term, oestrogen replacement might be advisable to prevent osteoporosis. Hypothyroidism should be corrected with thyroxine replacement.

Asherman's syndrome
Cervical stenosis can be treated by dilatation of the cervix. Intra-uterine adhesions should be divided hysteroscopically. Insertion of an intra-uterine contraceptive device is advisable for at least three months to prevent redevelopment of adhesions. Stimulation of endometrial re-growth using exogenous oestrogens i.e. hormone replacement therapy is sometimes necessary.

Hormone-secreting tumours
Ovarian and adrenal hormone secreting tumours should be surgically removed. As much ovarian tissue as possible should be preserved especially in younger women.

Prescribed drugs that can cause hyperprolactinaemia	
Types of drug	**Drug class**
Antipsychotic drugs	Phenothiazines
	Haloperidol
Antidepressants	Tricyclic antidepresssants
Antihypertensive drugs	Methyldopa
	Reserpine
Oestrogens	Combined oral contraceptive pill
H_2-receptor antagonists	Cimetidine
	Ranitidine
	Metoclopramide and domperidone
Don't forget chemotherapy for malignancy or immunological disorders	

Fig. 19.3 Prescribed drugs that can cause hyperprolactinaemia

Sheehan's syndrome
Postpartum infarction of the pituitary gland due to massive obstetric haemorrhage (Sheehan's syndrome) requires oestrogen replacement in the form of the combined contraceptive pill or HRT to prevent osteoporosis. In addition, replacement of other pituitary hormones might be necessary.

Menorrhagia

Menorrhagia is defined as menstrual blood loss (MBL) of more than 80 mL per period. This represents two standard deviations above the mean MBL, which is about 40 mL per period. Two-thirds of women with genuine menorrhagia will have iron-deficiency anaemia.

Incidence of menorrhagia
The incidence of true menorrhagia is reported to be 9–15% of population samples in Western Europe, however, as many as one-third of women regard their menstrual loss as heavy. Early menarche, late menopause, reduction in family size with concurrent reduction in periods of lactational amenorrhoea have all contributed to an almost tenfold increase in the number of periods that women experience during their reproductive life. This, combined with the changing role of women within society whereby many are involved in work outside the home, has meant that excessive menstrual bleeding has become one of the most common causes of concern for health in women.

Diagnosing menorrhagia
Menorrhagia can be diagnosed using the following techniques:
• Subjective assessment.
• Pictorial blood loss assessment charts (Fig. 19.4).
• Objective assessment.

As only half of women complaining of heavy periods will have menorrhagia, reliance on subjective assessment alone will mean that many women are treated for a condition that they do not suffer from. A visual method of assessing menstrual blood loss using pictorial charts has been shown to be more effective at diagnosing menorrhagia than subjective assessment alone. They take into account the degree to which each item of sanitary protection is soiled with blood as well as the quantity used but, unfortunately, are not frequently used in practice.

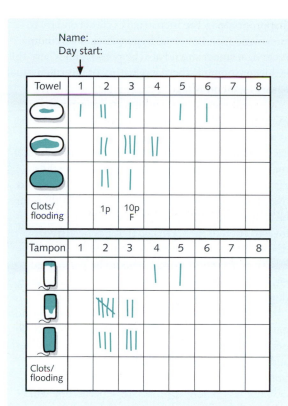

Fig. 19.4 Pictorial blood loss assessment chart.

Aetiology of menorrhagia	
Types of disorder	**Specific problem**
Systemic disorders	Thyroid disease
	Clotting disorders
Local causes	Fibroids
	Endometrial polyps
	Endometrial carcinoma
	Endometriosis/adenomyosis
	Pelvic inflammatory disease
	Dysfunctional uterine bleeding
Iatrogenic	Intrauterine contraceptive devices
	Oral anticoagulants

Fig. 19.5 Aetiology of menorrhagia.

Objective measurement of menstrual blood loss is rarely performed and usually only during clinical trials. The idea of collecting and storing soiled sanitary protection for measurement of menstrual blood loss is distasteful to most and is the main reason why objective assessment is rarely performed.

Aetiology of menorrhagia

There are three categories for the aetiology of menorrhagia (Fig. 19.5):

- Systemic conditions.
- Local pathology.
- Iatrogenic causes.

Systemic conditions

The relationship between hypothyroidism and menorrhagia has not been confirmed because of insufficient objective data, although individual cases have been reported.

Up to 90% of women with bleeding disorders have been shown to have menorrhagia. Coagulation disorders are found in up to one-third of young women admitted to hospital with profound menorrhagia.

Local pathology

Fibroids can increase menstrual loss in two ways. First, they can enlarge the uterine cavity, thereby increasing the surface area of the endometrium from which menstruation occurs and second, they can produce prostaglandins, which have been implicated in the aetiology of menorrhagia. In a similar way, endometrial polyps can increase the surface area of the endometrium and are also hormonally active.

Measured MBL in the presence of pelvic pathology, such as endometriosis and PID, is very variable and often in the normal range. Menorrhagia is therefore associated with, not necessarily caused by, these conditions.

Dysfunctional uterine bleeding (DUB) is the most common cause of menorrhagia and is the term used when there are no local or systemic causes for menorrhagia. It is therefore a diagnosis made by exclusion. Altered endometrial prostaglandin metabolism would appear to have an important role in the aetiology of DUB. Further evidence is given by the fact that prostaglandin inhibitors are known to decrease menstrual blood loss in women with DUB.

Premalignant and malignant endometrium can present with menorrhagia and must always be excluded in women who complain of excessive MBL.

Iatrogenic causes

The presence of an IUCD has been shown to increase menstrual blood loss and is the most common iatrogenic cause of menorrhagia. Menorrhagia and anaemia are up to five times more common in IUCD users than with other forms of contraception.

Roughly one half of women taking oral anticoagulants will be found to have objective evidence of menorrhagia.

Investigating menorrhagia

Investigation (Fig. 19.6) is aimed at excluding the systemic and local causes of menorrhagia and include:

- Full blood count and, where clinically indicated, thyroid function tests and clotting tests.
- Pelvic ultrasound (vaginal ultrasound is particularly sensitive).
- Endometrial biopsy.
- Hysteroscopy.

A full blood count should be performed in all cases. Thyroid function and clotting studies should be performed only where indicated by the clinical history.

A pelvic ultrasound has become almost mandatory and will identify uterine enlargement due to fibroids as well as adnexal masses. Endometrial polyps or submucous fibroids should be suspected where the endometrial thickness is increased.

An endometrial biopsy should be performed in all women over 40 and in women under 40 if there are suspicious findings on ultrasound scan. This can be performed either in the outpatient clinic or under general anaesthesia. It might show endometrium inappropriate to the menstrual cycle secondary to anovulation, endometrial hyperplasia or carcinoma. A cervical smear should also be performed where this is due, or sooner if there is a history of intermenstrual or postcoital bleeding.

Current methods of endometrial sampling, for example pipelle suction tubing, appear to be at least as accurate as D&C, have high levels of patient acceptability, lower complication rates and do not require inpatient admission or general anaesthesia. However, they have been shown to miss benign and malignant endometrial pathology and must therefore be considered inadequate for the further investigation of menorrhagia that has persisted despite medical therapy. In this instance, a hysteroscopy plus sampling should be performed either as an outpatient or under general anaesthesia depending on facilities and patient preference.

The most effective way of excluding intrauterine pathology is by diagnostic hysteroscopy. This can be performed in the outpatient setting without analgesia and will identify endometrial polyps, submucous fibroids, endometritis and most endometrial carcinomas. Where appropriate, laparoscopy will be indicated to exclude pelvic pathology.

There would appear to be enough evidence to suggest that blind D&C, used as a diagnostic or therapeutic tool in the management of menorrhagia, is one of the most inappropriately used surgical procedures of our time.

Complications of menorrhagia

Apart from the effect on the quality of life and interference with both social life and work, which can be profound, the most common complication of menorrhagia is iron-deficiency anaemia.

Treatment of menorrhagia

The treatment of menorrhagia should be tailored to the patient's needs and also to the findings of the relevant investigations. Practically, this usually includes the following:

- Correction of iron-deficiency anaemia.
- Treatment of systemic disorders or focal pathology.
- Attempted control of menorrhagia by medical treatment and, if this fails.
- Surgical treatment of menorrhagia.

Medical treatment of menorrhagia

It is generally believed, by doctors and patients alike, that most drugs used to treat menorrhagia are not only ineffective but produce intolerable side-effects.

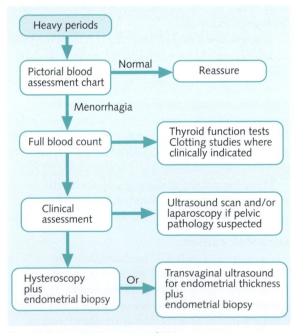

Fig. 19.6 Investigating menorrhagia.

This has led to their inappropriate use and a greater reliance on surgical techniques in the management of menorrhagia. For instance, progestogens are the most commonly prescribed drug for menorrhagia and yet are the least effective. The reduction of mean MBL for different medical therapies is shown in Fig. 19.7.

Prostaglandin inhibitors

A wide range of non-steroidal anti-inflammatory drugs (NSAIDs), including aspirin, indomethacin, flufenamic and mefenamic acid, are potent inhibitors of the cyclo-oxygenase enzyme system, which is a controlling step in the production of cyclic endoperoxides from arachidonic acid. Three-quarters of women treated with NSAIDs will find an improvement in MBL, with a mean reduction of 50%. Dysmenorrhoea and menstrual headaches are also improved. As medication is taken with menstruation, side-effects are usually better tolerated than with those drugs that are taken daily.

Antifibrinolytics and haemostatics

Tranexamic acid is an antifibrinolytic that inhibits the activation of plasminogen to plasmin. The rationale for its use is to reduce the excessive fibrinolytic activity found in the endometrium of menorrhagic women. Rare anecdotal but potentially fatal intracranial thrombosis might account for its lack of popularity in the UK. In women with menorrhagia who have no history or family history of thrombosis it should be regarded as the first line of treatment.

Ethamsylate, a haemostatic agent with antihyaluronidase activity and possibly a prostaglandin inhibitor, is thought to maintain capillary integrity. The reduction in mean MBL appears to be proportional to the severity of menorrhagia. Ethamsylate is not a popular medical treatment of menorrhagia in the UK.

Hormonal therapy
Progestogens

Oral progestogens are the most commonly used drugs for the treatment of menorrhagia and are probably the least effective. Early studies showed an improvement in subjective MBL but objective studies have shown no statistical improvement. They are most effectively used in anovulatory menorrhagia to produce cycle control.

Intrauterine systems

Intrauterine contraceptive systems impregnated with either progesterone or levonorgestrel have been shown to dramatically reduce MBL as well as acting as a very reliable contraception. The Mirena intrauterine system releases 20 µg of levonorgestrel every 24 h into the endometrium from a silicone barrel. As a result of minimal systemic absorption, side-effects are usually limited to irregular spotting in the initial year of usage and, as a safe long-term medical treatment for menorrhagia, this method seems extremely encouraging. Amenorrhoea is induced in up to 50% of long-term users because of endometrial atrophy. Contraceptively, it is as effective as sterilization and yet fertility returns almost immediately on removal of the system. It has recently been granted its license in the UK for the treatment of menorrhagia for up to 5 years per system.

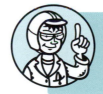

The most effective long-term medical therapy for menorrhagia is currently the levonorgestrel intrauterine system.

Mean per cent reduction in measured menstrual blood loss in women with menorrhagia treated with medical therapy	
Drug	**Mean % MBL reduction**
Non-steroidal anti-inflammatory drugs (NSAIDs)	
Mefenamic acid	47
Antifibrinolytics	
Tranexamic acid	54
Hormonal therapy	
COCP	50
Danazol	60
Levonorgestrel IUS	97
Luteal phase progestogen	15

Fig. 19.7 Mean per cent reduction in measured menstrual blood loss in women with menorrhagia treated with medical therapy.

The combined oral contraceptive pill

When taken in a cyclical fashion, the COCP inhibits ovulation and produces regular shedding of a thin endometrium. This makes it an effective and acceptable longer-term medical treatment for some women with menorrhagia. Thrombogenic side-effects restrict its therapeutic use to younger women, especially in smokers.

Danazol

Danazol is a testosterone derivative producing a number of effects on the hypothalamic–pituitary–ovarian axis. The optimum dosage in the treatment of menorrhagia appears to be 200 mg daily, significantly reducing mean MBL as well as reducing dysmenorrhoea. The androgenic properties of danazol produce unacceptable side-effects in some women.

Gonadotrophin-releasing hormone agonists

GnRH agonists suppress pituitary–ovarian function and effectively produce a temporary, reversible menopausal state. Because of the subsequent bone density loss their long-term use as a primary medical treatment for menorrhagia is limited unless add-back hormone therapy is given. This relegates their clinical use to that of preoperative adjunct allowing correction of iron-deficiency anaemia, reduction in the size of fibroids and reduction in surgical blood loss (see Chapter 20).

The management of menorrhagia using medical therapies should be tailored to the patient's individual needs. Guidelines are shown in Fig. 19.8.

Surgical treatment of menorrhagia

Surgical treatment of menorrhagia depends on the diagnosis. Intrauterine pathology such as endometrial polyps and submucous fibroids can be removed hysteroscopically. Following hysteroscopic myomectomy, MBL has been shown to reduce by 75%. Open myomectomy may be required in the presence of large fibroids and where the uterus is to be conserved. Endometrial ablation and hysterectomy are the most common operations performed for menorrhagia and these will be discussed in detail.

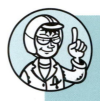 Endometrial ablative methods are becoming increasingly popular due to rapid recovery and the possibility of outpatient treatment.

Endometrial ablation

Endometrial ablation techniques aim to reduce menstrual loss by producing an 'iatrogenic' Asherman's syndrome. Endometrium is destroyed using laser, resection or thermal ablation techniques and the ensuing intrauterine adhesions reduce endometrial regrowth from deep within crypts or glands. Although not guaranteeing amenorrhoea as hysterectomy does, advantages include speed of surgery, quicker recovery, rapid return to work and the use of local as opposed to general anaesthesia. Following endometrial ablation, MBL has been shown to be reduced by up to 90%

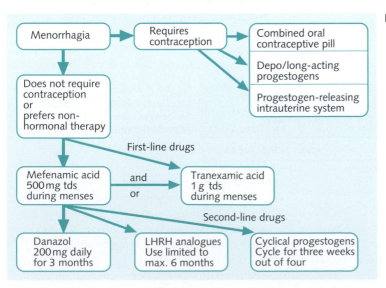

Fig. 19.8 Algorithm for menorrhagia.

Complications of endometrial ablation

Deaths have occurred after endometrial ablation; these have been due to air embolism during laser ablation, toxic shock following endometrial resection, sepsis from bowel perforation and from haemorrhage following major vessel transection. The most common operative complications are:

- Uterine perforation.
- Fluid overload.
- Haemorrhage.
- Infection.

Uterine perforation

Uterine perforation is potentially one of the most serious complications of endometrial ablation as it is associated with fluid overload as well as trauma to the gastrointestinal and genitourinary tracts and major blood vessels resulting in peritonitis or haemorrhage. Perforation commonly occurs where the uterine wall is thinnest, such as the cornual regions and the cervical canal.

Fluid overload

The use of non-electrolytic solutions, such as 1.5% glycine, for electrosurgery and the relatively high pressures needed to distend the non-compliant uterine walls predispose to the absorption of large quantities of fluid, which can result in hyponatraemia due to dilutional effects of the irrigating fluid. Congestive cardiac failure, hypertension, hyponatraemia, neurological symptoms, haemolysis, coma and even death can develop.

Haemorrhage

Haemorrhage is likely to occur if the myometrium is resected too deeply and in the event of perforation of the uterus.

Infection

The true incidence of pelvic infection following endometrial ablation is difficult to quantify. Infection can be overwhelming and might cause long-term pelvic pain.

Hysterectomy

Hysterectomy is one of the most commonly performed operations in the UK. In 1993–4, 73 517 hysterectomies were performed in NHS hospitals and approximately two-thirds of these were performed for menorrhagia. The overall lifetime risk of having a hysterectomy in the UK is 20%.

Complications of hysterectomy

The mortality rate following hysterectomy for benign disease is very low – approximately 6 per 10 000 – and is usually a consequence of cardiovascular disease and sepsis.

Morbidity associated with hysterectomy is common and occurs in almost half the women undergoing abdominal hysterectomy and one-quarter of those undergoing vaginal hysterectomy. Although conditions such as thromboembolic disease should not be forgotten, the following are some of the more likely complications to be encountered:

- Febrile morbidity.
- Haemorrhage requiring transfusion.
- Unintended major surgery because of:
  - Urinary tract damage.
  - Bowel damage.
- Long-term complications.

Febrile morbidity

Febrile morbidity accounts for most of the overall morbidity following hysterectomy, with one in three women experiencing this following the abdominal approach. In one-quarter of cases the source of infection is not identifiable; the most common identifiable infection is urinary tract infection, followed by wound or vaginal cuff infection. The use of prophylactic antibiotics is associated with a lower rate of infection of the urinary tract, abdominal wound and vaginal cuff.

Urinary tract damage

Damage to the ureter occurs in approximately 1 in every 200 hysterectomies. The ureter is likely to be damaged at the infundibulopelvic ligament, beneath the uterine artery and adjacent to the cervix. Predisposing factors to ureteric damage include congenital anomaly of the renal tracts and distortion of normal anatomy from pelvic inflammatory disease, endometriosis and malignancy.

Trauma to the bladder occurs in approximately 1 in 100 hysterectomies and is much higher following vaginal hysterectomy. Predisposing factors include previous surgery and obesity.

Bowel damage

The incidence of bowel trauma is approximately 1 in 200 hysterectomies. Risk factors predisposing to bowel damage are obesity, previous laparotomy, adhesions, intrinsic bowel problems (e.g. chronic inflammatory bowel disease) and irradiation.

Bowel dysfunction following hysterectomy is well documented, with constipation occurring in up to half the patients during the first 2 weeks of the abdominal approach. One in five patients will continue to complain of constipation in the first three postoperative months.

Long-term complications of hysterectomy

During the removal of the uterus, the pelvic floor and its nerve supply are disrupted. This can predispose to pelvic floor laxity with subsequent prolapse, as well as bladder and bowel dysfunction. Even when the ovaries are conserved, disruption of their blood supply is thought to interfere with their function, and might even predispose to premature ovarian failure, a risk factor for cardiovascular disease and osteoporosis.

Postmenopausal bleeding

Postmenopausal bleeding (PMB) is vaginal bleeding occurring more than 6 months after the menopause. In clinical practice, the menopause is a retrospective diagnosis and it is therefore important to keep in mind, and exclude, causes of secondary amenorrhoea such as pregnancy. PMB is a common disorder and requires prompt investigation to exclude malignancy.

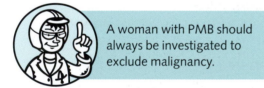
A woman with PMB should always be investigated to exclude malignancy.

Causes of postmenopausal bleeding

There are many causes of PMB and the simplest way of remembering them all is by anatomy (Fig. 19.9). However, although atrophic changes to the genital tract are the most common cause of PMB, malignancy of the endometrium, cervix and ovary must always be remembered and excluded.

Disease of the ovary in postmenopausal women is uncommon but can present with PMB. An oestrogen-secreting tumour causes PMB by stimulating the endometrium in the absence of progesterone. This is likely to cause hyperplasia and even carcinoma of the endometrium. Ovarian carcinoma usually causes PMB by direct invasion through the uterine wall.

Submucous fibroids can cause PMB, although these are likely to have been present from before the menopause. The endometrium should be inactive in the postmenopausal years and atrophic endometritis

Causes of postmenopausal bleeding	
Structure affected	**Specific cause**
Ovary	Carcinoma of the ovary
	Oestrogen-secreting tumour
Uterine body	Myometrium:
	• submucous fibroid
	Endometrium:
	• atrophic changes
	• polyp
	• hyperplasia - simple or atypical carcinoma
	(Pregnancy)
Cervix	Atrophic changes
	Malignancy:
	• squamous carcinoma
	• adenocarcinoma
Vagina	Atrophic changes
Urethra	Urethral caruncle
	(Haematuria)
Vulva	Vulvitis
	Dystrophies
	Malignancy

Fig. 19.9 Causes of postmenopausal bleeding.

is a common consequence. Endometrial polyps might be benign, contain areas of atypical hyperplasia or be malignant. Endometrial hyperplasia can arise de novo, or be secondary to oestrogen stimulation. Exogenous unopposed oestrogens and endogenous oestrogens arising from peripheral conversion of precursors in adipose tissue, or from oestrogen-secreting ovarian tumours, can result in endometrial hyperplasia and adenocarcinoma. Adenocarcinoma of the endometrium is an important cause of PMB and must always be considered in the differential diagnosis.

Atrophic changes to the genital tract due to oestrogen deficiency can cause bleeding and, in fact, are the most common cause of PMB. Atrophic changes can occur to the endometrium, cervix and vagina. Urethral caruncle (prolapse of the urethral mucosa) is also associated with oestrogen deficiency.

Cervical carcinoma and squamous carcinoma of the vulva can present with PMB and although the non-neoplastic epithelial disorders of the vulva (vulva dystrophies) do not themselves usually cause PMB, scratching because of pruritus vulvae can.

Investigating PMB

Clinical examination should reveal lesions of the vulva, vagina and cervix as well as identifying pelvic

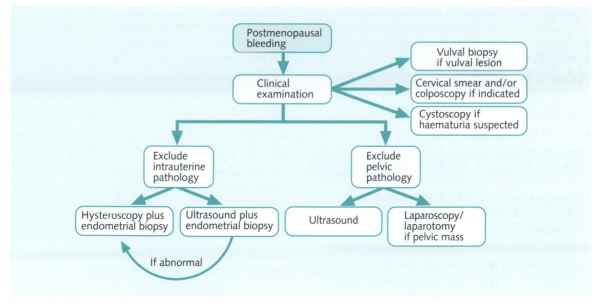

Fig. 19.10 Algorithm for postmenopausal bleeding.

masses. The most common cause of PMB is atrophic vaginitis and, although this might be evident on clinical examination, it must not be assumed to be the cause of the PMB until other more serious causes have been excluded.

Investigation depends on the clinical findings. Vulval and vaginal biopsies should be performed when abnormal lesions are present. Cervical pathology can be excluded by cytology or colposcopic examination (Fig. 19.10).

Intrauterine pathology is best excluded by hysteroscopic examination of the uterine cavity with endometrial biopsy, although ultrasound estimation of the endometrial thickness combined with endometrial sampling can be used. The endometrial thickness in a postmenopausal woman should be less than 5 mm. Although a negative endometrial sample is reassuring, the commonest method of taking the sample in the outpatient setting is by using the 'pipelle' endometrial sampler, which samples only 4% of the uterine cavity. Ultrasound with biopsy can therefore miss early focal pathology. Although D&C can be performed at the same time as hysteroscopy as a method of endometrial biopsy, there is no place for D&C alone in the management of PMB. The ovaries can be assessed using ultrasound and if an

oestrogen-secreting tumour is suspected, circulating oestradiol levels should be measured.

Treating PMB

Treatment obviously depends on the pathology. The most commonly encountered cause of PMB is atrophic change and therefore oestrogen replacement is indicated, not only to prevent a recurrence of PMB but also treat other symptoms associated with oestrogen deficiency. Most women in this situation prefer to use topical oestrogen. The newer 17β oestradiol-releasing creams, rings and vaginal tablets avoid the risk of endometrial hyperplasia because of minimal systemic absorption. If systemic HRT is requested then oestrogen therapy must be combined with a progestogen or progesterone in women who have a uterus.

The treatment of urethral caruncle is by surgical excision of the prolapsed urethral mucosa and is a painful and unpleasant procedure. It should therefore be reserved for those cases in which recurrent PMB or pain occur. Small caruncles might recede with oestrogen cream.

The treatment of vulval, cervical and ovarian malignancy is discussed in detail in Chapter 23.

- What are the possible diagnoses in a woman presenting with primary amenorrhoea?
- What are the possible diagnoses in a woman presenting with secondary amenorrhoea?
- What are the effective medical treatments for menorrhagia?
- What are the surgical options for treatment of menorrhagia?

Further reading

Llewellyn-Jones, D (1999) *Fundementals of Obstetrics & Gynaecology* 7th edn (Mosby, London)

McKay Hart, D & Norman, J (2000) *Gynaecology Illustrated* 5th edn (Churchill Livingstone, London)

Shaw RW, Soutter WP, Stanton SL (1997) *Gynaecology* 2nd edn (Churchill Livingstone, London)

http://www.rcog.org.uk/guidelines

20. Fibroids

Uterine fibroids are benign tumours of the myometrium. They are the most common benign tumours found in women, occurring in approximately 20% of women over the age of 30 years. Histologically they are composed of whorling bundles of smooth muscle cells that resemble the architecture of normal myometrium.

Although their aetiology is unknown, fibroids are associated with exposure to oestrogens. Factors influencing the incidence of fibroids are shown in Fig. 20.1. The hyperoestrogenic state of pregnancy might stimulate the growth of fibroids already present. Fibroids can be categorized by the their position within the myometrium (Fig. 20.2).

Symptoms of uterine fibriods

Symptoms associated with uterine fibroids are shown in Fig. 20.3.

No symptoms

Approximately 50% of women with fibroids are asymptomatic, diagnosis being made during incidental clinical or ultrasound assessment of the pelvis and during pregnancy.

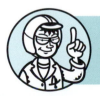 Up to 50% of women with fibroids will be completely asymptomatic.

Menstrual abnormalities

Menstrual abnormalities occur in about one-third of women with fibroids, usually heavy periods. Submucous fibroids can also cause intermenstrual bleeding, postcoital bleeding, continuous vaginal bleeding or dysmenorrhoea. Increased menstrual blood loss due to fibroids is associated with:
- Increased endometrial surface area.
- Prostaglandin production.

Abdominopelvic mass

Large fibroids growing into the abdominal cavity can cause abdominal swelling or distension.

Pain

Abdominopelvic pain can be caused by:
- Degeneration of uterine fibroids.
- The presence of associated pelvic varicosities.
- Stretching of the uterine ligaments.

Subfertility

Fibroids compressing the cornual region of the fallopian tubes can cause infertility. Submucous fibroids, especially those that are hormonally active, can affect implantation and might result in miscarriage. There is now evidence that even intramural fibroids that are not distorting the endometrial cavity can still lead to reduced embryo implantation and pregnancy rates, possibly because of interference with the endometrial blood supply.

Pressure symptoms

Urinary frequency, nocturia and urgency can be caused by pressure on the bladder from an enlarged uterus and incarceration of a pelvic fibroid can result in urinary retention. Pressure on the rectum might also be noticed.

Complications

Red degeneration occurring in pregnancy can present with acute pain and the subsequent massive release of prostaglandins can cause miscarriage or premature labour. Pedunculated fibroids can undergo torsion and present with an acute abdomen. Urinary retention might occur with impaction of a pelvic fibroid. Hyaline, cystic and calcific degenerative changes can also occur. Sarcomatous (malignant) change, usually within very large or rapidly growing fibroids, is a rare (approximately 1:1000) but potentially fatal complication.

In pregnancy, fibroids situated low in the uterus can result in malpresentation of the fetus and obstruct delivery. Fibroids can also restrict

Factors influencing the incidence of fibroids	
Increased incidence with:	**Decreased incidence with:**
African–Caribbean women	Cigarette smoking
Increasing age	Use of combined oral
Nulligravidity	contraceptive pill
Obesity	Full term pregnancy

Fig. 20.1 Factors influencing the incidence of fibroids.

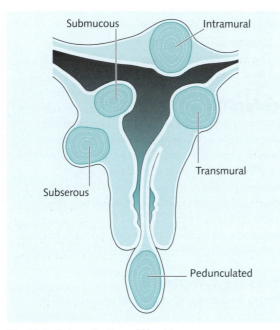

Fig. 20.2 Categorization of fibroids.

Symptoms associated with uterine fibroids
• Asymptomatic
• Menstrual abnormalities
• Abdominopelvic mass
• Subfertility
• Pressure symptoms
• Pregnancy complications

Fig. 20.3 Symptoms associated with uterine fibroids.

postpartum involution of the uterus and predispose to postpartum haemorrhage.

Clinical evaluation and investigations

The presence of fibroids can be elicited by abdominopelvic examination; classically the uterus feels firm and irregular. If a fibroid is moved on bimanual examination the uterus moves with it, although this can also occur with an ovarian mass adherent to the uterus. Pelvic ultrasound might show characteristic diffuse changes associated with the presence of fibroids. Individual larger fibroids can be seen and measured by ultrasound but the best method of excluding submucous fibroids in the presence of menstrual abnormalities is by hysteroscopy. MRI has become the gold standard imaging method for differentiating fibroids from other pelvic masses. However, laparotomy might be required to be 100% certain in some cases.

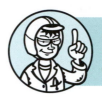
Diagnosis is usually confirmed by ultrasound scan, which will define size and location.

Indications for treatment

Small, asymptomatic fibroids do not require intervention. Indications for treatment include:

- Symptomatic fibroids.
- Rapidly enlarging fibroids.
- Fibroids that are thought to be causing infertility.

Fibroids need treatment only if they are causing symptoms or if there is subfertility.

Medical therapy

Medical therapy is only useful as an adjunct to surgery and as an aid to correction of anaemia prior to surgery. Fibroids regrow to their original size within 3 months of ceasing medical therapy without surgical intervention.

Gonadotrophin-releasing hormone analogues

Gonadotrophin-releasing hormone (GnRH) analogues produce a hypogonadotrophic hypogonadal state; that is, they produce a temporary, reversible, chemical menopause that results in a reduction in fibroid volume by up to 50% with a maximum benefit within 3 months of starting therapy.

GnRH analogues have several different uses prior to surgery:

- They reduce surgical blood loss and the need for blood transfusions.
- They increase the likelihood of performing surgery through a transverse suprapubic incision rather than a midline incision.
- They reduce the risk of hysterectomy when myomectomy is planned.

The long-term use of GnRH analogues has been limited because of their side-effects, which include menopausal symptoms and bone density reduction (osteoporosis). However, recent data have indicated that low-dose hormone replacement therapy (HRT), used concomitantly as 'add back', can avoid menopausal side-effects and prevent loss of bone density while maintaining the benefits of the GnRH analogues. GnRH analogues are currently licensed for 6 months use. More data are required before GnRH analogues with add back are licensed for longer-term use.

Surgical treatment

Definitive surgery includes one of:

- Myomectomy.
- Hysterectomy.

Myomectomy is the removal of fibroids with preservation of the uterus and can be performed either at laparotomy (open myomectomy), hysteroscopically or laparoscopically. Complications include haemorrhage, which might require blood transfusion, and – rarely – hysterectomy. Adhesion formation can impair future fertility and is most common after open myomectomy, especially for posterior wall fibroids. Fibroid regrowth is likely to occur in 40% of patients with a reoperation rate of up to one-fifth of cases. Hysterectomy is the surgical procedure of choice in women who have completed their families.

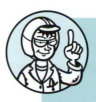

Surgical treatment with hysterectomy often causes less morbidity than myomectomy, the latter is performed in women who wish to preserve their fertility.

Advances in fibroid treatment

Techniques for the treatment of fibroids are currently being developed to reduce the need for laparotomy, postoperative adhesion formation and the avoidance of large uterine scars. These include:

- Interstitial laser photocoagulation: laser probes are inserted into the fibroid laparoscopically to produce tissue degeneration and subsequent fibroid shrinkage.
- Laparoscopic diathermy.
- Radiological embolization of fibroids via uterine artery catheterization using tiny silicone microbeads.
- Directed high energy ultrasound.

- What are the different types of fibroid degeneration?
- What are the possible locations for fibroids?
- What symptoms can be caused by fibroids?
- How can fibroids be managed medically?
- How can fibroids be managed surgically?
- What are the new techniques for dealing with fibroids?

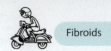
Further reading

Anderson J ed (1997) *Gynaecological Imaging* (Churchill Livingstone, London)

Llewellyn-Jones D, (1999) *Fundementals of Obstetrics & Gynaecology* 7th edn (Mosby, London)

McKay Hart, D & Norman, J (2000) *Gynaecology Illustrated* 5th edn (Churchill Livingstone, London)

Monaghan, JM (1992) *Bonney's Gynaecological Surgery* 9th edn (Balliere Tindall)

http://www.rcog.org.uk/guidelines

21. Endometriosis

Endometriosis is the presence of functional endometrium outside the uterine cavity. Endometriosis occurring in the myometrium is known as adenomyosis. The true incidence of endometriosis is difficult to ascertain as not all women with endometriosis complain of gynaecological symptoms. Endometriosis occurs in about 10% of the female population in their reproductive years but has been defined in up to 25% women undergoing gynaecological laparoscopy.

Endometriosis is the most common gynaecological condition after fibroids.

Aetiology

The aetiology of endometriosis is unknown but several theories have been suggested (Fig. 21.1).

Retrograde menstruation/implantation theory

During menstruation, endometrial tissue spills into the pelvic cavity through the fallopian tubes, resulting retrograde menstruation. This ectopic endometrium then implants and becomes functional, responding to the hormones of the ovarian cycle. This theory is supported by the association between endometriosis and increased menstruation occurring with a short menstrual cycle and prolonged periods, and by the fact that the most common sites for endometriosis are the ovaries and the uterosacral ligaments – areas in which retrograde menses spill. The implantation theory would also account for the rare cases of endometriosis found in the surgical incision following surgery on the uterus. Imperforate hymen and other outflow obstructions that exacerbate retrograde menstruation are also associated with severe endometriosis.

However, this theory does not account for the existence of endometriosis at the distant sites in the body (e.g. lungs). There is growing laparoscopic evidence to suggest that most women experience retrograde menstruation, in which case the incidence of endometriosis would be expected to be higher. This would suggest that this theory, as it stands, is too simplistic.

Lymphatic and venous embolization

This theory hypothesizes that endometrial tissue is transported through the body by the lymphatic or venous channels and would explain the rare cases of distant sites for endometriosis. However, distant endometriotic deposits would be expected to be more common if the lymphatic and venous embolization theories were the only mechanism for the development of endometriosis.

Coelomic metaplasia

This theory relies on the principle that tissues of certain embryonal origin maintain their ability to undergo metaplasia and differentiate into other tissue types. This is certainly true of peritoneum of coelomic origin, which can undergo metaplasia and differentiate into functional endometrium. Although this is an attractive theory, it does not explain the distribution of endometriosis within the peritoneal cavity itself (most common in the lower part of the peritoneal cavity) or the presence of endometriosis in sites of the body that are not of coelomic origin.

Genetic and immunological factors

The role of a genetic influence is supported by the strong family history seen in endometriosis sufferers. What exactly that role is has not yet been ascertained. It is possible that those women with a genetic predisposition to endometriosis have an abnormal response to the presence of ectopic endometrium, which results in the development of endometriosis. There is some evidence that an altered or defective cell-mediated response is implicated.

Composite theories

None of the above theories will alone account for all cases of endometriosis, however, together all the theories could play a role in some way. Whereas an abnormal response to the presence of ectopic

Fig. 21.1 Suggested theories for the aetiology of endometriosis.

endometrium might result in functioning endometrium responding to the ovarian cycle, this in turn could trigger coelomic metaplasia and further development or advancement of the disease process in response to the local release of endometrial hormones and/or the inflammatory response.

Sites of endometriosis

The most common sites for the development of endometriosis are the ovaries and the uterosacral ligaments. These and other pelvic sites are show in Fig. 21.2. Although endometriosis has been reported in nearly every organ except the spleen, extrapelvic endometriosis is rare. Assessment of the severity of pelvic endometriosis can be made using the American Fertility Society Classification (Fig. 21.3), which takes into account the site and size of endometriotic lesions, and the presence and consequences of adhesions.

Symptoms

The key to the diagnosis of endometriosis is the presence of cyclical pain associated with menstruation. Cyclical pain occurs because the deposits of endometriosis, whatever their location in the body, respond to the ovarian cycle and bleeding from these deposits causes local irritation and inflammatory responses (Fig. 21.4). The exact location of type of pain depends on the sites of ectopic endometrium. If the endometriosis is severe, pain can be continuous, with exacerbations at the time of menstruation. Neural and intracranial endometriosis produce continuous pain.

Endometriosis of the lung, bladder, bowel or umbilicus will produce bleeding from these sites associated with the menstruation.

Rupture of an ovarian endometrioma will cause severe lower abdominal pain. The release of the very irritant 'chocolate' material from the cyst causes peritonitis.

Infertility

An association between infertility and endometriosis exists, with as many as one-third of infertile women being diagnosed as having endometriosis. Dense adhesions and the resultant tubal and ovarian damage and distortion caused by severe endometriosis will obviously contribute to the lack of conception. The

Fig. 21.2 Sites of endometriosis.

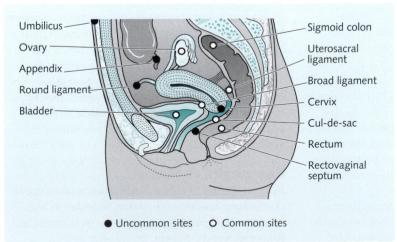

Umbilicus — Sigmoid colon
Ovary — Uterosacral ligament
Appendix — Broad ligament
Round ligament — Cervix
Bladder — Cul-de-sac
— Rectum
— Rectovaginal septum

● Uncommon sites   ○ Common sites

American Fertility Society Classification of Endometriosis						
Anatomical Site	Score	1	2	3	4	6
Peritoneum	Endometriotic lesion size	<1 cm	1–3 cm	>3 cm		
	Adhesions	Flimsy	Dense with partial pouch of Douglas occlusion	Dense with complete pouch of Douglas occlusion		
Ovary [points for each side involved]	Endometriotic lesion size		<1cm		1–3 cm	>3 cm
	Adhesions		Filmy		Dense with partial ovarian coverage	Dense completely enclosing ovary
Fallopian tubes [points for each side involved]	Endometriotic lesion size		<1cm		>1cm	Tubal occlusion
	Adhesions		Filmy		Dense and distorting tubes	Dense and completely enclosing tubes
		Stage I (Mild) <5 Stage II (Mod) 6–15			Stage III (Severe) 16–30 Stage IV (Extensive) >31	

Fig. 21.3 American Fertility Society Classification of Endometriosis.

association with mild endometriosis, in which no mechanical damage has occurred, is less easy to understand. Release of substances from the ectopic endometrium, such as prostaglandins, which can affect ovulation or tubal motility has been implicated. There is evidence that treatment of even mild disease can lead to an improvement of fertility prospects.

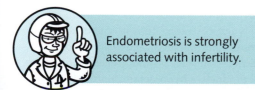

Endometriosis is strongly associated with infertility.

Clinical evaluation

Endometriosis should be considered in any woman who presents with any of the symptoms shown in Fig. 21.4. The classic 'quartet' of symptoms of endometriosis is:

- Secondary dysmenorrhoea.
- Deep dyspareunia.
- Pelvic pain.
- Infertility.

The dysmenorrhoea associated with endometriosis typically starts prior to the beginning of the period and is exacerbated by menstrual flow.

Pelvic examination can reveal a tender, retroverted, retroflexed, fixed uterus with thickening of the cardinal or uterosacral ligaments. Endometriotic nodules might be palable in the posterior vaginal fornix and ovarian endometriomata might be evident on bimanual palpation. The pelvic anatomy might be normal with mild disease and a useful sign is to elicit pain on moving the cervix anteriorly. This stretches the uterosacral ligaments, which is painful in the presence of endometriosis. In the presence of adenomyosis, the uterus is typically smoothly enlarged (globular) and tender.

Diagnosis and severity of disease can only effectively be assessed through the laparoscope. The classic 'powder-burn' lesions of endometriosis might be seen but these areas of haemosiderin pigmentation might represent 'burnt-out' endometriosis. Non-pigmented lesions can appear as opaque white areas of peritoneum, red lesions or glandular lesions. If there is doubt about the macroscopic appearance then a peritoneal biopsy should be taken. Ovarian endometrioma can be seen by ultrasound but differentiation from other ovarian pathology can be difficult.

Fig. 21.4 Symptoms of endometriosis.

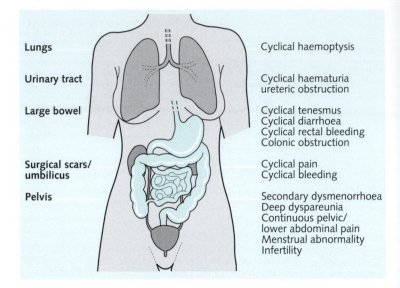

Lungs — Cyclical haemoptysis

Urinary tract — Cyclical haematuria
ureteric obstruction

Large bowel — Cyclical tenesmus
Cyclical diarrhoea
Cyclical rectal bleeding
Colonic obstruction

Surgical scars/umbilicus — Cyclical pain
Cyclical bleeding

Pelvis — Secondary dysmenorrhoea
Deep dyspareunia
Continuous pelvic/lower abdominal pain
Menstrual abnormality
Infertility

Differential diagnosis

Complications

Complications of endometriosis are often due to the resultant fibrosis and scarring and can affect not only the reproductive organs but might cause colonic and ureteric obstruction. Rupture of an endometrioma and the subsequent release of the very irritant 'chocolate' material contents can cause peritonitis. Malignant change within endometriotic lesions is rare and most commonly occurs in ovarian endometriosis.

Treatment

Treatment of endometriosis is indicated to:
- Alleviate symptoms.
- Stop progression of disease and development of complications.
- Improve fertility.

Treatment depends on the severity of the disease and should be tailored to the woman's needs; it can be medical or surgical.

 Endometriosis is a recurring disease and initial treatment should be followed by maintenance therapy.

Medical treatment

The lesions of endometriosis regress in response to pregnancy and the menopause. Medical treatment is therefore aimed at mimicking one of these two physiological processes (Fig. 21.5).

Progestogens

Continuous progestogen therapy can effectively induce a state of pseudopregnancy, causing decidualization of endometriotic deposits, which then regress. Progestogens can be taken orally or as depot preparations, and treatment should be for 6 months.

Danazol

Danazol is a testosterone derivative and used to be the most common medical treatment for endometriosis. As well as its androgenic properties, Danazol produces a hypo-oestrogenic and hypoprogestogenic state, and it is this pseudomenopausal state that induces endometrial regression and atrophy. The mode of action of Danazol is complex; it acts at pituitary, ovarian and target tissue levels. It should be taken for 6–9 months and the dose should be titrated to the patient's response and presence of side-effects. Patients should be warned to stop treatment if they develop deepening of the voice, as this could be irreversible.

Summary of medical treatment of endometriosis		
Drug	Mode of action	Side-effects
Progestogens	Pseudopregnancy	Break-through bleeding, weight gain, oedema, acne, abdominal bloating, increased appetite, decreased libido
Danazol	Pseudomenopause	Increase weight, break-through bleeding, muscle cramps, decreased breast size, hot flushes, emotional lability, oily skin, acne, hirsutism, headache, increased libido, hoarseness or deepening of the voice
Gestrinone	Pseudomenopause	Similar to Danazol
LHRH-analogues	Pseudomenopause	Hot flushes, break-through bleeding, vaginal dryness, headaches, decreased libido, bone density loss

Fig. 21.5 Summary of medical treatment of endometriosis.

Gestrinone
Gestrinone is a synthetic steroid that has mild androgenic, marked antioestrogenic and antiprogestogenic activity. It exhibits similar endocrine effects to those of Danazol without significantly reducing basal levels of gonadotrophins. Clinical response is also similar to Danazol.

GnRH analogues
This class of synthetic drugs are GnRH superagonists. Continued administration desensitizes pituitary gondotrophes and result in a temporary, reversible state of hypogonadotrophic hypogonadism, in other words, a temporary, reversible, chemical menopause. GnRH analogues are as effective as Danazol in reducing the symptoms and severity of endometriosis and are usually used for 3–6 months. Their menopausal side-effects are often better tolerated than the androgenic side-effects of Danazol and can be reduced by using 'add-back' continuous combined hormone replacement therapy (see Chapter 20).

Combined oral contraceptive pill
The COCP suppresses ovulation and the normal cyclical ovarian production of oestrogen and progesterone. Mild symptoms of endometriosis can be controlled by using the COCP but it is more often used as maintenance therapy following initial treatment. Endometriosis is a recurring disease, with up to 40% women developing recurring symptoms within 1 year of stopping treatment. Initial treatment should therefore be followed by maintenance therapy to reduce the chance of recurrence. Maintenance therapy aims to suppress or reduce the frequence of periods and this can be achieved by tricycling a continuous dose combined oral contraceptive pill.

Surgical therapy
Surgical treatment of endometriosis can be conservative or radical. Which method is used depends on the patient's:
- Age.
- Fertility requirements.
- Response to medical treatment.

Conservative surgery
Conservative surgery can be performed through a laparoscope or at laparotomy and aims to:
- Return the anatomy of the pelvis to normal.
- Destroy visible lesions of endometriosis.
- Improve fertility.
- Conserve ovarian tissue.

Necessary procedures can include division of adhesions, destruction of endometriotic lesions using diathermy or laser, and excision of deep-seated endometriomas, which are known not to respond well to medical therapy. Complications include damage to other pelvic structures including bowel, bladder and ureters. Recurrence of symptoms might occur not only because endometriosis is a recurring disease but because endometriotic deposits not visible to the naked eye will not have been destroyed. Diffuse peritoneal endometriosis might be better treated medically. Pregnancy rates following conservative surgery are directly related to the severity of the disease.

Radical surgery

Definitive radical surgery for endometriosis is reserved for women who no longer wish to maintain fertility and in whom other forms of treatment have failed. Total abdominal hysterectomy with bilateral salpingo-oophorectomy is the procedure of choice. It is the removal of the ovaries, the main source of oestrogens, that produces an hypo-oestrogenic state and effectively treats the endometriosis. As many of these women are relatively young, HRT is advised. Oestrogen replacement can cause a recurrence of endometriosis in a small percentage of women and should therefore be kept to a minimum. Continuous combined oestrogen and progesterone replacement might further reduce the rate of recurrence because of the effects of progestogens on endometriosis.

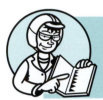

- What are the theories for the genesis of endometriosis?
- What are the most common sites of endometriosis?
- What are the typical symptoms of endometriosis?
- How is endometriosis thought to cause subfertility?

Further reading

Llewellyn-Jones, D (1999) *Fundementals of Obstetrics & Gynaecology* 7th edn (Mosby, London)

McKay Hart, D & Norman, J (2000) *Gynaecology Illustrated* 5th edn (Churchill Livingstone, London)

Shaw RW, Soutter WP, Stanton SL (1997) *Gynaecology* 2nd edn (Churchill Livingstone, London)

http://www.rcog.org.uk/guidelines

22. Benign Ovarian Tumours

Incidence

Benign ovarian cysts are common and often asymptomatic, resolving spontaneously. Therefore, despite being a frequent cause for admission to hospital, their exact incidence is unknown. About 90% of ovarian tumours overall are benign, but this changes with age. Malignant tumours are most common in the postmenopausal age-group.

Aetiology

Ovarian tumours can be physiological or pathological. Classification depends on the ovarian tissue from which they arise (Fig. 22.1). Excluding the physiological group, a germ cell tumour is the more common diagnosis in a woman less than 40 years of age, whereas an epithelial cell tumour is more likely in an older woman.

Physiological cysts

These are often asymptomatic and occur commonly in younger women.

Follicular cysts

These are the result of either non-rupture of the dominant follicle during the normal cycle or from failure of atresia of a non-dominant follicle. Smaller cysts might resolve spontaneously but intervention could be necessary if the cyst causes symptoms or if ultrasound follow-up shows failure of resolution or an increase in size.

Luteal cysts

In contrast to follicular cysts, luteal cysts are more likely to present with intraperitoneal bleeding secondary to rupture.

Benign germ cell tumours

Such tumours arise from totipotential germ cells and thus can contain elements of all three layers of embryonic tissue – ectodermal derivatives such as teeth and hair, endodermal tissue such as intestine and mesodermal structures such as bone.

Mature cystic teratoma

Also known as a dermoid cyst, this type of tumour has a median age of presentation of 30 years with about 10% being bilateral. Most are asymptomatic but they can undergo torsion or, rarely, rupture.

Mature solid teratomas

Much less common than a dermoid cyst, these tumours must be distinguished from an immature solid teratoma which is malignant.

Benign epithelial tumours

The majority of ovarian cysts arise from the ovarian epithelium. They develop from the coelomic epithelium over the gonadal ridge of the embryo and might therefore be derived from any of the pelvic organs or the renal tract.

Serous cystadenoma

This is the most common tumour in this group. Again, they are bilateral on about 10% of cases and they contain thin serous fluid, usually within a unilocular cavity. Histologically, they appear to have a tubal origin.

Mucinous cystadenoma

In contrast to the serous cystadenomas, these tumours are usually unilateral, larger in size and multilocular with thick mucoid fluid. The mucus-secreting cells are likely to indicate an endocervical derivation.

Endometrioid tumours

These are mostly malignant tumours arising from endometrial cells.

Brenner tumours

The majority of these tumours are benign. They arise from uroepithelial cell lines and contain transitional epithelium; 10–15% are bilateral, usually small in size, and some might secrete oestrogen.

Benign sex cord stromal tumours

Such tumours account for only about 4% of benign ovarian tumours. Many secrete hormones and thus

Classification of benign ovarian tumours	
Type of tumour	**Name**
Physiological	Follicular cysts Luteal cysts
Benign germ cell tumours	Mature cystic teratoma (dermoid cyst) Mature solid teratoma
Benign epithelial tumours	Serous cystadenoma Mucinous cystadenoma Endometrioid cystadenoma Brenner
Benign sex cord stromal tumours	Theca cell tumours Fibroma Sertoli–Leydig cell tumour

Fig. 22.1 Classification of benign ovarian tumours.

Differential diagnoses for ovarian tumours	
Symptom	**Differential diagnosis**
Pain	Ectopic pregnancy Spontaneous miscarriage Pelvic inflammatory disease Appendicitis Diverticulitis
Abdominal swelling	Pregnancy Fibroid uterus Full bladder
Pressure effects	Constipation Urine frequency Vaginal prolapse
Hormonal effects	Menstrual irregularity Postmenopausal bleeding Precocious puberty

Fig. 22.2 Differential diagnoses for ovarian tumours.

present at any age with hormonally mediated symptoms.

Theca cell tumours

These cysts are nearly always benign solid tumours presenting over the age of 50 years (in contrast granulosa cell tumours are always malignant).

Fibroma

These tumours are rare and can be associated with ascites.

Diagnosis

History

Benign ovarian tumours can be asymptomatic, detected by routine bimanual palpation during a cervical smear test or on routine antenatal ultrasound scan, for example. The presenting symptoms include:

- Pain secondary to torsion/rupture/haemorrhage/infection.
- Abdominal swelling.
- Pressure effects on bowel or bladder.
- Hormonal effects secondary to secretion of oestrogens or androgens.

Figure 22.2 shows the differential diagnoses that need to be considered for the history, examination and investigations. The history must include the date of the LMP and the regularity of the menstrual cycle, as well as current contraception, if appropriate. Any history of gastrointestinal symptoms might be important, for example, a patient with an ovarian torsion might present with sudden onset of right-sided abdominal pain associated with nausea and vomiting, and appendicitis must be excluded.

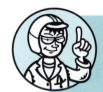 Benign ovarian cysts that undergo an accident (rupture or torsion) can present as an acute abdomen.

Examination

Initial examination must include the pulse and blood pressure; rupture of an ovarian cyst can result in intraperitoneal bleeding that leads to hypovolaemia. In a young patient, this might present at first with tachycardia and cold peripheries, with hypotension showing as a relatively late sign.

Distension might be seen on abdominal inspection, resulting from the cyst itself or from ascites if the cyst is malignant. If the cyst has torted, or if there is haemorrhage into the cyst so that the capsule stretches, abdominal palpation will elicit tenderness, typically in the iliac fossa, which might be associated with signs of peritonism. A large ovarian tumour might rise up out of the pelvis and be palpated in the abdomen; this is done using the left hand and moving distally from the xiphisternum towards the pelvis (see Chapter 46). Ascites, associated with malignant tumours, should be excluded by testing for shifting dullness.

Bimanual palpation of the pelvic organs, as described in Chapter 46, is essential. If the tumour has presented acutely with abdominal pain then adnexal tenderness or an adnexal mass will assist in excluding gastrointestinal aetiology. Assessing the size of the uterus will help to exclude a fibroid uterus or intrauterine pregnancy. If there seems to be an adnexal mass, then its approximate size, consistency and the presence of any tenderness should be elicited.

Investigations

In line with the list of differential diagnoses in Fig. 22.2, investigations include:
- Haemoglobin.
- White blood cell count.
- Urine pregnancy test and/or serum β-hCG level.
- Pelvic ultrasound scan.
- Serum CA125 level.
- Chest X-ray and intravenous urogram if malignancy is suspected (see Chapter 23).

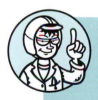 The epithelial tumour marker (CA125) is almost always checked in the presence of an ovarian cyst to aid in the differential diagnosis.

Management of a benign ovarian tumour

The patient's management depends on the:
- Severity of presenting symptoms.
- Patient's age.
- Future fertility needs.
- Risk of malignancy.

Asymptomatic cysts

Treatment might not be warranted if an ovarian cyst is asymptomatic; this depends on the patient's age and the size of the cyst (Fig. 22.3). In a younger woman (usually taken as less than 40 years of age), the risk of the tumour being malignant is reduced and therefore the cyst can be monitored with pelvic ultrasound scans. A physiological cyst is likely to

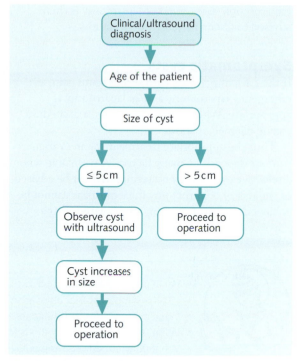

Fig. 22.3 Management of an asymptomatic benign ovarian tumour.

resolve spontaneously but, if it persists or increases in size, then a laparoscopy or laparotomy might be indicated.

 Simple ovarian cysts < 5 cm diameter can be managed conservatively with repeat ultrasound scans every 6 months.

In a woman who is older, for example at or nearing the menopause, the issue of maintaining fertility is usually less important and the diagnosis of a physiological cyst is unlikely. If the cyst is above a certain size (5 cm has been suggested), malignancy must be excluded by:
- Measuring tumour markers.
- Ultrasound scan to distinguish solid elements within the cyst.
- Colour Doppler studies of the blood flow around the cyst.

Laparoscopic assessment or laparotomy is then advised to obtain histological specimens.

Symptomatic cysts

If the patient presents with severe acute pain, an emergency laparoscopy and/or laparotomy is appropriate. With chronic symptoms, a procedure can be planned as above.

Thus the appropriate treatment for an ovarian tumour depends on many factors. A woman in whom a selective cystectomy is attempted must be advised of the risk of oophrectomy if haemostasis cannot be achieved or if the cyst cannot be isolated. If the patient is young, with minimal risk of malignancy, a laparoscopic procedure might be an option. In an older woman, it might be more advisable to perform a laparotomy, possibly including bilateral oophrectomy, hysterectomy and infracolic omentectomy (see Chapter 23).

An ovarian cyst thought to be benign can be managed by observation, ultrasound-guided drainage, laparoscopic or open ovarian cystectomy.

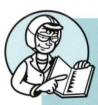

- What are the potential origins of the tissue that forms an ovarian cyst?
- List the symptoms that an ovarian cyst can cause the patient.
- What are the differential diagnoses for an ovarian cyst?
- What are the treatment options for a patient with an ovarian cyst?
- What ultrasound features would increase suspicion for malignancy within an ovarian cyst?

Further reading

Shaw RW, Soutter WP, Stanton SL (1997) *Gynaecology* 2nd edn (Churchill Livingstone, London)

23. Gynaecological Malignancy

Ovarian malignancy

Ovarian malignancy is the most common gynaecological malignancy and over 50% of ovarian cancer occurs in women aged 45–65. Ovarian tumours can be divided into different groups according to their cell of origin: epithelial, sex cord stromal or germ cell, and whether they are benign (see Chapter 22), borderline or malignant. Most tumours are derived from epithelial cells; their particularly unpleasant characteristic is that they cause non-specific symptoms and therefore women often present 'late', when spread has already occurred. Their staging, treatment and survival rates are summarized in Fig. 23.1.

 There are 6000 new cases of ovarian cancer diagnosed each year in England and Wales; 75% of those diagnosed will die of the disease.

Aetiology
The life factors that increase and reduce the risk of developing ovarian cancer are shown in Fig. 23.2. Women with a familial predisposition to ovarian cancer probably account for around 10% of cases, and most of these will have either the BRCA1 or BRCA2 mutations (chromosomes 17 and 13), or the Lynch II syndrome (an autosomal dominant inherited disorder that predisposes to breast, endometrial, colonic and ovarian cancer).

Presentation
Ovarian tumours are relatively 'silent', producing vague symptoms. Pain is rare but could occur if the ovary twists (torsion) or if there is bleeding into the tumour. More common are abdominal distension, urinary frequency due to pressure on the bladder and gastrointestinal upset (e.g. vague diarrhoea or constipation symptoms).

Investigations
Ultrasound
Ultrasound scans will identify an ovarian mass. Features suspicious of malignancy include:
- A solid rather than a cystic mass, or a cyst containing septae.
- Mass measuring more than 5 cm.
- Presence of ascites.
- Bilateral tumours.

If cancer is suspected an ultrasound of the liver is performed to look for metastatic disease.

CA125
This tumour marker is often raised with epithelial tumours of the ovary, although it can also be high in the presence of fibroids, diverticular disease and pregnancy, thus giving false-positive results. False negatives are also possible: some malignant tumours, especially mucinous tumours, will not secrete high levels of CA125.

Management
Surgery
Surgery is performed unless there are distant metastases, the aim being to remove as much tumour mass as possible. A midline incision is used. Uterus, tubes, ovaries and omentum are removed. The pelvis is carefully explored, looking for and biopsying any deposits. Peritoneal fluid is sent for cytology.

Staging will determine further management. Unless distant metastases have been seen on scans prior to surgery, it is the operation that will define the stage, on the basis of what is found at laparotomy and the ensuing pathology report.

Stage I tumours are treated with surgery alone but stage II and III tumours will require chemotherapy. Stage IV tumours (distant metastases present) can be operated upon but this will not be for cure – surgery is performed for staging or to relieve bowel obstruction only.

Fig. 23.1 Staging of ovarian carcinoma.

Stage	Description	Treatment	Success rate (%)
I A B C	Limited to the ovaries: One ovary, capsule intact, no ascites Both ovaries, capsules intact, no ascites Breached capsule(s) or ascites present	Surgery	80
II A B C	Presence of peritoneal deposits in pelvis: On uterus or tubes On other pelvic organs With ascites	Surgery then chemotherapy	60
III	Peritoneal deposits outside pelvis: Microscopic deposits Macroscopic < 2 cm diameter Macroscopic > 2 cm diameter	Surgery then chemotherapy	25
IV	Distant metastases	Surgery for palliation only	5–10

Staging of ovarian carcinoma

Risk factors for ovarian carcinoma	
Increased risk	**Reduced risk**
Few or no pregnancies Treatment with ovulation-induction drugs White Caucasian Blood group A Higher socioeconomic status Late age of first conception Family history	Pregnancies Treatment with the combined pill Black/Asian Blood group O

Fig. 23.2 Risk factors for ovarian carcinoma.

Chemotherapy

Another option for treatment might be to give chemotherapy prior to surgery to shrink the tumour mass – studies are ongoing to look into this further.

Combination therapy is used, for example cyclophosphamide + carboplatin or Taxol + carboplatin. Common side-effects include:
- Myelosuppression.
- Nausea and vomiting.
- Peripheral neuropathy.
- Alopecia.

Taxol gives severe hypersensitivity reactions so a 'pre-med' of corticosteroid and antihistamine is needed.

Platins are also toxic to the kidney, ear and eye. Cisplatin, an older platin drug, had a poor side-effect profile so has been largely superseded by carboplatin.

Radiotherapy is not very practical in ovarian malignancy because of the large area involved.

Screening

The rationale for screening for ovarian cancer is to reduce the late presentation that currently results in poor survival. Unfortunately, screening for this condition is very difficult, partly because there is no premalignant stage but also because there is no one test to diagnose ovarian cancer. Large studies have looked at using CA125 and ultrasound (with or without Doppler), but the non-specificity of CA125 adds to the confusion and, at present, there is no screening programme.

Uterine endometrial tumours

Incidence

Endometrial carcinoma affects 20 women per 100 000 women per year in the UK. The median age of women affected is 61, and 80% are postmenopausal.

Risk factors

Predisposing factors are shown in Fig. 23.3 and include women who have high oestrogen levels (obesity, polycystic ovarian syndrome, tamoxifen therapy) and those who have had many menses (nulliparous, late menopause). The COCP protects against endometrial carcinoma, halving the user's risk. The protective effect is most marked where the COCP has been used for more than 10 years and it continues for at least 20 years after the woman stops taking the pill. A family history of breast or colon cancer might point to the Lynch II syndrome.

Endometrial hyperplasia is recognized as being a premalignant condition. Simple (also called cystic) hyperplasia and complex (adenomatous) hyperplasia are unlikely to progress to carcinoma but can be treated with progesterone to encourage regression. Atypical hyperplasia, however, is likely to progress, and in many cases might indicate that a carcinoma is already present in another part of the uterus.

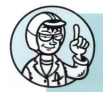

Of all women with postmenopausal bleeding, 12% will have cancer or atypical hyperplasia.

Pathology and spread

Endometrial cancer is an adenocarcinoma, the most common type being endometrioid. Other subtypes are adenocanthoma, papillary serous and clear cell adenocarcinomas. The latter two have a particularly poor prognosis.

Spread is initially local myometrial invasion and then transperitoneal. Lymphatic spread occurs to the para-aortic nodes. Staging is shown in Fig. 23.4.

Presentation

Most women present with bleeding that is either abnormal perimenopausal or postmenopausal.

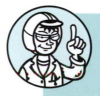

Women with atypical hyperplasia of the endometrium are treated as if they have endometrial carcinoma due to the high likelihood of progression and coexisting malignancy.

Investigation

Women with postmenopausal or suspicious perimenopausal bleeding should be investigated with

Risk factors for endometrial carcinoma
• Obesity
• Nulliparity
• Late menopause
• PCOS
• Unopposed oestrogen therapy
• Tamoxifen therapy
• Diabetes
• Personal or family history of breast or colon cancer

Fig. 23.3 Risk factors for endometrial carcinoma.

Fig. 23.4 Staging of endometrial cancer.

Staging of endometrial cancer		
Stage	**Structures involved**	**Survival rates**
I A B C	Body of uterus: Endometrium only Extension into inner half of myometrium Extension into outer half of myometrium	85
II A B	Extension from body of uterus to cervix: Endocervical glands only Cervical stroma	60
III A B C	Spread to adnexae, or positive peritoneal cytology Metastases in vagina Pelvic or para-aortic lymphadenopathy	40
IV A B	Involvement of bladder or bowel mucosa Distant metastases	10

ultrasound to measure the endometrial thickness and some form of endometrial sampling. Endometrial cancer causes thickening of the endometrium. Pipelle sampling involves the passage of a thin plastic tube through the cervix into the uterine cavity and uses aspiration to obtain an endometrial biopsy. It is done as an outpatient without the need for anaesthetic but causes period-type pain during and after the procedure. The pipelle can be expected to miss a number of tumours but in combination with ultrasound it is a useful tool. Alternatively, endometrial tissue can be sampled at the time of hysteroscopy under general anaesthetic, either under direct vision (using a resectoscope) or blind, with a curette.

Once a tissue diagnosis is obtained, ideally an MRI scan is performed to assess the extent of myometrial involvement and thus differentiate between stages Ia and Ib and those above (see Fig. 23.4). Stages Ia and Ib can be treated in a cancer unit; higher stages should be treated in a regional cancer centre.

Treatment

Stages Ia and Ib are treated by total abdominal hysterectomy and bilateral salpingo-oophrectomy (TAH BSO). The vaginal route of hysterectomy is not suitable for the treatment of cancer. The role of lymphadenectomy for treatment of these stages is unclear and is being investigated. Washings are taken from the peritoneum for cytology.

Stages Ic and IIa are treated by TAH BSO followed by radiotherapy. This might be external beam or intravaginal (brachytherapy).

Stage IIb is treated first with radiotherapy. Stage III needs debulking surgery prior to radiotherapy. Stage IV tumours are incurable, so the woman will need palliative care and treatment as necessary.

Prognosis

The overall recurrence rate is 30%; cases with positive lymph nodes or peritoneal cytology are more likely to recur than those without (50% versus 10%). Most recurrence occurs within 2–3 years and the earlier recurrences are harder to treat, and therefore carry a poorer prognosis. Isolated vaginal recurrences can be treated with radiotherapy. Later recurrence can be treated with progestogens in the first instance. If hormonal treatment fails chemotherapy is used.

Survival rates are shown in Fig. 23.4; the overall survival rate is 60%.

Uterine sarcoma

Stromal sarcoma

Tumours of stromal cells can be divided into the following categories:
- Low grade sarcomas: look like fibroids, are slow-growing. Treatment is TAH BSO with wide excision of the parametria.
- High grade sarcomas: aggressive tumours with less than 50% survival rates, treated with radiotherapy.
- Mixed Mullerian tumours: derived from the glandular cells within the stroma, these are aggressive tumours that commonly spread to cervix and lymph nodes. Treatment is TAH BSO with postoperative radiotherapy.

Myometrial sarcoma

Leiomyosarcoma could be described as a 'malignant fibroid', although only 5–10% of them arise within an existing fibroid they are macroscopically very similar, being tumours of smooth muscle cells. Often diagnosis is not made until a TAH specimen is examined histologically but lymph node sampling and BSO must be performed.

Atypical myometrial tumours

Leiomyoblastoma, clear cell leiomyoma and epithelioid leiomyoma are tumours of smooth muscle that occur most often in premenopausal women and are oestrogen dependent. Treatment is therefore TAH BSO and the issue of HRT is difficult.

Cervix

Cervical intraepithelial neoplasia

Cervical intraepithelial neoplasia (CIN) is a premalignant condition of the cervix. CIN is divided into three grades, although the disease itself is a continuum. CIN grading is shown in Fig. 23.5.

The national screening programme was designed to detect CIN on smear tests, thus allowing intervention before the condition progressed to cancer. The first smear is performed at age 25, then smears are taken at intervals of 3–5 years, stopping at age 64 if the previous two smears have been negative.

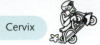

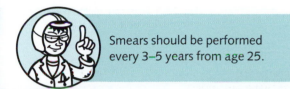

Smears should be performed every 3–5 years from age 25.

The success of screening is seen in the fact that the incidence of cervical carcinoma has decreased by 25% since 1986, and mortality is decreasing. However, many women still die and those who are missed by screening are often women who have a much higher chance of having and dying from cervical cancer because of their high-risk factor profile. Around 85% of women in the UK are screened.

The smear test does have its limitations; the result is governed by subjective cytological assessment, the technique is subject to sampling errors, and it has false negative (2–20%) and false positive (10–13%) rates. Screening for Human Papilloma Virus (HPV) increases sensitivity and specificity (see Fig. 23.6, page 122)

Aetiology of CIN

The risk factors for CIN are the same as those for cervical carcinoma (see Fig. 23.9, page 123). HPV is described more fully in Fig. 23.6.

Management of CIN

Figure 23.7 provides an algorithm for management of CIN based on the smear result and on the patient's smear history. The first smear showing mild dyskariosis does not merit referral because, especially if the woman is a non-smoker, there is a good chance that over 6 months the cells will revert to normal. The moderate and severe dyskariosis cases (fewer than 2% of smears) should be referred for colposcopy.

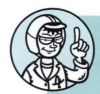

Smoking makes it less likely that low grade CIN will resolve, and more likely that CIN will recur after treatment.

At colposcopy the cervix is washed with acetic acid and then with iodine. The cervix is inspected for suspicious features (Fig. 23.8). Abnormal areas can be biopsied, meaning that the patient will be invited back at a later date for treatment if appropriate, or treatment can be performed at this point.

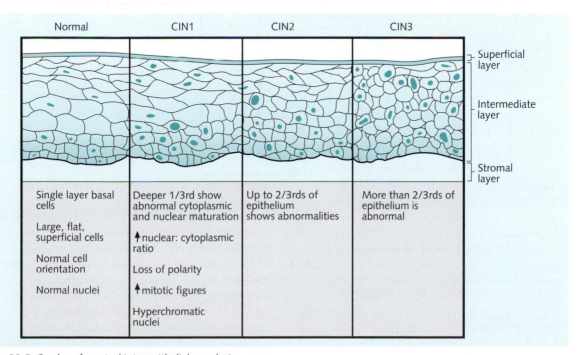

Normal	CIN1	CIN2	CIN3
Single layer basal cells	Deeper 1/3rd show abnormal cytoplasmic and nuclear maturation	Up to 2/3rds of epithelium shows abnormalities	More than 2/3rds of epithelium is abnormal
Large, flat, superficial cells	↑nuclear: cytoplasmic ratio		
Normal cell orientation	Loss of polarity		
Normal nuclei	↑mitotic figures		
	Hyperchromatic nuclei		

Superficial layer
Intermediate layer
Stromal layer

Fig. 23.5 Grades of cervical intraepithelial neoplasia.

Fig. 23.6 Human papilloma virus information box.

Human papilloma virus information box

- Double-stranded DNA viruses
- Over 90 different types identified, 30 of which present in the human genital tract
- Most lead to focal epithelial proliferation, some are linked to cervical cancer
- Low-risk virus types: associated with benign warts and occasionally CIN1 – HPV6, HPV11, HPV42, HPV43 and HPV 44
- Intermediate-risk virus types: associated with CIN2 and CIN3 but rarely seen with invasive cancer – HPV33, HPV35, HPV39, HPV45, HPV51, HPV52 and HPV56
- High-risk virus types: commonly detected in women with CIN2, CIN3 or invasive cancer – HPV16, HPV18 and HPV31
- High-risk HPV types lead to increased degradation of p53, a tumour suppressor
- Higher viral load is associated with a higher risk of developing invasive cancer
- The prevalence of HPV in sexually active women under 30 is 20–40% but most women will clear themselves of HPV within 6–8 months
- Smoking and increasing age make it less likely that the virus will be cleared.

Fig. 23.7 Algorithm for abnormal smears.

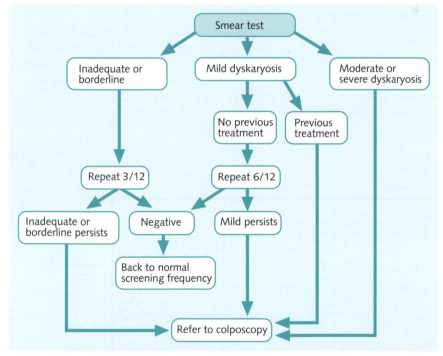

Suspicious features at colposcopy

- Intense acetowhite, pale on iodine staining
- Mosaicism and punctation due to atypical vessel formation
- Raised or ulcerated surface

Fig. 23.8 Suspicious features at colposcopy.

Treatment consists of either excising or destroying the transformation zone. Excision techniques include LLETZ (large loop excision of transformation zone), NETZ (needle excision of transformation zone) and cone biopsy; these allow the tissue removed to be sent for histology and examined to confirm the diagnosis and to check the margins, ensuring complete excision. Destructive techniques include cold coagulation, diathermy or laser.

Risk factors for cervical cancer
• Early age of first intercourse
• Higher number of sexual partners
• HPV (human papilloma virus) infection
• Lower socioeconomic group
• Smoking
• Partner with prostatic or penile cancer

Fig. 23.9 Risk factors for cervical cancer.

Staging of cervical cancer	
Stage	**Description**
0	Carcinoma in situ
I	Confined to the cervix:
A	• Visible only under a microscope:
A1	• <3mm in depth
A2	• >3mm in depth
II	Beyond the cervix:
A	• No parametrial involvement
B	• Parametrial involvement
III	Spread to the pelvic side wall, or affecting the kidney, or spread to the lower third of the vagina
IV	
A	Involving the rectal or bladder mucosa
B	Beyond the true pelvis

Fig. 23.10 Staging of cervical cancer.

Initial treatment has 95% success rate. Patients are followed up with a smear (see Fig. 23.7).

Cervical carcinoma

Cervical cancer affects 20 per 100 000 women per year in the UK. There is a 'double peak' in terms of age group affected as it is most common in 40–44 and 70–74-year-olds. The risk factors for cervical cancer are shown in Fig. 23.9.

Pathology
Squamous cell tumours account for 90–95% of cervical cancers, the other 5–10% are adenocarcinomas derived from cervical glands. The national cervical screening programme aims to detect changes in the cervix that occur before squamous cell tumours develop – it was not designed to look for adenocarcinomas.

Presentation and investigation
Women can present with symptoms of abnormal bleeding, particularly intermenstrual and postcoital, or might be asymptomatic but have had an abnormal smear result. At colposcopy suspicious features are noted (see Fig. 23.8).

Staging
Staging is shown in Fig. 23.10. The procedures necessary to stage the tumour are:
• Cone biopsy, to assess depth of invasion.
• Chest X-ray.
• Intravenous urogram (IVU).
• Cystoscopy and sigmoidoscopy or MRI to look for bladder/bowel involvement.

Management
Patients with cervical tumours that have progressed beyond the microinvasive stage should be referred to a regional cancer centre for treatment by a specialist multidisciplinary team.

Treatment is summarized in the algorithm in Fig. 23.11. Early-stage disease (stages I and IIa) can be treated equally well with surgery or radiotherapy, although surgery is preferred because it leads to fewer sexual, bowel and bladder problems in the long term. Later-stage disease is treated with radical radiotherapy. At present chemotherapy use is only experimental. When the disease has spread (stage IVb) palliative treatment is appropriate.

Vulval tumours

Vulval intraepithelial neoplasia
Vulval intraepithelial neoplasia (VIN) is a premalignant condition but the risk of progression to invasive carcinoma seems to be far less than that of CIN to cervical carcinoma. If VIN is present, CIN is often seen too, and HPV is an underlying factor. Treatment of VIN is not clear-cut, partly due to the lack of knowledge about the danger of not treating. Presentation is usually vulval irritation and, although vulval colposcopy is practised, diagnosis is based on the histopathological study of a biopsy.

Incidence and aetiology
Vulval tumours are uncommon, affecting around 1 in 100 000 women per year. The peak incidence is from the age of 63–65. Predisposing factors include:

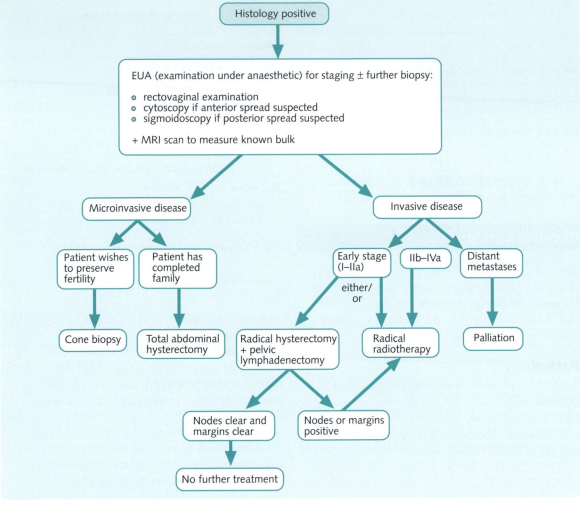

Fig. 23.11 Management of cervical cancer.

Lichen sclerosis information box

Lichen sclerosis is a benign skin condition, with white plaques and atrophy seen in a figure-of-eight pattern around the vulva and anus. Extragenital plaques on the trunk and back might be seen. It is associated with autoimmune disorders, e.g. vitiligo. It can be classed as premalignant, as around 4% will go on to develop vulval squamous cell carcinoma

Fig. 23.12 Lichen sclerosis information box.

- Smoking.
- Immunosuppression.
- Vulvar maturation disorders, e.g. lichen sclerosus (Fig. 23.12).
- History of CIN, VIN or HPV.

Pathology
The majority of vulval tumours are squamous cell carcinomas. Non-squamous cell tumours include melanoma, sarcoma, adenocarcinoma and basal cell tumours. Paget's disease of the vulva is a malignant change in cells of the epidermal layer, which have a characteristic appearance. The presence of vulval Paget's disease is associated with an adenocarcinoma elsewhere in the body in one in four cases, with the most common sites being breast, urinary tract, rectum and genital tract.

Presentation
The most common presenting symptoms are:
- Pruritus.
- Lump/ulcer.
- Bleeding.
- Pain.

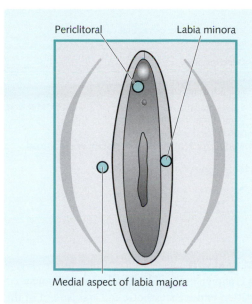

Periclitoral

Labia minora

Medial aspect of labia majora

Fig. 23.13 Squamous cell carcinoma of the vulva – most common sites.

Staging of vulval cancer	
Stage	**Description**
I	Confined to vulva:
A	<1 mm invasion
B	<2 cm diameter, no groin nodes
II	Confined to vulva, <2 cm diameter, no groin nodes palpable
III	Confined to vulva, suspicious nodes or beyond vulva with no suspicious nodes
IV	Obvious groin nodes *or* involving rectum, bladder, urethra or bone *or* pelvic or distant metastases

Fig. 23.14 Staging of vulval cancer.

Complications of vulvectomy and radiotherapy	
Type of treatment	**Complication**
Vulvectomy	Haemorrhage
	Thromboembolism
	Infection – wound, urinary tract
	Wound breakdown
Radiotherapy	Erythema
	Necrosis of the femoral head or pubic symphysis
	Fistula formation (urethrovaginal, vesiculovaginal or rectovaginal)

Fig. 23.15 Complications of vulvectomy and radiotherapy.

Urinary symptoms or unusual discharge can also be symptoms. The most common sites are shown in Fig. 23.13. The tumour can be multifocal.

Spread
Local spread occurs to the vagina, perineum, clitoris, urethra and pubic bone. Lymphatic spread is to the superficial inguinal, deep inguinofemoral and iliac nodes. Unless the tumour is central only the nodes on the affected side are involved.

Investigation
Biopsy is performed, and at the time of biopsy the vagina and cervix are thoroughly inspected for signs of involvement. Positive nodes are detected by CT or MRI scan.

Staging
Stages are shown in Fig. 23.14 but the disease can be more broadly divided into 'early' and 'late', with those having nodal involvement or large, multifocal lesions being in the latter group.

Management
The aim of treatment is to excise the cancer and minimize the risk of recurrence while preserving as much function as possible. Patients should be treated in a regional cancer centre.

The management plan depends on the stage; early tumours are treated by wide local excision. If the initial biopsy showed the depth of invasion to be more than 1 mm, the nodes on the affected side must be dissected, if less than 1 mm nodal dissection is unnecessary.

Larger tumours are treated by radical vulvectomy, with ipsilateral node dissection if the tumour is less than 2 cm in diameter and bilateral if it is more than 2 cm. If groin nodes are not obviously involved the operation can be performed using either one incision (en bloc) or three separate incisions (the butterfly method); the latter seems to reduce the postoperative complications without increasing mortality or recurrence.

Radiotherapy is necessary if histology reveals the nodes to be positive. Chemotherapy has not been shown to be helpful.

Complications of treatment are shown in Fig. 23.15. Due to the large area involved, wound breakdown is, sadly, relatively common. With the en bloc method it occurs in up to 80% of cases, whereas rates for the butterfly incision are between 5 and 50%. Some surgeons advocate performing skin grafts at the time of initial surgery. Radiotherapy adds extra complications.

Prognosis

The most important factor is nodal involvement, and in particular whether the pelvic nodes are positive. Overall survival rates are:

- Node negative: 70–90%.
- Node positive: 25–40%.

Patients with positive pelvic nodes, as opposed to groin nodes only, very rarely survive.

Staging of vaginal cancer	
Stage	**Description**
0	Vaginal intraepithelial neoplasia
I	Limited to the vaginal wall
IIA	Subvaginal tissue, but not the parametrium, involved
IIB	Parametrial involvement
III	Spread to the pelvic side wall
IV	Bladder/rectum involved or distant organ spread

Fig. 23.16 Staging of vaginal cancer.

Vaginal tumours

Vaginal tumours are rare and are usually either primary squamous carcinoma or spread from vulval or cervical squamous cancers. Even rarer tumours include endodermal sinus tumours, rhabdomyosarcoma (both seen in children, but the latter also seen in older women) melanoma, clear cell adenocarcinoma and leiomyosarcoma.

Aetiology

Associations are with CIN and HPV, and with a history of another gynaecological malignancy in the past.

Presentation

The upper third of the vagina is the most common site, and women usually present at an early stage with abnormal bleeding.

Investigation

Staging is shown in Fig. 23.16 and requires biopsy, examination under anaesthetic and assessment of the bladder and rectum either at operation or on MRI. Chest X-ray is performed as part of the evaluation.

Management

Treatment is a combination of external beam and intravaginal radiotherapy, with the complications being fistulae (as with vulval radiotherapy) and stenosis of the vagina and rectum.

Prognosis

Seventy per cent of women who present have stage I or II disease, with 5-year survival rates of around 70%.

- Name three features of an ovarian cyst seen on ultrasound that raise the suspicion of malignancy
- Give an example of a chemotherapy drug used to treat ovarian cancer, and a common side-effect
- Which age group of women is most affected by endometrial carcinoma, and how do they usually present?
- Who has smears, and how often are they performed?
- What is the treatment of a large vulval carcinoma?

Further reading

Govan, Macfarlane, Callander *Pathology Illustrated* (Churchill Livingstone, London)
Miller AWF & Hanretty KP *Obstetrics Illustrated* (Churchill Livingstone, London)

McKay Hart, D & Norman, J (2000) *Gynaecology Illustrated* 5th edn (Churchill Livingstone, London)
Monaghan, JM (1992) *Bonney's Gynaecological Surgery* 9th edn (Balliere Tindall)

24. Vulval Disease

Diseases of the vulva are, to some, difficult to understand. This is likely to be due to a combination of the lack of information or understanding of the aetiology of and the classification of these diseases. Although the vulval dystrophies have recently been renamed (Fig. 24.1), to avoid confusion the more familiar names will be used here.

Please take heed of the new nomenclature as this can be very confusing.

Histology of the vulva

The whole surface of the vulva up to the inner aspect of the labia minora is covered by stratified, keratinized squamous epithelium with a superficial cornified layer. The cornified layer is absent in the vagina and there is a decreasing degree of keratinization (Fig. 24.2). The anatomy of the vulva is shown in Fig. 24.3.

Vulval dystrophies

Histologically, the vulval dystrophies are divided into atrophic and hypertrophic or a mixed picture of both. Atrophic vulval dystrophy is better known as lichen sclerosis.

Most vulval lesions should ideally have colposcopic examination and biopsy to exclude malignancy.

Women with recurrent disease should be seen in a special multidisciplinary vulva clinic.

Lichen sclerosis

Lichen sclerosis is the most common of the vulval dystrophies. It usually develops in postmenopausal women although any age group can be affected, including prepubertal girls (Fig. 24.4). The cause of lichen sclerosis is not understood.

Skin affected by lichen sclerosis is typically thin, shiny and can be white (leucoplakia) or red due to inflammation. Anatomical changes associated with lichen sclerosis include shrinkage or loss of the labia minora and shrinkage of the introitus. Adhesions can fuse the labia together. Lichen sclerosis can affect the perineum and perianal region.

Diagnosis is made histologically from vulval biopsies. Treatment is aimed at relieving the itching and soreness and, as this is a chronic relapsing condition, treatment is usually intermittent. Simple emollient creams can relieve mild symptoms but, if severe, short courses of potent topical steroids might be needed. Testosterone cream is sometimes used but probably acts more as an emollient than hormonally.

Complications are unusual and include anatomical changes and the risk of malignancy. Anatomical changes can cause dyspareunia and, if fusion of the labia occurs in the midline, difficulty in micturition, which might require separation of the labia. Long-term follow-up of women with lichen sclerosis is important as up to 5% will develop squamous carcinoma of the vulva.

Hyperplastic vulval dystrophy

Histologically, squamous cell hyperplasia occurs which is distinguishable from vulval intra-epithelial neoplasia by the absence of atypia. Clinically, the two conditions have a similar presentation. Typical lesions are raised, thickened and can be white, grey or red depending on the degree of inflammation. Treatment is with topical steroids and the condition is likely to recur.

Neoplasia

Neoplastic conditions of the vulva include what is, effectively, the carcinomas-in-situ, VIN and Paget's disease of the vulva, and malignant squamous carcinoma.

Vulval intraepithelial neoplasia

This is a relatively uncommon condition, although the incidence is increasing in young women. Human papilloma virus (specifically HPV 16) has been implicated in the aetiology. Histologically, neoplastic cells are contained within the basement membrane

and the degree of dysplasia is divided into mild, moderate and severe (VIN 1, VIN 2 and VIN 3, respectively).

Symptoms include pruritus, pain, soreness and palpable lesions but many are asymptomatic and found incidentally. Lesions can be papular (like genital warts) or macular with irregular borders. They can be red, brown or black (pigmented), or white (leucoplakia) and ulceration might be present. Unifocal lesions are more common postmenopausally. The diagnosis is made histologically from vulval biopsies.

New nomenclature for the vulval dystrophies	
Old name	New name
Vulval dystrophy	Non-neoplastic epithelial disorders of the vulva
Lichen sclerosus et atrophicus	Lichen sclerosis
Hypertrophic vulval dystrophy	Squamous cell hyperplasia

Fig. 24.1 New nomenclature for the vulval dystrophies.

 Any of the vulval conditions (including vulval carcinoma) can present purely as a mild pruritus vulvae so the symptom should not be underestimated.

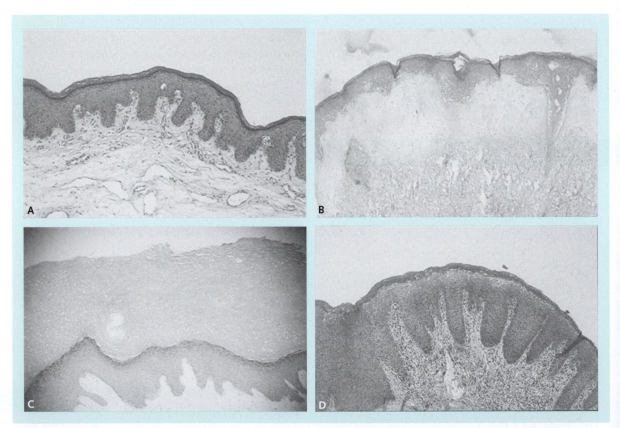

Fig. 24.2 Histology. (A) normal, (B) lichen sclerosis, (C) squamous hyperplasia and (D) dysplasia. Reproduced with kind permission from *Fundamentals of Obstetrics and Gynaecology* (7th edn), published by Mosby.

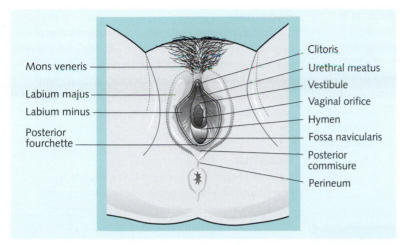

Fig. 24.3 Vulval anatomy.

Mons veneris
Labium majus
Labium minus
Posterior fourchette

Clitoris
Urethral meatus
Vestibule
Vaginal orifice
Hymen
Fossa navicularis
Posterior commisure
Perineum

Characteristics of some important vulval diseases					
	Age at presentation	Incidence	Mode of treatment	Recurrence rate	Malignant potential
Vulval dystrophies					
Lichen sclerosis	Any age but usually postmenopausal	Common	Topical steroids and emollients	Frequent	<5% Develop squamous carcinoma of the vulva
Neoplasias					
Vulval intraepithelial neoplasia	Any age but increasing in the young	Relatively uncommon, but increasing	Usually surgical more conservative in young women	Up to 80% will recur	Overall low, but higher in the elderly and immunosuppressed
Paget's disease of the vulva	Postmenopausal women	Rare	Surgical	Up to 33% will recur	Associated with adenocarcinoma in 25% Malignant change in lesion is rare

Fig. 24.4 Characteristics of some important vulval diseases.

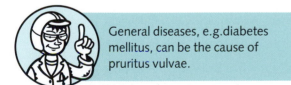

General diseases, e.g. diabetes mellitus, can be the cause of pruritus vulvae.

Treatment is usually surgical, either by ablating the lesion with laser or cryotherapy or by local excision. VIN will recur in up to 80% of treated women and as the risk of malignant change is small, especially in younger women, major mutilating surgery should be avoided. Surgical treatment is recommended when the risk of malignant change is increased:

- Excessively hyperkeratotic lesions.
- In postmenopausal women.
- In the immunosuppressed.
- If the severity of dysplasia is seen to worsen on serial biopsy.

Where conservative treatment is planned, topical steroids may give symptomatic relief.

Squamous carcinoma of the vulva

Squamous carcinoma of the vulva is discussed in Chapter 23.

Paget's disease of the vulva

Paget's disease of the vulva is uncommon; it is usually seen in postmenopausal women. The aetiology is unknown although the lesion is thought to be of glandular origin. In 25% of cases, there is an underlying adenocarcinoma (breast, urinary, genital or colonic).

Lesions can be unifocal or multifocal and are typically clearly defined, scaly, erythematous plaques with varying degrees of ulceration and leucoplakia. The main symptom is pruritus and the diagnosis is made histologically. Treatment is surgical using laser ablation or local excision and up to one-third will recur. Although associated with adenocarcinoma, malignant change within the lesion is rare.

Dermatological conditions

Many dermatological conditions can affect the vulva often with a confusing clinical picture, especially if the vulva is the only area affected.

Psoriasis

The typical raised, erythematous, scaly lesions of psoriasis can occur on the vulva, although here they might appear smooth and without the scaling. The presence of psoriasis elsewhere on the body will suggest the diagnosis, which can be confirmed histologically. Treatment is with topical steroids but the relapse rate is high.

Eczema

Eczema of the vulva is rare. More commonly, eczematous reactions occur due to contact with irritant substances such as soaps and detergents. Treatment is by identifying and removing the source of irritation and topical steroids.

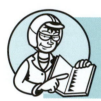

- What is the most common cause of pruritus vulvae in a postmenopausal woman?
- What are the possible treatments of lichen sclerosis?
- How should the vulval skin be investigated in the clinic?
- What possible infections could present as vulval disease?

Further reading

Llewellyn-Jones, D (1999) *Fundementals of Obstetrics & Gynaecology* 7th edn (Mosby, London)

McKay Hart, D & Norman, J (2000) *Gynaecology Illustrated* 5th edn (Churchill Livingstone, London)

Monaghan, JM (1992) *Bonney's Gynaecological Surgery* 9th edn (Balliere Tindall)

Shaw RW, Soutter WP, Stanton SL (1997) *Gynaecology* 2nd edn (Churchill Livingstone, London)

http://www.rcog.org.uk/guidelines

25. Pelvic Inflammatory Disease

Definition

Pelvic inflammatory disease (PID) is defined as the clinical syndrome associated with ascending spread of microorganisms from the vagina or cervix to the endometrium, fallopian tubes and/or contiguous structures. It usually begins with an acute infection; this might resolve completely or develop a chronic course with repeated acute or subacute episodes.

Incidence

The true incidence of PID is difficult to determine because of the lack of a precise clinical definition or a specific diagnostic test. However, the incidence is strongly correlated with the prevalence of sexually transmitted infections, and has increased in most countries. In the USA, the highest annual incidence is among sexually active women in their teenage years; 75% of cases occur in women under the age of 25. Figure 25.1 outlines risk factors for the development of PID.

Aetiology

- *Chlamydia trachomatis*.
- *Neisseria gonorrhoeae*.
- Non-specific.

Chlamydia trachomatis is the most common cause of PID in the UK. Along with *Neisseria gonorrhoeae*, this microorganism is responsible for at least 60% of cases of PID. They are thought to act as primary pathogens, causing damage to the protective mechanisms of the endocervix and allowing endogenous bacteria from the vagina and cervix into the upper genital tract as secondary invaders (Fig. 25.2). A variety of endogenous aerobic and anaerobic bacteria have been isolated from women with PID, such as *Mycoplasma* species, but their exact role is uncertain.

Occasionally, PID develops secondary to another disease process, such as appendicitis, or rarely, as part of more generalized disease such as tuberculosis.

Diagnosis

The diagnosis of PID is sometimes a difficult one to make, since it does not rely on one particular sign or symptom or combination of these. However, it is thought that the benefits of early diagnosis and appropriate treatment outweigh the possible overuse of antibiotics in a patient who might seem to have only mild disease.

The differential diagnosis (see Chapter 2) includes:
- Appendicitis.
- Endometriosis.
- Ectopic pregnancy.
- Ovarian cyst accident.

History

The history might include one or more of the following symptoms:
- Pelvic pain/lower abdominal pain, usually bilateral.
- Deep dyspareunia.
- Dysmenorrhoea.
- Increased vaginal discharge.
- Fever.

PID can also be asymptomatic, presenting many years after the acute infection with subfertility.

Examination

At least three of the following signs should be present to make the diagnosis of acute PID:
- Raised temperature > 37.5°C.
- Abdominal tenderness.
- Purulent vaginal discharge.
- Cervical excitation (pain or discomfort on moving the cervix).
- Adnexal tenderness.
- Adnexal swelling.

Pelvic inflammatory disease risk factors	
Risk factor	**Description**
Age	75% of patients are below 25 years of age
Marital status	Single
Sexual history	Young at first intercourse
	High frequency of sexual intercourse
	Multiple sexual partners
Medical history	Past history of sexually transmitted disease in patient or partner
	Past history of PID in patient
	Recent instrumentation of uterus, e.g. termination of pregnancy
Contraception	Use of intrauterine contraceptive device, especially insertion within 3 weeks

Fig. 25.1 Risk factors for the development of pelvic inflammatory disease.

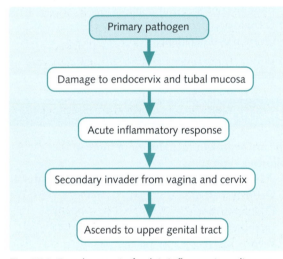

Fig. 25.2 Development of pelvic inflammatory disease.

Investigations

Appropriate investigations include:
- White blood cell count (WBC).
- C reactive protein (CRP).
- Blood cultures, depending on the level of the pyrexia.
- Full screen for sexually transmitted infections, including high vaginal swab, endocervical swabs and possibly urethral swabs and an MSU specimen.
- Pregnancy test (urinary β-hCG) depending on date of LMP.
- Ultrasound scan, which might be appropriate to exclude an ovarian cyst complication.

Complications of acute pelvic inflammatory disease	
Type of complication	**Description**
Short term	Pelvic abscess formation
	Septicaemia
	Septic shock
Long term	Infertility
	Ectopic pregnancy
	Chronic pelvic pain
	Dyspareunia
	Menstrual disturbances
	Psychological effects

Fig. 25.3 Complications of acute pelvic inflammatory disease.

Laparoscopy may be considered in some cases, for example if there is doubt about the diagnosis or if the patient fails to respond to antibiotic therapy.

Complications

The long-term morbidity associated with acute PID is considerable (Fig. 25.3) and thus the need for appropriate treatment, especially to cover chlamydial infection, is important. Moderately severe disease is associated with inflammation and oedema in the fallopian tubes, with deposits of fibrin and subsequent adhesion formation between the pelvic and abdominal organs. Thus, tubal morphology and function are affected resulting in subfertility and an increased risk of ectopic pregnancy. Adhesions in the pelvis may lead to chronic pain, either as a sole feature, or in relation to menstruation or sexual intercourse.

 Early diagnosis and treatment are important to reduce the risk of long-term complications.

Treatment

- Antibiotic therapy.
- Contact tracing.
- Surgery.

The aim of treatment is to prevent the long-term sequelae of PID mentioned above. First,

Antibiotic therapy for the treatment of pelvic inflammatory disease	
Infecting agent	Therapy
Chlamydia	Tetracyclines, e.g. doxycycline Erythromycin if the patient is pregnant Azithromycin if single-dose treatment is preferable
Gonorrhoea	Ciprofloxacin Ofloxacin
Anaerobes	Metronidazole

Fig. 25.4 Antibiotic therapy for the treatment of pelvic inflammatory disease.

administration of broad-spectrum antibiotics is indicated once the diagnosis of PID is suspected and should be started prior to obtaining the results of microbiology specimens (Fig. 25.4).

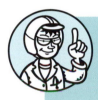

Antibiotic therapy must include treatment for *Chlamydia* because this microorganism is most commonly implicated in PID and its sequelae.

If a patient resumes sexual intercourse with a partner who is infected but untreated, there is obviously a high chance of reinfection. It is therefore important to trace all recent contacts of the patient so that they can be given treatment, either empirically or as a result of microbiology results. This

can be done more effectively by referring the patient to a genitourinary medicine clinic.

Apart from diagnostic laparoscopy, there is rarely a need for more invasive surgery in the management of PID. Laparoscopy or laparotomy might be necessary to drain a tubo-ovarian abscess.

Prevention

PID and its sequelae are responsible for a substantial amount of morbidity, both physical and psychological, as well as having considerable financial implications. Therefore, primary prevention of the disease is of great importance and needs the help of both the media and health care professionals. Government educational programmes are currently in progress:

- Educational campaigns to increase awareness of at-risk behaviour.
- Opportunistic screening of those at risk, e.g. termination of pregnancy (TOP) clinic, patient having evacuation of the retained products of conception (ERPC).
- Knowledge of up-to-date treatment regimens with locally agreed protocols.
- Understanding the importance of contact tracing.

Effective treatment for PID must include contact tracing and treatment of the patient's partners.

- What are the two main causes of PID?
- What are the differential diagnoses of PID?
- What are the investigations necessary to exclude PID?
- What are potential sequelae of PID?
- Discuss the treatment options for PID.

Further reading

Shaw RW, Soutter WP, Stanton SL (1997) *Gynaecology* 2nd edn (Churchill Livingstone, London)

26. Urinary Incontinence

Incidence

Female urinary incontinence is a very common problem, with up to one-quarter of women leaking urine occasionally. The prevalence of regular female urinary incontinence increases with increasing age; 8.5% of women under 65 years of age rising to 11.6% over 65 years and 43.2% over 85 years.

The most common cause of urinary incontinence is genuine stress incontinence (GSI), followed by detrusor overactivity (DO), which account for almost 50% and 40% of incontinent women, respectively. These and other causes are shown in Fig. 5.1 (page 26).

Aetiology

The bladder has two major roles; the retention of urine and expulsion of urine. Failure to retain urine, or loss of normal voiding control, give rise to two distinct aetiologies of incontinence.

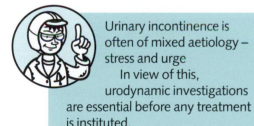

Urinary incontinence is often of mixed aetiology – stress and urge
In view of this, urodynamic investigations are essential before any treatment is instituted.

Genuine stress incontinence

The bladder acts as a low-pressure reservoir. As the volume increases, the bladder pressure rises only slightly. Urethral closure pressure, produced by the passive effect of elastic and collagen fibres and active striated and smooth muscle, causes the urethra to close. Continence requires a positive pressure gradient from the urethra to the bladder. In the resting state the urethral closure pressure is higher than the relatively low bladder pressure and continence is maintained.

Intra-abdominal pressure is transmitted to the bladder and raised intra-abdominal pressure, such as during coughing or straining, increases the bladder pressure. Intra-abdominal pressure is also transmitted to the bladder neck and that part of the proximal urethra which is intra-abdominal (above the pelvic floor) maintaining the positive pressure gradient and hence continence (Fig. 26.1B). If the bladder neck and proximal urethra are situated below the pelvic floor then the raised intra-abdominal pressure is no longer transmitted to these structures, the positive pressure gradient is lost and incontinence occurs (Fig. 26.1C).

GSI increases with increasing age as maximal urethral closure pressure decreases. Also, older women are more likely to be parous and postmenopausal. GSI increases with increasing parity being associated with the process of vaginal delivery. Prolapse is commonly thought to be associated with GSI although this is only true if the proximal urethra has descended below the pelvic floor (see above). Atrophic changes associated with the post-menopausal state and vaginal surgery to cure prolapse are also associated with GSI.

Detrusor overactivity

In women with DO, the urethra functions normally, but if the uninhibited detrusor activity increases bladder pressure above maximal urethral closure pressure, urinary leakage occurs.

The majority of women with DO have an idiopathic aetiology with no demonstrable abnormality to be found. DO can occur following surgery to the bladder neck and proximal urethra, especially following surgery for GSI, during which dissection around these structures occurs. Multiple sclerosis, autonomic neuropathy and spinal lesions can allow uninhibited detrusor contractions, although these women with neurological lesions are more correctly said to have detrusor hyperreflexia.

Increasing age and a history of nocturnal enuresis are associated with DO and diuretics will obviously exacerbate this condition.

Sensory urgency

Irritation of the bladder mucosa, due either to infection (cystitis), bladder stones or tumours, can cause sensory urgency. The aetiology of primary

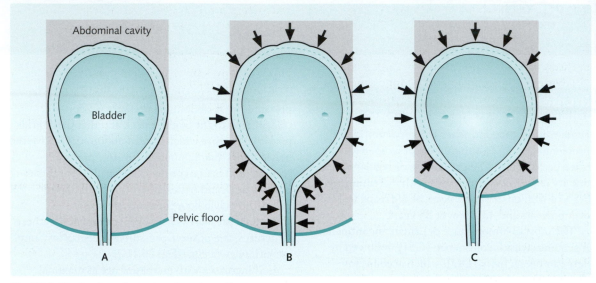

Fig. 26.1 Mechanism of genuine stress incontinence.

vesical sensory urgency is not well understood but accounts for almost 4% of incontinent women.

Voiding disorders

Voiding difficulties can present as acute or chronic urinary retention with overflow incontinence. Chronic overdistension of the bladder is likely to exacerbate and can itself cause voiding difficulties due to detrusor ischaemia and denervation.

Central, spinal and peripheral neurological lesions can produce voiding difficulties (Fig. 26.2). Approximately 25% of women with multiple sclerosis will present with acute urinary retention. Postoperative pain can cause reflex inhibition of micturition, as can severe inflammation of the bladder, urethra and vulva.

Drugs can cause voiding difficulties, epidural anaesthesia in labour being the most common encountered. Tricyclic antidepressants, anticholinergic agents, α-adrenergic agonists and ganglion blockers can all cause voiding difficulties.

Voiding difficulties can occur secondary to mechanical obstruction. Impaction of a pelvic mass, for instance the gravid uterus or fibroids, might obstruct the urethra, as can bladder polyps or malignancy. Oedema following bladder neck surgery causes voiding difficulties frequently enough to

Neurological causes of voiding difficulties	
Type of lesion	Neurological cause of voiding difficulty
Central lesions (suprapontine)	Cerebrovascular accident Parkinson's disease
Spinal lesions	Spinal cord injury Multiple sclerosis
Peripheral lesions	Prolapsed intervertebral disc Peripheral autonomic neuropathies (e.g. diabetic)

Fig. 26.2 Neurological causes of voiding difficulties (acute and chronic retention).

warrant prophylactic drainage of the bladder following these procedures. Surprisingly, it is rare for prolapse to cause retention.

Fistulae

The most common cause of fistula formation worldwide is obstructed labour. In the UK, avoiding prolonged labour has almost eradicated this complication of labour. Although uncommon, fistulae are likely to be secondary to malignancy, surgery and radiation to the pelvis or a combination of these. Fistulae can occur from the ureter, bladder or urethra to the vagina.

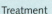

Investigation policy

Having excluded urinary tract infection, the mainstay of investigation are urodynamic studies. Urodynamic studies are important for diagnosing the causes of incontinence as symptoms are often multiple and do not correlate well with the underlying disorder (see Chapter 5). Cystoscopy can be helpful by inspecting the anatomy of the bladder and urethra and hence excluding mechanical causes of incontinence but does not allow assessment of their function. Bimanual pelvic examination and pelvic ultrasound will identify pelvic masses. Uretero-vaginal fistulae will require radiological investigations. Infusing coloured dyes into the bladder and observing vaginal leakage may confirm the presence of vesico- or urethro-vaginal fistulae.

A urinary tract infection and neurological defect must always be excluded.

Complications

Although incontinence itself is not life threatening, it does cause major psychosocial problems. Changes in lifestyle are common and occasionally symptoms are so severe as to render the woman housebound. Excoriation and soreness of the vulva occurs secondary to continual dampness and chronic urinary tract infection can lead to long-term damage of renal function. Acute and chronic overdistension of the bladder can cause denervation and necrosis of the detrusor muscle thereby causing further voiding difficulties.

Treatment

Treatment is determined not only by the underlying condition but also by the severity of the symptoms. Some women might be happy to undergo a trial of oral medication but not major abdominal surgery for the same degree of symptoms. Similarly, depending on lifestyle, some women can live with their symptoms whereas others find the same symptoms intolerable. A sympathetic approach and detailed counselling of the pros and cons of treatment are essential in treating women with incontinence.

Genuine stress incontinence

Physiotherapy is the mainstay of conservative treatment of GSI. Women are taught to use the pelvic floor muscles to achieve better urinary control and up to 60% will have improvement of symptoms. Techniques include simple pelvic floor exercises or insertion of vaginal cones, which can be retained only by contraction of the relevant pelvic floor muscles. Problems include return of symptoms if exercises are stopped and a spontaneous worsening of symptoms associated with the menopause. Oestrogen replacement has been shown to improve the symptom of stress incontinence in postmenopausal women although long term use is required to maintain the effect.

The majority of women with GSI can be cured by surgery. This is achieved by lifting and supporting the bladder neck and urethra, thereby restoring their intra-abdominal position. This also increases the urethral pressure by increasing outflow resistance. Abdominal procedures have been shown to be far more effective than vaginal procedures and colposuspension is the surgical procedure of choice achieving a success rate of up to 90%. Performed through a suprapubic incision, this involves placing sutures from the vagina, adjacent to the bladder neck, to the ligaments at the back of the symphysis pubis. This results in the vagina being elevated and this 'platform' supports the bladder neck in an intra-abdominal position. Slings can be placed under the bladder neck and sutured to the lateral pelvic side wall or rectus muscles to produce a similar effect. There is a current vogue for use of tension-free vaginal tape (TVT) – initial 5-year results suggest an efficacy approaching that of colposuspension.

Vaginal procedures, such as anterior colporrhaphy, can achieve continence in the short term but will have failed in up to 60% by 5 years. In the presence of poor detrusor activity, the bladder might not produce high enough pressures to overcome the relative outflow obstruction produced by abdominal procedures and self-intermittent catheterization might be necessary. Urodynamic studies will help to identify this group of women, although all women undergoing abdominal surgery for GSI should be warned of this complication.

Where GSI and DO coexist it is sensible to treat the DO in the first instance. A significant percentage of women will have a satisfactory enough response to simple medical treatment and avoid major surgery.

 The treatment of stress incontinence is surgical – tension free vaginal tape or colposuspension.

Detrusor overactivity

DO is treated medically except in the uncommon situations where symptoms are severe enough to warrant surgery. Behavioural and drug therapy are the mainstay of medical treatment.

Behavioural therapy

Bladder re-training aims to increase the voiding intervals and may be successful in up to 80% of women with DO, although there is a significant relapse rate. Having explained how the bladder functions, subjects are taught to micturate by the clock rather than desire and encouraged to increase voiding intervals incrementally. Other techniques include hypnotherapy and acupuncture.

Drug therapy

There is a strong placebo effect in the drug treatment of DO. Drugs that are effective in treating DO rely on their antimuscarinic properties (less correctly termed 'anticholinergics'). Antimuscarinic drugs effectively increase bladder capacity by:
- Delaying initial desire to void.
- Decreasing the strength of detrusor contractions.
- Decreasing the frequency of detrusor contractions.

Although improving symptoms in many women, the use of antimuscarinics is limited by their atropine-like side-effects (Fig. 26.3). Oxybutynin is currently widely used, although the recent introduction of a new drug with antimuscarinic properties that are highly selective for the bladder (Tolterodine) has proved popular. Tolterodine shows good efficacy with far fewer antimuscarinic side-effects and now can be given as a once daily formulation.

Tricyclic antidepressants also have antimuscarinic properties as well as a central sedative effect. They are useful for incontinent women who suffer from anxiety.

Sensory urgency

Removal of the source of bladder mucosal irritation (infection, bladder stones, tumours) is likely to relieve symptoms.

Voiding difficulties

The symptoms of urinary obstruction can be treated by drug therapy but where retention has occurred catheterization is necessary.

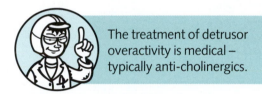 The treatment of detrusor overactivity is medical – typically anti-cholinergics.

Drug therapy

Drugs used to treat the symptoms of voiding difficulties are often ineffective or have limited use due to side-effects. They work in two ways:
- Relax the sphincter mechanism or.
- Produce detrusor contractions.

The selective α-blocker indoramin produces an increase in flow rate and improvement in obstructive symptoms by relaxing the sphincter mechanism. Side-effects include sedation, dizziness, tachycardia and hypotension and must be used with extreme caution in the elderly and in anti-hypertensive users.

The parasympathomimetics (bethanechol, carbachol and distigmine) exhibit muscarinic activity which improves voiding by increasing detrusor contraction. Side-effects include sweating, bradycardia and intestinal colic.

Catheterization

Acute retention of urine requires catheterization. If caused by a gravid uterus, the catheter may need to be left in situ until the uterus has become abdominal. An ovarian cyst or fibroid will need to be removed

Atropine-like side-effects	
Type of side-effect	Description
Peripheral	Dry mouth
	Reduced visual accommodation
	Constipation
	Glaucoma
Central	Confusion

Fig. 26.3 Atropine-like side-effects.

surgically, although disimpaction from the pelvis is sometimes possible as a palliative measure. Postoperative or postpartum retention usually resolve with bladder drainage. A suprapubic catheter is preferred as residual volumes can be measured to assess progress. If the bladder has been overdistended then normal bladder function is unlikely to occur immediately and free bladder drainage is required until normal function returns.

Chronic retention may require long term indwelling catheters which has a significant risk of sepsis. Intermittent self-catheterization might be more appropriate in those who are able to perform this technique. Subclinical sepsis is common although treatment is usually given only if symptoms are present.

Fistula

Small fistulae might close spontaneously by providing continuous free drainage of urine. This might require stenting of the ureters or catheterization of the bladder. If spontaneous closure does not occur, or if the fistulae are large, then surgical closure by a surgeon experienced in such techniques is required.

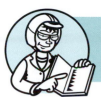

- What are the main treatments for stress incontinence?
- What are the main treatments for detrusor instability?
- What investigations are essential before any surgery is undertaken?

Further reading

Cardozo, I & Staskin, D (eds) *Textbook of Female Urology and Urogynaecology* (Martin Dunitz)
Llewellyn Jones, D *Fundamentals of Obstetrics & Gynaecology* Chapter 40 7th edn (Mosby)

Stanton, S & Monga, A *Clinical Urogynaecology* 2nd edn (Churchill Livingstone)

http://www.rcog.org.uk/guidelines

27. Genital Prolapse

Definition

A prolapse is the protrusion of an organ or a structure beyond its normal anatomical site. Genital prolapse involves weakness of the supporting structures of the pelvic organs so that they descend from their normal positions. The type of prolapse depends on the organ involved and its position in relation to the anterior or posterior vaginal wall (Fig. 27.1). Descent of the uterus is graded according to the position of the cervix on vaginal examination:

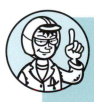 Genital prolapse is common and requires a basic knowledge of pelvic anatomy to help you understand how it develops and how it can be repaired.

- First degree: descent of the cervix within the vagina.
- Second degree: descent of the cervix to the introitus.
- Third degree: descent of the cervix outside the introitus (also known as a procidentia).

Incidence of genital prolapse

Genital prolapse is common; a cystourethrocoele is the most common type, followed by uterine descent and then rectocoele. The incidence increases with increasing age. Prolapse is seen less commonly in Afro-Carribean women than in Caucasian women.

Pelvic anatomy

Some knowledge of the pelvic anatomy, with particular reference to the pelvic floor muscles, fascia and ligaments, is necessary to understand the development of genital prolapse. Weakness of these tissues, either congenital or acquired, results in descent of the pelvic viscera.

Pelvic floor

The pelvic floor consists of a muscular, gutter-shaped, forward sloping diaphragm formed by the:

- Levator ani muscles.
- Internal obturator and piriform muscles.
- Superficial and deep perineal muscles.

The levator ani consists of two parts, the pubococcygeal part anteriorly and the iliococcygeal part posteriorly and is covered by pelvic fascia. The vagina and urethra pass through the urogenital aperture formed by the medial border of the levator ani. The rectum passes posteriorly with muscle fibres from the pubic bone uniting behind the anorectal junction. Thus, the muscles provide an indirect support for these structures (Fig. 27.2).

Pelvic ligaments

Condensations of the pelvic fascia form strong ligaments that act to support the upper part of the vagina, the cervix and the uterus. Those that support the uterus include the:

- Transverse cervical or cardinal ligaments.
- Uterosacral ligaments.
- Round ligaments.

The transverse cervical and uterosacral ligaments consist of smooth muscle and elastic tissue. They support the pelvic side wall and the sacrum, respectively. The round ligaments pass from the cornu of the uterus through the inguinal canal to the labium majus. They contain smooth muscle and maintain flexion of the uterus with only minimal role in support.

Aetiology of genital prolapse

 In terms of aetiology, obstetric factors are particularly important, and if prolapse is to be prevented, good intrapartum management of the patient is essential.

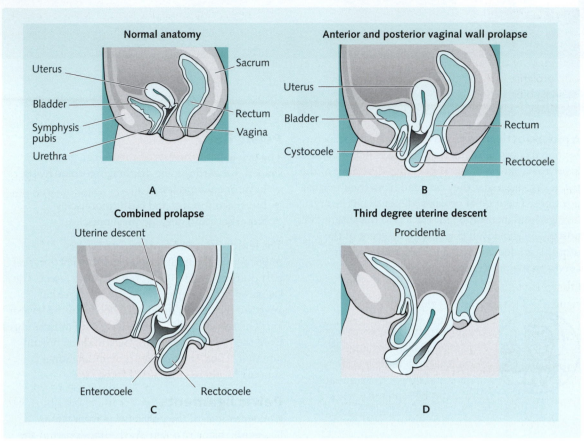

Fig. 27.1 Types of prolapse.

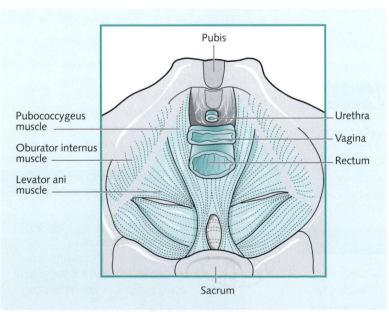

Fig. 27.2 Anatomy of the pelvic floor muscles.

Congenital

Some women are born with a predisposition to genital prolapse, which is probably secondary to abnormal collagen production. Conditions associated with prolapse include:
- Spina bifida.
- Connective tissue disorder.

Acquired

Although most women with genital prolapse have a degree of congenital predisposition, the following factors are also important:
- Obstetric factors.
- Postmenopausal atrophy.
- Chronically raised intra-abdominal pressure.
- Iatrogenic.

Obstetric factors

Figure 27.3 lists the factors that can cause prolapse secondary to denervation and muscular trauma of the pelvic floor.

Postmenopausal atrophy

The incidence of prolapse increases with age. This is due to atrophy of the connective tissues secondary to the hypo-oestrogenic state following the menopause.

Chronically raised intra-abdominal pressure

Any factors that raise intra-abdominal pressure in the long term can predispose to prolapse, including:
- Intra-abdominal or pelvic tumour.
- Chronic cough.
- Constipation.

Iatrogenic

Hysterectomy predisposes to future prolapse of the vaginal vault because, in order to remove the uterus, the transverse cervical and uterosacral ligaments have to be divided and the upper vaginal supports are weakened.

Colposuspension predisposes to development of an enterocoele because the anterior vaginal wall is lifted anteriorly, which in turn pulls the upper posterior vaginal wall forwards.

Clinical features of genital prolapse

History

Most commonly, the patient presents with a history of local discomfort or a feeling of 'something coming down', as the prolapsed organ pushes into the vagina and bulges towards the introitus. This can be exacerbated if the intra-abdominal pressure is increased, for example by coughing. It can interfere with sexual function.

Uterine descent often gives symptoms of backache, although other causes of backache must be excluded, especially in this older patient group. A procidentia causes discomfort as it rubs on the patient's clothing and this can cause a bloody, sometimes purulent, discharge.

Other symptoms depend on the organ/organs involved. Urinary symptoms occur with a cystocoele or a cystourethrocoele, such as frequency of micturition. The patient might notice incomplete emptying of the bladder, which predisposes her to urinary infection and even possibly overflow incontinence. Stress incontinence might be present if there is descent of the urethrovesical junction (bladder neck).

A rectocoele can cause incomplete bowel emptying. This can be relieved if the patient pushes back the prolapse digitally.

Examination

- General examination.
- Abdominal palpation.
- Sims speculum examination.
- Bimanual pelvic examination.

Obstetric factors that may predispose to genital prolapse

- Prolonged labour
- Precipitate labour
- Instrumental delivery
- Fetal macrosomia
- Increasing parity

Fig. 27.3 Obstetric factors that may predispose to genital prolapse.

 Examination of the patient with a prolapse must include abdominal palpation and bimanual pelvic examination to exclude an abdominal or pelvic mass as the cause of the prolapse.

A general examination should be performed, particularly if the patient's medical history might influence future management options. Abdominal palpation is essential to exclude a mass that might be causing the pelvic organs to prolapse.

Inspection of the vulva might reveal an obvious genital prolapse. The patient should be examined in the left lateral position using a Sims' speculum. With the posterior vaginal wall retracted, any anterior wall prolapse will be demonstrated if the patient is asked to bear down. This can extend anteriorly as far as the urethral orifice, distinguishing between a cystocoele and a cystourethrocoele. Conversely, if the anterior vaginal wall is retracted, then an enterocoele or rectocoele will be seen. A bulging rectocoele can be reduced digitally to exclude an enterocoele.

Uterine descent can be assessed using the Sims' speculum but this might be difficult in the outpatient setting; unless the cervix is at or protuding through the introitus, then the degree of uterine prolapse might be better determined under general anaesthesia when traction can be applied to the cervix. There might be combined prolapse, most commonly uterine descent associated with anterior vaginal wall prolapse.

If the patient has a full bladder, stress incontinence can be demonstrated by asking her to cough. A bimanual pelvic examination is mandatory to exclude a pelvic mass as the cause of the prolapse.

Management

The aim is to replace the prolapsed organs to their normal anatomical site. The options can be categorized into:
- Prevention.
- Conservative measures.
- Surgery.

Always remember to consider the patient's general health and other conservative measures, such as HRT, as well as the need for surgery.

Prevention

Because obstetric factors are most commonly involved in the development of a genital prolapse, it is important that damage to the supporting structures of the pelvis is minimized. Appropriate management of labour should include:
- Avoid prolonged first and second stages.
- Postnatal pelvic floor exercises.

The current decline in parity, as well as the increasing use of caesarean section might reduce the incidence of prolapse.

Conservative measures

Improvement in general health should aim to treat the underlying cause of chronically raised intra-abdominal pressure, including:
- Weight loss.
- Advising the patient to stop smoking to reduce cough.
- Treat constipation.

Pelvic floor exercises

Pelvic floor exercises can improve symptoms of minor degrees of genital prolapse sufficiently to avoid surgery. However, their use is probably more important in prevention.

Hormone replacement therapy

In the presence of atrophic pelvic tissues, HRT can help in minor degrees of prolapse by increasing skin collagen content. Preoperative use of HRT reduces the friability of atrophic tissues, making tissue handling easier during surgery.

Vaginal pessaries

The most commonly used pessary is a ring pessary made of inert plastic. The diameter is measured in millimetres and the appropriate size is assessed by vaginal examination. The pessary is passed into the vagina so that it sits behind the pubic bone anteriorly and in the posterior fornix of the vagina posteriorly, enclosing the cervix. The other less common type of pessary is the shelf pessary.

The indications for the use of a vaginal pessary include:
- The patient has not completed her family.
- The patient prefers conservative management.
- The patient is medically unfit for surgery.
- While the patient is on the waiting list for surgery.

With major degrees of prolapse, especially where the introitus is lax and the perineal body deficient, the pessary might not stay in situ. The main complications of a pessary are vaginal discharge or bleeding, particularly if the pessary is not replaced every 6 months. Vaginal ulceration can occur if the ring is too large and the pessary might simply fall out if it is too small. Granulation tissue might develop, incarcerating the pessary, if it is not changed regularly.

Surgical treatment

Surgery should be considered with a severe degree of prolapse or if conservative management fails. Prior to surgery it is important to know whether a woman is sexually active, because the vagina might be narrowed and shortened, potentially causing dyspareunia.

Surgery is not recommended in a woman who has not completed her family. Caesarean section is indicated following pelvic floor repair; vaginal delivery is likely to result in soft tissue trauma and recurrence of prolapse.

Anterior colporrhaphy

This operation, also known as an anterior repair, is indicated for the repair of a cystocoele or a cystourethrocoele. A portion of redundant anterior vaginal wall mucosa is excised and the exposed fascia is plicated to support the bladder.

Posterior colporrhaphy

Also known as a posterior repair, this operation is used to repair a rectocoele or a rectocoele combined with an enterocoele. Using a similar technique to the operation described above, a triangle of posterior vaginal wall mucosa – its apex behind the cervix and the base at the introitus – is removed. The underlying levator ani muscles are plicated to support the perineum. If an enterocoele is present, the pouch of Douglas is opened and the enterocoele sac of redundant peritoneum is excised.

Vaginal hysterectomy

This operation is performed for uterine prolapse, although it might be indicated for other gynaecological pathology. It can be combined with one or both of the operations mentioned above.

Manchester repair (Fothergill procedure)

This operation is much less commonly performed for uterine prolapse – in cases where there is a reason to preserve the uterus. It consists of amputation of the cervix and then apposing the cardinal ligaments to lift the uterus, followed by anterior and posterior colporrhaphy if necessary.

Sacrospinous fixation

Using the transvaginal approach, the prolapsed vaginal vault is fixed to sacrospinous ligament, which runs from the ischial spine to the lower lateral aspect of the sacrum. Care must be taken to avoid the pudendal nerve and vessels, as well as the sacral plexus and the sciatic nerve.

Sacral colpopexy

This abdominal procedure involves suspending the vaginal vault from the sacrum or from the sacral promontory, using either strips of fascia or synthetic mesh. The main complications are intraoperative haemorrhage and infection of the mesh.

- What are the common presenting symptoms of genital prolapse?
- What are the different types of prolapse?
- Describe how a patient complaining of prolapse should be examined.
- Discuss the conservative management of prolapse.
- For which patients is conservative management appropriate?

Further reading

McKay Hart, D & Norman, J (2000) *Gynaecology Illustrated* 5th edn (Churchill Livingstone, London)

Monaghan, JM (1992) *Bonney's Gynaecological Surgery* 9th edn (Balliere Tindall)

Shaw RW, Soutter WP, Stanton SL (1997) *Gynaecology* 2nd edn (Churchill Livingstone, London)

Studd, J (1994) *Progress in Obstetrics and Gynaecology* vol 11

28. Subfertility

If a cause for a couple's subfertility is discovered (see Chapter 8), treatment can be aimed at the problem, but many couples suffer unexplained subfertility. They can still be helped by the methods described below.

Anovulation

The absence of ovulation should be suspected if a woman's cycle is irregular and is confirmed if there is no rise of progesterone in the luteal phase of the cycle. If the woman is not ovulating:

- Maximize general health (correct thyroid disease, diabetes, etc.).
- Consider BMI (ovulation is less likely at the extremes of weight).
- Discuss psychological stress levels.
- Prescribe clomiphene (see below) to induce ovulation.

There is no evidence that the use of temperature charts or LH 'ovulation predictor' kits to time intercourse around ovulation improves the chance of conception; body temperature is a poor predictor of ovulation and LH kits, although better, are expensive. Also, timing intercourse is psychologically stressful and can be counterproductive.

Clomiphene is an antioestrogen that occupies oestrogen receptors in the hypothalamus, thereby increasing GnRH release, which leads to increased release of LH and FSH. This induces follicular development and ovulation. It is given on days 2–6 of the cycle. Ovulation should be confirmed by a raised progesterone level. If ovulation does not occur the dose can be increased the next month.

The patient must be warned of the risk of multiple pregnancy. Some units arrange to scan the ovaries during the cycle to see whether follicles are developing and, when there are many follicles, to advise couples to use barrier contraception for that month.

All procedures that involve ovarian stimulation will lead to a risk of multiple birth. Why worry? Miscarriage is more common, cerebral palsy is three times more common, perinatal mortality is five times more common, and the mother is more likely to suffer from hyperemesis, pre-eclampsia and premature labour.

Uterine and pelvic problems

Submucous fibroids, polyps and uterine septae, which all distort the uterine cavity, do not cause infertility but are thought to impair fertility and cause miscarriage. They should be removed prior to in vitro fertilization (IVF) to maximize the chances of success. Hydrosalpinges reduce the implantation rate and can be removed or drained for this reason. Endometriosis is associated with infertility. Surgical treatment of mild endometriosis (i.e. diathermy or laser at time of laparoscopy) has been shown to temporarily improve fertility.

Tubal problems

Tubal problems can be diagnosed on hysterosalpingogram but blocked tubes are usually confirmed at laparoscopy, using the dye test. If the tubes are not patent the choice is between tubal surgery and IVF.

Tubal surgery
Some centres perform tubal surgery, usually using microsurgical techniques, for selected patients. The patient must be aware that her risk of ectopic

pregnancy will be increased as the tubes are scarred. Success rates vary, with the best results being seen where tubal damage was proximal. Distal damage can be treated by laparoscopic salpingostomy. Midtubal damage has the poorest prognosis, unless it is due to Filshie clip sterilization, in which case there is a relatively good outlook.

In vitro fertilization

Some patients are referred directly for IVF. As the success of IVF is influenced by age, if the woman is older it might be better not to wait for tubal surgery and then wait to see if it works, because by the time she gets to IVF her chance of conception will be lower. If there is severe tubal damage, or tubal blockage in association with other pathology (e.g. adhesions) referral for IVF is more sensible. IVF involves several steps:

- Down-regulation of the woman's own hormones using nafarelin, goserelin or buserelin, which are GnRH agonists. They initially stimulate LH and FSH but then cause down-regulation, leading to reduction in oestrogen production and 'menopausal' side-effects. These drugs are given by nasal spray or subcutaneous injection.
- Induction of multiple follicular development using gonadotrophins such as human menopausal gonadotrophin (hMG), which contains FSH and LH and is prepared from the urine of menopausal

women, hCG, which is obtained from the urine of pregnant women and has a similar action to LH, or recombinant FSH, an expensive but pure form of FSH.
- Egg collection: performed transvaginally using ultrasound, under sedation (Fig. 28.1).
- Sperm preparation.
- In vitro fertilization of the oocytes with sperm.
- Transfer of the healthy embryos (maximum of three) back into the uterine cavity (Fig. 28.2).

New techniques making IVF more specialized are being developed all the time. If a couple is affected by a hereditary disorder that can be detected using gene probes, the embryos can be subjected to preimplantation diagnosis. Cells from each embryo are removed and analysed so that only unaffected embryos are replaced. In some cases of genetic abnormality or advanced maternal age, eggs can be collected from a healthy donor, then mixed with the man's sperm in vitro. New techniques of 'assisted hatching', where the zona pellucida of the embryo is breached before reimplantation, are said to improve the chances of successful implantation.

Male infertility

If the semen analysis is persistently abnormal despite advice regarding loose underwear and reduction of

Fig. 28.1 Egg collection.

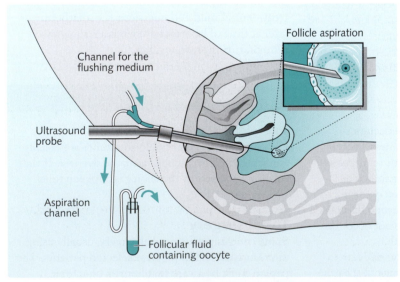

Follicle aspiration

Channel for the flushing medium

Ultrasound probe

Aspiration channel

Follicular fluid containing oocyte

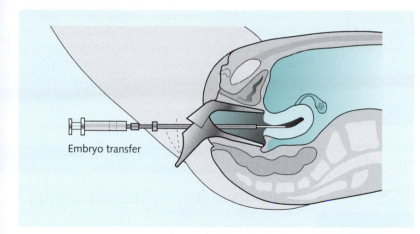

Fig. 28.2 Embryo transfer.

Embryo transfer

alcohol and nicotine intake, assisted fertility can be considered. Intrauterine insemination may be tried before IVF or intracytoplasmic sperm injection (ICSI) because it involves less intervention.

Intrauterine insemination

Intrauterine insemination (IUI) usually involves inducing follicular development and ovulation in the woman as for IVF. The process can be carried out with spontaneous ovulation but the success rate is lower. However, the incidence of multiple pregnancy is also lower. Thirty-six hours after ovulation, prepared sperm is placed into the uterine cavity using an intrauterine catheter.

Donor insemination (DI) is an option for couples where the sperm is of poor quality. Its use has fallen since the advent of ICSI (see below), but ICSI is not always successful.

Intracytoplasmic sperm injection (ICSI)

ICSI is an advanced form of IVF where one sperm is injected into the egg (Fig. 28.3). This technique has revolutionized treatment for couples where the man's sperm count is very low or showing lots of abnormal forms. If there are no sperm in the semen at all (due to obstruction or to congenital absence of the vas) sperm can sometimes be extracted from the vas, the epididymis, or even from a testicular biopsy. It has recently been suggested that spermatids (i.e. immature spermatozoa) could be used, but at present this has not been licensed by the Human Fertilization and Embryology Authority (HFEA).

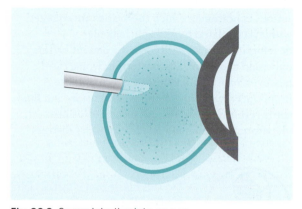

Fig. 28.3 Sperm injection into an egg.

 The Human Fertilisation and Embryology Authority (HFEA) was established in 1991 and regulates all centres in the UK that offer assisted conception.

Surgical options for male infertility

If the sperm count is suboptimal because of epididymal blockage, surgery can be performed to restore patency. If a varicocoele is present this can be repaired. This has not been proven conclusively to improve spermatogenesis but it is known that the incidence of varicocoele in the male partner of couples with subfertility is 40% compared with 15% in the general population.

Unexplained infertility

Couples with unexplained infertility are helped by IUI with controlled ovarian stimulation, and if this is unsuccessful may try IVF.

Ovarian hyperstimulation syndrome

Gonadotrophin therapy can lead to ovarian hyperstimulation syndrome (OHSS), which is a serious condition in which the ovaries are enlarged with cysts, related to multiple follicular development. In its mild form the patient suffers only mild abdominal discomfort. In worse cases, however, nausea and vomiting develop, there is pronounced, painful abdominal distension, and fluid shifts resulting in ascites and pleural effusions. Hepatorenal failure and adult respiratory distress syndrome (ARDS) can ensue and the patient is at greatly increased risk of thromboembolism. Hospitalization and careful fluid balance are necessary. There is no real treatment for OHSS, which is why its prevention by careful ultrasound monitoring of the ovaries and serial blood tests for serum oestradiol is so important.

Prognosis for the infertile couple

As a result of developments in infertility treatment, couples have a 30% greater chance of a live birth than they did at the beginning of the 1990s. However, the reality is that the majority of couples undergoing a cycle of fertility treatment will not have a baby, which is why the role of the counsellor in the infertility team is so important.

IUI and DI with ovarian stimulation give around a 9.5% chance of live birth per treatment cycle. The results are age dependent.

IVF success rates (i.e. live birth) are around 15–20%. If the mother is under 30 the results are better; once over 35 there is a marked decrease, and over 40 the chance is around 12%. ICSI improves the chances of live birth to around 21%.

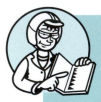

- What is the desired effect of clomiphene and which blood test can be used to investigate for this effect?
- Pregnancies conceived after tubal surgery are more at risk of which complication?
- Prior to egg collection for IVF, what treatment is given to the woman?
- Which factor most affects the likelihood of live birth following IVF?
- What are the two options available when the man has a low sperm count that is not due to a cause that can be treated surgically?

Further reading

Gonick & Wheelis *The Cartoon Guide to Genetics* (Harper & Row)

McKay Hart, D & Norman, J (2000) *Gynaecology Illustrated* 5th edn (Churchill Livingstone, London)

http://www.rcog.org.uk/guidelines

29. Early Pregnancy Failure

Miscarriage

Miscarriage is the most common complication of pregnancy and will be experienced by 1 in 4 women at some point in their lives. It is defined as the loss of a pregnancy before 24 weeks.

Aetiology

It is often difficult to identify the cause of a miscarriage but factors that have contributed can be noted. These include:

- Fetal abnormality: 50% of miscarried fetuses are genetically (e.g. trisomy, monosomy) or structurally (e.g. neural tube defect) abnormal. Multiple pregnancies are more likely to be affected in these ways.
- Infection: *Toxoplasma* species, the rubella virus, tuberculosis, *Listeria* species, malaria, *Salmonella* species and cytomegalovirus are just a few of the potential causes. Bacterial vaginosis, where there is a change in the natural flora of the vagina, has been linked to second trimester miscarriage.
- Maternal age: the miscarriage rate begins to increase when the mother reaches the age of 35.

Risks of miscarriage in relation to mother's age:
- under 35:   6.5%
- 35–40:   15%
- over 40:   23%

- Abnormal uterine cavity: the presence of an intrauterine contraceptive device (IUCD or 'coil'), submucous fibroids, a congenital septum or adhesions (Ashermann's syndrome).
- Maternal illness, including Wilson's disease, poorly controlled diabetes, thyroid or renal disease.
- Intervention: e.g. amniocentesis, chorionic villus sampling.
- Antiphospholipid antibodies and cervical weakness ('incompetence') can result in second trimester loss (see the section 'Recurrent miscarriage', below).

Investigation of the cause of miscarriage is usually delayed until the woman has had three miscarriages (see the section 'Recurrent miscarriage', below).

Investigation of miscarriage

Ultrasound is used to aid diagnosis where women present with bleeding and the os is closed on examination. If the os is open a miscarriage is inevitable and a scan is unnecessary, but is sometimes performed at the request of the patient.

Management of miscarriage

Once the fetus has died, the uterus will expel the products of conception. This process can take some weeks if left to happen spontaneously. Because of the fear of infection of retained products women have traditionally been advised to have a surgical evacuation to empty the uterus (a procedure that many women still think of as a 'D&C'). Studies comparing the operative route with expectant management have now confirmed no difference in infection rates. Evacuation of retained products of conception (ERPC) is a simple operation that takes 5–10 min; the cervix is dilated to allow suction or sharp curettage. The pregnant uterus is easily perforated, so curettage must be gentle. Syntocinon can be given intravenously during the procedure to encourage uterine contraction and to minimize blood loss. Products of conception are sent for histology.

If the patient is offered the choice of expectant management she should be booked for follow-up scans to confirm that the uterus is empty. They, and women who have had an ERPC, should be warned of the possibility of endometritis and told of the symptoms and signs to watch out for. These are: fever, feeling unwell, lower abdominal pain and a change in vaginal bleeding, which can become offensive smelling and suddenly heavy.

If the woman is Rhesus negative she might need anti-D. This is given at any gestation if the woman has an ERPC, and after 12 weeks even if no ERPC is performed.

Unless investigation for recurrent miscarriage is needed, no follow-up in hospital is necessary. Before going home the woman should be given a contact number for a local support group that can help her answer the questions that will arise after the miscarriage (Fig. 29.1). If she is not going to try to get pregnant again in the near future, methods of contraception should be discussed.

Recurrent miscarriage

This is currently defined as three or more consecutive miscarriages and affects 1 woman in 100. In many cases no specific cause will be found but the investigations below can be used to guide the treatment of other women, leading to a happy outcome.

 Incidence of miscarriage:
- overall, any pregnancy: 15%
- After one miscarriage: 20%
- After two miscarriages: 30%
- After three miscarriages: 40%

Aetiology of recurrent miscarriage
- Parental genetic abnormality (e.g. balanced translocation): found in 3–5% of partners in couples affected by recurrent loss. Those diagnosed are referred to a clinical geneticist.

- Uterine abnormality (e.g. septum, submucosal fibroid): the incidence of these in women with recurrent miscarriage has not been shown to be significantly different from women with normal pregnancies, but once diagnosed it may be difficult to dissuade the woman from seeking surgery.
- Polycystic ovarian syndrome: the higher rate of miscarriage in these women has been attributed to their higher levels of LH. Unfortunately, suppression of LH does not improve the live birth rate.
- Antiphospholipid antibodies: this family of autoantibodies includes lupus anticoagulant and anticardiolipin antibodies. Their presence impairs trophoblast function, partly by causing thrombosis of the uteroplacental vessels. Some affected patients might have only a 10% chance of a live birth if untreated.
- Thrombophilic defects (e.g. factor V Leiden mutation): women who have thrombophilia due to protein C resistance (most commonly due to a mutation of the factor V Leiden gene), or abnormalities of protein S or antithrombin, are more prone to recurrent miscarriage.
- Cervical weakness ('incompetence'): this is usually secondary to cervical trauma caused by damage in childbirth or at operation (e.g. forcible dilatation for late termination of pregnancy), but in some cases can be congenital. It causes mid-trimester miscarriage.

Why has this happened?
She should be reassured that she has done nothing wrong and is not to blame, but told that in most cases we do not find the cause for early miscarriage. Flying, working, having smear tests, using mobile phones and VDUs and making love when pregnant do not cause miscarriage.

Will it happen again?
Many women who have had a miscarriage will go on to have a healthy term pregnancy. Realising how common early miscarriage is may reassure her.

When can I start trying to get pregnant again?
Physically there is no reason why she cannot conceive with her next cycle, and this has no adverse effects on a resulting pregnancy, but mentally it may be better to have a few months to recover from the miscarriage. Couples can be advised to use condoms if they wish to wait for this time, as condoms are an instantly reversible form of contraception.

When will my next period come?
The next period may be early or late, but should be expected in roughly one month (or sooner or later depending on her usual cycle length). If she does not use contraception after the miscarriage and the next period is late she should seek a pregnancy test.

Fig. 29.1 Common questions asked by women who have suffered a miscarriage.

- Bacterial vaginosis: an imbalance in vaginal flora – with a lack of lactobacilli, which are usually commensal – results in bacterial vaginosis. The cause of this change is unknown. It is not linked to early miscarriage but it does predispose to mid-trimester miscarriage.

Treatment of recurrent miscarriage

The treatment must be aimed at the cause. If no cause is found (as is the case for a significant proportion) support and reassurance should be offered:

- Couples affected by genetic abnormality might opt for prenatal diagnosis, or even IVF with preimplantation testing (see Chapter 28).
- Uterine septae and submucous fibroids are best treated hysteroscopically and treatment does not always improve the chances of a successful pregnancy.
- Maintaining a normal BMI in polycystic ovarian syndrome has been shown to improve pregnancy outcome, whereas hormonal manipulation has not.
- Women with antiphospholipid antibodies are given 75 mg aspirin daily as soon as the pregnancy test is positive and 5000 iu subcutaneous heparin once fetal heart activity is seen on scan (around 6.5 weeks). The treatment is stopped at 34 weeks. The same treatment for women with thrombophilias has yet to be proved to be effective in trials.
- Cervical cerclage (suture) for weakness can be performed in pregnancy using the transvaginal route at around 12 weeks, or before conception by the transabdominal route (see Chapter 38). With the former the suture is removed at around 36 weeks to allow vaginal delivery. Abdominal sutures are left in situ and the woman is delivered by caesarean section.
- Bacterial vaginosis is simply treated with metronidazole or intravaginal antibiotic cream.

Treatments not proven to be effective include progesterone pessaries/tablets/injections in the first trimester, LH suppression, immunotherapy for women said to be 'allergic' to their fetus, oral/systemic steroids for women with antiphospholipid antibodies and hCG supplementation.

Ectopic pregnancy

This is a pregnancy that has implanted outside the uterine cavity (see Fig. 29.2 for likely sites). The incidence of ectopic pregnancy is increasing due to the rising number of cases of pelvic inflammatory disease (PID) and as IVF pregnancies increase in number. Currently in the UK the incidence is around 1 per 150 term deliveries; 10–15% of ectopics occur after IVF.

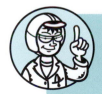

If a woman has a positive pregnancy test with bleeding or pain, ectopic pregnancy must be ruled out.

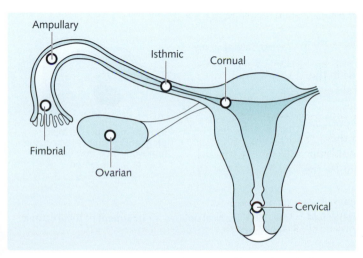

Fig. 29.2 Implantation sites of ectopic pregnancy.

Ampullary

Isthmic

Cornual

Fimbrial

Ovarian

Cervical

Aetiology of ectopic pregnancy

Ectopic pregnancy is caused by conditions that damage the uterine tubes or their ciliary lining, thus hindering the passage of the fertilized egg towards the uterine cavity, and anything that distorts the cavity itself or predisposes to abnormal implantation. These include:

- PID.
- Tubal surgery, e.g. sterilization, reversal of sterilization, previous ectopic pregnancy.
- Peritonitis or pelvic surgery in the past (e.g. appendicitis).
- IUCD ('coil') in situ.
- IVF.
- Endometriosis.
- Progesterone-only ('mini') pill – this does not cause ectopic pregnancy but if a woman conceives when using it the pregnancy is more likely to be ectopic than if she is using no contraception at all.

Clinical evaluation of ectopic pregnancy

In a few cases the patient will require immediate resuscitation and, as soon as possible, laparotomy. Those who have an acute abdomen but who are stable can have a laparoscopy to confirm the diagnosis. Treatment can then be performed laparoscopically or at laparotomy, depending on the surgeon's skill.

If, as in most cases, the presentation is subacute – it is not necessary to head straight for the operating theatre. An ultrasound scan can be arranged; this may not identify the ectopic pregnancy but will demonstrate the fact that the uterus is empty. If there has been bleeding from the ectopic the scan will show free fluid in the pelvis. In some cases a mass in the adnexae can be visualized and, uncommonly, this might contain a live ectopic, with a fetal heartbeat present.

The appearance of an empty uterus on scan in the presence of a positive pregnancy test should always raise the strong suspicion of ectopic pregnancy, which can be confirmed at laparoscopy. However, in some cases there might be uncertainty about the dates of LMP, meaning that the pregnancy could still be a very early gestation, which might account for the 'empty' appearance of the uterus.

In other cases the history might not be clear cut and there could be suspicion that the woman has had a complete miscarriage, which also gives the appearance of an empty uterus on scan, and, as β-hCG does not return to a non-pregnant level immediately, can cause confusion. In these cases, if the patient is stable and there is doubt about the diagnosis it is reasonable to delay laparoscopy by performing two blood tests for β-hCG 48 h apart. If the pregnancy is viable the level will double. In the case of miscarriage it will fall significantly. With an ectopic the level will plateau or rise, but not as much as double – the patient can then be booked for laparoscopy.

Treatment of tubal pregnancy

The aim is to eliminate the ectopic pregnancy in such a way as to minimize the risk of future pregnancies being ectopic. Various methods are used.

Surgical management

These techniques can all be performed at laparotomy, through a low transverse incision, or at laparoscopy. The skill of the operator will dictate the choice (Fig. 29.3).

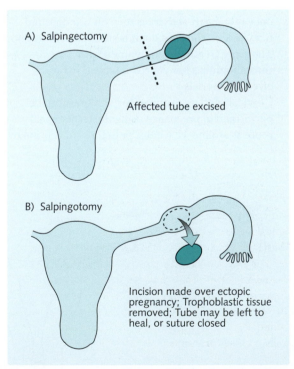

A) Salpingectomy

Affected tube excised

B) Salpingotomy

Incision made over ectopic pregnancy; Trophoblastic tissue removed; Tube may be left to heal, or suture closed

Fig. 29.3 Surgical options for treatment of tubal ectopic pregnancy.

Salpingectomy, complete or partial

Where the affected tube, or part of it, is removed. This might be the only option if the ectopic has ruptured because the tubal anatomy will have been destroyed. In the event that an ectopic has occurred following IVF where the tubes are scarred, the patient and surgeon might decide that it would be wise to remove both tubes at operation so that future IVF attempts do not lead to further tubal pregnancies.

Salpingotomy

An incision is made over the ectopic, which is removed, and the tube is usually allowed to heal.

Salpingostomy

An incision is made over the ectopic, which is removed, and the tube is left open and will heal by secondary intention.

'Milking' the tube

When the ectopic is near the ampulla it is sometimes possible to squeeze it out of the end of the tube without needing to cut the tube at all.

Medical treatment

The use of the cytotoxic drug methotrexate to treat ectopic pregnancy is increasing but it is not available in all hospitals. It can be given as intramuscular injections or by injection directly into the ectopic pregnancy either at laparoscopy or transvaginally under ultrasound control.

Patients are carefully selected for medical management – it is only suitable if the pregnancy is small and the tube is intact. The sac is measured on ultrasound scan as less than 4 cm in size, and the β-hCG level should be less than 1500 iu/L.

Follow-up of ectopic pregnancy

Patients treated with methotrexate or by conservative surgery (i.e. salpingostomy, salpingotomy or milking out the ectopic) must have serial β-hCG levels performed to ensure the resolution or removal of all trophoblastic tissue. Around 5% of patients treated medically will require further treatment with either methotrexate or a surgical procedure.

Prognosis after ectopic pregnancy

The chance of a repeat ectopic pregnancy is dependent on the health of the remaining tubal tissue. If management was conservative the affected tube will have been scarred by the ectopic pregnancy. Rates of ectopic implantation in future pregnancies are around 11% after medical treatment, 12% after 'conservative' surgery and 9% after salpingectomy. The chance of conception after salpingectomy is obviously lower, so the risks must be weighed up when deciding on management.

Other sites of ectopic pregnancy

These have high rates of maternal mortality and morbidity. Cervical, interstitial and intramural pregnancies are best treated with methotrexate. The haemorrhage that can ensue from rupture or from attempted surgical treatment can be severe, necessitating hysterectomy and sometimes proving fatal. Cornual pregnancy is treated surgically, to remove the rudimentary horn in which the pregnancy has implanted and the tube on the affected side. Ovarian pregnancy can be treated surgically, performing wedge resection of the ovary, or medically. Abdominal pregnancy, if the fetus survives, should be delivered as soon as the fetus is viable.

Heterotopic pregnancy

The extremely rare combination of intra- and extrauterine pregnancy is becoming more common with the increase in IVF pregnancies where at least two embryos are replaced. Treatment is usually surgical, with the procedure being performed laparoscopically but avoiding instrumentation of the uterus. There is an increased risk of miscarriage for the intrauterine pregnancy, being around 25%.

Trophoblastic disease

This term covers partial and complete molar pregnancies and the choriocarcinoma that can follow them.

Definitions

- Complete mole: a pregnancy within the uterus consisting of a multivesicular mass of trophoblastic tissue with hydropic change (looking like a bunch of grapes on ultrasound), and no evidence of a fetus, formed by mono or dispermic fertilization of an oocyte which has deleted all maternal genetic material, i.e. all genes are paternal (see below)

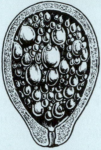

Fig. 29.4 Definitions. Reproduced with kind permission from *Gynaecology Illustrated* (5th edn), published by Churchill Livingstone.

- Partial mole: a pregnancy within the uterus consisting of some trophoblastic proliferation and some hydropic change, where a fetus (usually non-viable) may also be seen. Formed by dispermic fertilization of an oocyte resulting in triploidy i.e. maternal and paternal genes
- Choriocarcinoma: a tumour of trophoblastic cells which secrete hCG occurring when molar pregnancies do not regress after surgical evacuation or, more rarely, after a non-molar pregnancy

Incidence of molar pregnancy

In the UK, complete mole occurs around 1 per 1000 normal pregnancies. Partial mole is more common but the exact incidence is harder to calculate as many go unreported. Three per cent of molar pregnancies do not regress spontaneously and therefore require chemotherapy – this is more common with complete moles than partial moles.

Some ethnic groups are more prone to molar pregnancy – it is more common in the Far East – but the incidence there is decreasing prompting the suspicion that there is a nutritional element.

Women at the extremes of reproductive age are more likely to experience trophoblastic disease.

Diagnosis and clinical evaluation of molar pregnancy

There is likely to be bleeding early in the pregnancy, so the diagnosis can be made on ultrasound scan or perhaps picked up first by the histopathologist after the study of retained products of conception. The trophoblastic tissue secretes hCG, so serum levels are very high and might lead to exaggerated symptoms of pregnancy (e.g. hyperemesis).

Management of molar pregnancy

Molar pregnancies are treated with surgical evacuation in the same way as miscarriage. The products of conception are sent for histology. The patient must then be followed up with fortnightly serum samples for β-hCG to ensure that levels are falling, as this will confirm that the trophoblastic tissue is regressing. This follow-up is coordinated by the nearest specialist centre (Sheffield, Dundee or Charing Cross). Once the levels are normal, urine samples are tested every month for β-hCG in case of reactivation of trophoblast tissue.

If hCG levels return to normal within 8 weeks, follow-up is limited to 6 months. All other cases are followed for 2 years. Women are advised not to use hormonal contraceptives and not to become pregnant until levels have been normal for 6 months. In future pregnancies serum β-hCG will be measured at 6 and 10 weeks postpartum because of the possibility of choriocarcinoma occurring.

If hCG levels rise, plateau or are still abnormal 6 months after surgical evacuation, chemotherapy is started. Most are given methotrexate and folinic acid, although some with adverse prognostic factors might need different combinations of other chemotherapies.

The current survival rate of patients requiring chemotherapy is 94%. Metastases from choriocarcinoma are seen in the lung, liver and brain.

- What is the definition of recurrent miscarriage, and how common is this condition?
- Which hormone is measured when investigating the possibility of ectopic pregnancy, and after what interval should a repeat sample be sent?
- What are the surgical and medical options for treatment of ectopic pregnancy?
- What is the difference between the genetic make-up of complete and partial moles?
- How is choriocarcinoma treated?

Further reading

Why Mothers Die, Report on Confidential Enquiries into Maternal Deaths in the United Kingdom, 1996–1999

Gonick & Wheelis *The Cartoon Guide to Genetics* (Harper & Row)

Govan, Macfarlane, Callander *Pathology Illustrated* (Churchill Livingstone, London)

Miller, AWF & Hanretty KP *Obstetrics Illustrated* (Churchill Livingstone, London)

McKay Hart, D & Norman, J (2000) *Gynaecology Illustrated* 5th edn (Churchill Livingstone, London)

Nelson-Piercy, C *Handbook of Obstetric Medicine* (Isis Medical Media)

Smith & Smith *Obstetric Ultrasound Made Easy* (Churchill Livingstone, London)

www.swot.org.uk
www.rcog.org.uk/guidelines
www.hmole-chorio.org.uk
www.update-software.com/cochrane

30. The Menopause

Definitions

The term 'menopause' specifically refers to the last menstrual bleed that a woman experiences. It is a retrospective diagnosis, generally considered to have occurred after 1 year of amenorrhoea. The range of age at menopause is 45 to 55 years, with an average of 51 years; factors that affect this is cigarette smoking, which lowers the age, and an inherited genetic predisposition. A premature menopause is one that occurs before the age of 45 years. This can occur naturally, by surgery (bilateral oophrectomy), or by chemotherapy or radiotherapy.

The term 'climacteric' is used to describe the perimenopausal period, that is, the transitional phase around the time of a woman's last menstrual bleed when endocrine changes occur as ovarian follicular activity ceases.

With the average life expectancy of women today at 78 years, a woman can spend up to a third of her life in the postmenopausal phase. Therefore, an understanding of the physiological and psychological changes that take place is important.

Pathophysiology

The total number of oocytes is maximum at 20 weeks of in utero fetal development and progressively decreases to about 750 000 at the time of birth. From childhood through to adult life, the number of oocytes becomes further depleted by ovulation and atresia. Eventually, at the time of the climacteric, the remaining oocytes are increasingly resistant to stimulation by the gonadotrophins FSH and LH, and the Graafian follicles that form do not secrete sufficient oestrogen and progesterone to cause regular menstruation.

The endocrine changes that occur at the climacteric are:
- Hypothalamic–pituitary hyperactivity (raised FSH and later LH).
- Decreased or absent progesterone levels.
- Unopposed oestrogen secretion.

These changes result in dysfunctional uterine bleeding secondary to anovulatory cycles as the menopause approaches. In time, insufficient follicles develop with subsequent inadequate oestrogen to stimulate the endometrium; therefore menstruation ceases.

Clinical features of the menopause

Figure 30.1 illustrates the clinical feature of the menopause.

Immediate symptoms
The more short-term symptoms associated with the climacteric can begin prior to the menopause (Fig. 30.2).

Vasomotor symptoms
These include those characteristically associated with the menopause: hot flushes and night sweats, which are the result of poor peripheral vascular control secondary to oestrogen deficiency. Night sweats can result in insomnia, with lethargy and loss of concentration during the day.

End-organ atrophy
The genital tract and the lower urinary tract have the same embryological origin and thus both systems will be affected by loss of oestrogen.

The vulva and vagina become atrophic and the thinner epithelium is more susceptible to infection or trauma.

Vaginal dryness causes dyspareunia, which can contribute to the psychosexual symptoms that are another factor associated with the menopause.

The supporting tissues of the pelvic organs (see Chapter 27) become thinner and weaker, resulting in the development of vaginal and uterine prolapse. The epithelium of the urethra and the trigone also become atrophic, with weakening of the connective and elastic tissue of the lower urinary tract. Thus, post-menopausal women may complain of dysuria, frequency and urgency.

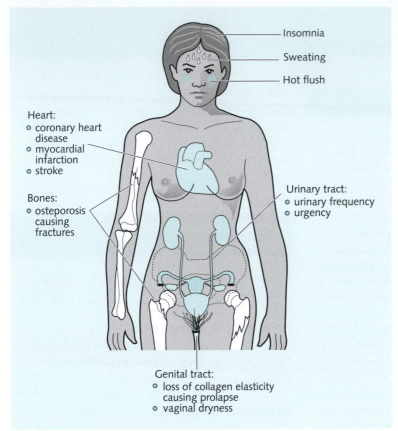

Fig. 30.1 The clinical features of the menopause.

Insomnia

Sweating

Hot flush

Heart:
- coronary heart disease
- myocardial infarction
- stroke

Bones:
- osteporosis causing fractures

Urinary tract:
- urinary frequency
- urgency

Genital tract:
- loss of collagen elasticity causing prolapse
- vaginal dryness

The immediate effects of the menopause

- Vasomotor symptoms
- End-organ atrophy
- Psychological symptoms

Fig. 30.2 The immediate effects of the menopause.

Psychological symptoms

These include depression, irritability, poor memory and loss of libido, which are particularly common prior to the woman's last period. It is thought that fluctuating hormone levels are important, as opposed to simply low hormone levels. Social and environmental factors can play a part in these symptoms but should not necessarily be taken as the diagnosis.

Long-term symptoms

With an increasingly elderly population, the long-term consequences of the menopause carry a high

morbidity and mortality, as well as being important social and economic factors.

Osteoporosis

Osteoporosis is a skeletal disease characterized by low bone mass and disruption of the normal bone architecture; this results in increased bone fragility and thus susceptibility to fractures. Bone mass in both men and women reaches a peak at 30–40 years of age and then starts to decline. However, in women, there is an acceleration in this decline immediately after the menopause. As a result, this increased bone loss, combined with the lower peak bone mass prior to the menopause, predisposes women to a greater risk of fracture compared with men.

Postmenopausal osteoporosis is caused by changes in bone remodelling, such that the rate of osteoclast bone resorption exceeding that of osteoblast bone formation. Other factors can contribute to this (Fig. 30.3), including – in particular – a family history of osteoporosis. It is important that postmenopausal

Factors which predispose to the development of osteoporosis
• Family history • Nulliparity • Late menarche and/or early menopause • Small build • Lack of exercise • Smoking • Drugs including corticosteroids and heparin

Fig. 30.3 Factors which predispose to the development of osteoporosis.

women with any of these associated risk factors should be counselled about treatment such as hormone replacement therapy to reduce their risk of fractures. The three most common sites for fractures in this group are the spine, the hip and the distal radius. In the UK, 130 000 vertebral fractures and over 50 000 hip fractures occur each year.

Cardiovascular disease

Ischaemic heart disease is about five times less common in a premenopausal woman than in a man. However, following the menopause, the incidence rises so that by the age of 70, there is no longer any sex difference. This is thought to be caused by a shift in lipoprotein metabolism with an increase in the serum LDL level, so that the HDL : LDL ratio is altered.

A similar pattern is seen in the incidence of strokes (cerebrovascular accidents). At the time of the menopause, there is a small rise compared with premenopausal women, but this is much less marked than in ischaemic heart disease.

Management

History

Presenting symptoms include:
- Vasomotor symptoms and mood changes.
- Menstrual history.
- Sexual history including contraception.
- Gynaecological history including recent smear.
- Family history, in particular of osteoporosis.

Examination

This should include blood pressure and a breast examination, as well as abdominal and pelvic examination.

Investigations

Plasma gonadotrophins and oestrogen levels vary markedly in the climacteric; thus, diagnosis of the menopause is usually made on clinical grounds, although it is confirmed by a raised serum FSH concentration.

Other investigations should be performed according to the patient's age and presenting symptoms including:
- Cervical smear.
- Mammogram.
- Pelvic ultrasound.
- Endometrial sampling.
- Bone mineral density measurement.

Treatment

General measures include:
- Diet, exercise and weight control.
- Treat any medical condition such as hypertension or diabetes.
- Psychological support if appropriate.

Hormone replacement therapy

Both the immediate and the long-term effects of the menopause have been shown to be improved by administering oestrogen and progesterone. Oestrogen therapy has been proven to improve the bone mineralization of osteoporosis and so reduce substantially the risk of fractures. With respect to cholesterol metabolism and the associated risk of vascular disease, giving oral oestrogen lowers total cholesterol and LDL levels and raises the HDL fraction. This effect might be negated somewhat by the concomitant administration of progesterone.

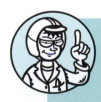

If the patient has a uterus, she needs a hormone replacement therapy with both oestrogen and progesterone.

All patients should be fully informed about the benefits and risks of HRT, so that they can decide whether to commence treatment. In particular, women in the menopause who are below 45 years of age and women with osteoporosis or with a combination of risk factors for the disease must discuss HRT thoroughly. Figure 30.4 lists the

Contraindications to hormone replacement therapy

- Endometrial carcinoma
- Breast carcinoma
- Undiagnosed vaginal bleeding
- Undiagnosed breast lump
- Suspected pregnancy
- Liver disease with impaired liver function
- Previous thromboembolic disease associated with hormonal contraception, pregnancy or oestrogen replacement

Fig. 30.4 Contraindications to hormone replacement therapy.

Patient choice is important; patient compliance can be difficult, especially if a woman does not want regular withdrawal bleeds or is asymptomatic.

contraindications to HRT. Particular controversy exists over the risk of HRT in the development of breast cancer; recently it has been proved that there is a slight increased risk, but this is likely to be offset by the improved morbidity from osteoporosis.

The most important point to remember in prescribing HRT is that giving a woman with an intact uterus long-term unopposed oestrogen will cause stimulation of the endometrium, which puts her at risk of endometrial hyperplasia or even endometrial carcinoma. She must therefore also be given concomittant progesterone therapy to prevent this.

The next decision in prescribing is whether the patient finds a monthly withdrawal bleed acceptable. If she does, then she can be given oestrogen with cyclical progesterone to protect the uterus. If she prefers not to have a regular bleed and has not had any bleeding for more than 1 year, the woman might be suitable for continuous combined oestrogen and progesterone therapy, which should avoid monthly bleeds.

Finally, the route of administration of the treatment must be discussed with the patient (Fig. 30.5).

Non-hormonal drug treatment

Clonidine is a central α-adrenergic stimulator that has been used in the past for the treatment of hot flushes and night sweats.

Other drug treatments are appropriate to offer protection against long-term consequences of the menopause, in particular osteoporosis, in those postmenopausal women for whom oestrogens are neither contraindicated nor desired.

Raloxifene (Evista™) is a newly developed selective oestrogen receptor modulator (SERM) with a similar structure to tamoxifen, a drug used to treat breast cancer. It has no effect on menopausal symptoms such as hot flushes but offers long-term protection against osteoporosis.

Other drug treatments such as bisphosphonates are also effective for osteoperosis treatment in asymptomatic woman. Increasing dietary calcium and vitamin D are also recommended.

Fig. 30.5 Routes of administration of hormone replacement therapy.

Routes of administration of hormone replacement therapy

Route	Advantages	Disadvantages
Oral	Cheap Effective	Partial metabolism in gut Peaks and troughs in plasma levels
Transdermal	Avoids liver Continuous absorption	Cost Skin reactions
Implant	Every 6 months	Cannot be removed Still need progesterone
Topical gel	Continuous absorption	Oestrogen-only preparation Messy
Vaginal cream	Specific local effect	Oestrogen-only preparation Long-term endometrial stimulation because of systemic absorption

- What is the definition of the menopause and how can it be diagnosed?
- What are the short term symptoms of the menopause?
- What are the possible long term sequelae of the menopause?
- Describe the various types and routes of administration of hormone replacement therapy (HRT).
- What are the potential risks of HRT?
- Describe some of the alternatives to HRT in the treatment of menopausal problems and compare their relative merits and risks.

Further reading

Current problems in pharmacovigilance Vol 28 (April 2002)

CMO's Update 33 (May 2002) (Department of Health May)

Abernethy K (ed) *The Menopause & HRT* (Balliere Tindall)

Andrews G, *Women's Sexual Health* 2nd edn (Bailliere Tindall/RCN)

Rees M & Purdie DW (eds) 'Management of the Menopause' *The Handbook of the British Menopause Society* (BMS Publications Ltd)

Studd J (ed) (1998) 'Management of the Menopause' *Annual Review* (Parthenon Publishing)

Studd J (ed) (2000) 'Management of the Menopause' *The Millenium Review* (Parthenon Publishing)

Whitehead M (ed) (1998) *HRT: The Prescriber's Guide to Hormone Replacement Therapy* (Parthenon Publishing)

Core Product Information for HRT: http://heads.medagencies.org/

31. Contraception, Sterilization and Unwanted Pregnancy

Introduction

The ideal contraceptive is one that is 100% effective, with no side-effects, is readily reversible and does not need medical supervision; this does not exist. Hence it is important that the doctor assesses the patient's requirements at the particular time in her life that she requests contraception, and reviews the advantages and disadvantages so that the patient can make an informed choice (see *Crash Course in Endocrinology*, p. 98).

Informed choice as to the method of contraception used by every individual patient is important.

The effectiveness of a particular method is measured by the number of unwanted pregnancies that occur during 100 women years of exposure; this is known as the Pearl Index (Fig. 31.1).

Natural family planning methods

Rhythm method

The rhythm method involves predicting the time of maximum fertility (3 to 4 days around ovulation) by:

- Using a menstrual calendar.
- Charting the basal body temperature, which rises 0.2–0.4°C when progesterone is released from the corpus luteum.
- Recognizing changes in cervical mucus.
- Using an ovulation predictor kit, e.g. Persona™.

Advantages

The rhythm method might be useful if other methods are unacceptable to the couple, such as in certain religious groups or because of unwanted side-effects.

Disadvantages

The method relies on a regular menstrual cycle, lengthy instruction and commitment.

Coitus interruptus

Advantages

Still widely practised, this method is free and without side-effects.

Disadvantages

The failure rate is high due to variable ejaculatory control and the fact that pre-ejaculatory fluid contains some sperm. There is no protection against sexually transmitted infections (STIs).

Barrier methods

These methods include the male condom and, for women, the diaphragm, the cervical cap and the female condom. Their effectiveness increases with concommitant use of a spermicide such as nonoxynol-9, which alters sperm membrane permeability resulting in sperm death (use of spermicides alone as contraception is not recommended).

Advantages

When used properly, these are effective, free from side-effects and widely available. They offer protection against STDs, in particular the male condom, which protects against HIV.

Disadvantages

They must be applied before penetration and can reduce the level of sensation. The diaphragm and the cap have to be fitted and checked regularly by a trained professional. In all methods, effectiveness is dependent on correct use and sustained motivation.

Hormonal contraception

Combined oral contraceptive pill

Since their introduction in 1961, various combinations of different oestrogens and

The relative effectiveness of contraception methods	
Method	Relative effectiveness
Sterilization: female	0–0.2
Sterilization: male	0–0.5
Combined oral contraception	0.2–3.0
Progesterone-only contraception	0.3–4.0
Depot injection	0–1.0
IUCD	0.3–2.0
Mirena IUS	0–0.2
Condoms: male	2.0–15.0
Diaphragm	2.0–15.0

Fig. 31.1 Methods of contraception and their relative effectiveness as measured by the Pearl Index.

Contraindications to the combined oral contraceptive pill	
Degree of contraindication	Description
Absolute	Pregnancy
	Arterial or venous thrombosis
	Liver disease
	Undiagnosed vaginal bleeding
	History of oestrogen-dependent tumour
	Recent hydatidiform mole
Relative	Family history of thrombosis (consider investigations for thrombophilia)
	Hypertension
	Migraine
	Varicose veins

Fig. 31.2 Contraindications to the combined oral contraceptive pill.

progestogens have been used to prevent pregnancy. Combined oral contraceptive pills (COCP) have the following modes of action:

- Inhibiting ovulation by:
  - Inhibiting FSH release.
  - Preventing follicular ripening.
  - Preventing the LH surge.
- Altering the endometrium.
- Altering the cervical mucus.

Contraindications
Figure 31.2 lists the contraindications to the COCP.

Advantages
This method is reliable if taken correctly, convenient and not intercourse related. Its use reduces dysmenorrhoea, menorrhagia and premenstrual syndrome (PMS) symptoms. It also controls functional ovarian cysts and is associated with a reduced incidence of carcinoma of the ovary and endometrium.

Disadvantages
The main risks of the COCP are thromboembolism and cardiovascular complications; these are exacerbated by:

- Age.
- Obesity.
- Cigarette smoking.
- Diabetes.
- Hypertension.
- Familial hyperlipidaemia.

Other more minor side-effects include weight gain, decreased libido, breast discomfort, mood

disturbance and breakthrough bleeding. The effectiveness of the COCP is limited by some antibiotics, hepatic-enzyme-inducing drugs and by vomiting and diarrhoea. Use is associated with an increase in cervical intraepithelial neoplasia and carcinoma of the cervix; the effect on breast cancer is uncertain.

The COCP should be discontinued 6 weeks before major surgery; otherwise heparin prophylaxis is necessary.

Progesterone-only pill
Although slightly less effective than the COCP, the progesterone-only pill (POP) is used in women in whom oestrogens are contra-indicated or who cannot tolerate the side-effects. This includes women aged over 35 who smoke and those who are breast-feeding.

The mode of action differs from the COCP in that ovulation is suppressed in only 50–60% of cycles, but with similar changes in cervical mucus and in the endometrium, as well as reduced tubal motility.

Advantages
Without oestrogen, few serious side-effects occur.

Disadvantages
Efficacy is reduced if the time of pill-taking is delayed by more than 3h. The main problem is a change in menstrual pattern, with spotting or

breakthrough bleeding that does not settle despite continued use.

Injectable progestogens
Intramuscular injection of medroxyprogesterone acetate given every 3 months ensures that high-dose progestogen is gradually released into the circulation and inhibits ovulation; it is almost as effective as the COCP.

Advantages
This method of contraception is highly effective and not intercourse related, it also does not require daily motivation.

Disadvantages
- Because it is injected, it cannot be removed and any side-effects must be tolerated for 3 months.
- Most women become amenorrhoeic but heavy, unpredictable bleeding patterns can sometimes occur.
- Being a slow-release depot preparation, there might be a delay in return to fertility of 12 to 18 months.

Postcoital contraception
Since 1984, the Yuzpe method has been used to reduce the risk of pregnancy by administering two doses of the following medication 12h apart and within 72h of unprotected intercourse:
- 100µg ethinyloestradiol *plus*.
- 500µg levonorgestrel.

The endometrium is made unfavourable for implantation and there is interference with normal corpus luteum function. If taken before the preovulation oestrogen surge, ovulation can be inhibited.

The medication is often administered with an antiemetic to reduce nausea and vomiting, which occurs in up to 50% of patients.

The failure rate is 2–5%, depending on the time in the cycle at which it is taken.

Counselling is essential so that the patient understands the implications of the failure rate and so that she makes sure she is followed up, especially if she has not had a period but also to decide on future long-term contraception.

More recently, this method has been superceeded by Levonelle-2 (×2 tabs of 750 mg Levonorgestrel) which is available over the counter.

Another method of emergency contraception is to insert an IUCD within 5 days of unprotected intercourse (see below for more details); this can be removed after the patient's next period or left in situ to provide ongoing contraception.

Postcoital or emergency contraception is not for routine use:
- High-dose oral contraceptive Levonelle-2 pill within 72 h.
- Insert an intrauterine contraceptive device within 5 days.

Intrauterine contraceptive devices (IUCD)

Insertion of one of a variety of synthetic devices into the uterine cavity (Fig. 31.3) is likely to ensure that blastocyst implantation is prevented. There is also some foreign body reaction to the IUCD in the endometrium, resulting in altered cell numbers and fluid compositions, which might affect gamete viability. There might also be changes in the cervical mucus; these reduce sperm penetration.

Contraindications
Figure 31.4 lists the contraindications to IUCD use.

Advantages
Once in situ, IUCDs can remain in place for 3 to 5 years and their effect on preventing conception is almost immediately reversible. The progestogen containing IUS (intruterine system), the Mirena™, has the extra advantages related to local secretion of progestogen, which acts on the endometrium; this results in amenorrhoea in up to 85% of patients at 6 months. Hence this type of IUCD has various gynaecological indications, such as treating menorrhagia and dysmenorrhoea.

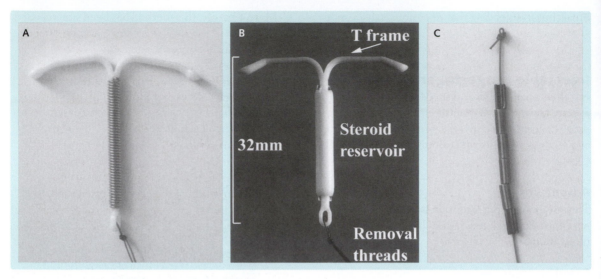

Fig. 31.3 Types of intrauterine contraceptive device: (A) Copper T (B) Mirena IUS (C) Gynefix.

Contraindications to the intrauterine contraceptive device

- Pregnancy
- Undiagnosed uterine bleeding
- Active and/or past history of PID
- Previous ectopic pregnancy
- Previous tubal surgery

Fig. 31.4 Contraindications to the intrauterine contraceptive device.

Disadvantages

- Infection.
- Uterine perforation.
- Expulsion of IUCD.
- Menorrhagia and/or abdominal pain.
- Ectopic pregnancy.

Introduction of infection at the time of insertion of the IUCD is one of the main risk factors for using this form of contraception; for this reason, it is usual to take a *Chlamydia* swab from the patient and/or give prophylactic antibiotics. The possibility of developing PID means that an IUCD is less commonly used in nulliparous women, especially if they have multiple partners.

Other disadvantages that the patient should be told about include risk of uterine perforation at the time of coil insertion or possibly at a later date. The woman should be taught to check that she can feel the threads of the coil to ensure that it has not fallen out. If either of these situations arises, attempts to locate the IUCD should be made by X-ray, ultrasound and possibly laparoscopy.

The most common reasons for a patient requesting removal of the IUCD are menorrhagia and abdominal pain; these symptoms are much less common with a Mirena™ than with other IUCDs. If a pregnancy does occur with a coil in situ, the risk of an ectopic pregnancy is higher than with other forms of contraception.

Female sterilization

The more commonly used techniques include the application of Falope rings or Filshie clips to each tube laparoscopically as a day-case procedure. At laparotomy, a modified Pomeroy tubal ligation is usually performed, for example at caesarean section. Rarely, in the presence of pelvic pathology, a hysterectomy is appropriate. It is now possible to perform sterilization hysteroscopically by insertion of microcoils into the tubal.

Counselling

Sterilization should be regarded as an irreversible procedure and therefore the patient must be sure that she has completed her family and that she has considered all other methods of contraception. The issues are particularly emotive if the patient makes the request at the time of termination of pregnancy or caesarean section.

Although the most successful form of contraception (see Fig. 6.1), there is still a failure rate of about 2 per 1000; this might be due to failure to exclude pregnancy preoperatively or incorrect application of a clip. If a pregnancy does occur, the risk of an ectopic pregnancy is higher than other forms of contraception.

Male sterilization

Compared to female sterilization, a vasectomy is a relatively easy operation, avoiding the risks of a general anaesthetic. The vas deferens is ligated via bilateral incisions in the scrotum. Another method of contraception must be used until two azospermic samples have been obtained 3 and 4 months after the procedure. The failure rate is similar to the female operation.

Termination of pregnancy

Since the Abortion Act of 1967 (amended in 1991 to reduce the upper limit of gestation from 28 weeks to 24 weeks), termination of pregnancy has been legal in England, Scotland and Wales. Two registered medical practitioners must agree on one of five circumstances relevant to the individual patient; this is most commonly clause C, which states that continuing the pregnancy involves greater risk to the woman's physical or mental health than termination.

Counselling

Alternatives to abortion should be discussed with the woman, including support if she continues the pregnancy or adoption. If she decides to proceed with the termination, the appropriate method must be agreed (see below) and future contraception should be arranged.

Surgical methods

Up to 12 weeks of pregnancy, vacuum aspiration is the most commonly used method. Preoperative prostaglandin to ripen the cervix is often used, especially in nulliparous women, followed by cervical dilatation and evacuation of the uterus using a plastic cannula.

After 12 weeks, dilatation and evacuation can be used; the uterine contents must be crushed as well as using curettage.

Medical methods

Increasingly, medical termination can be offered with up to 63 days of amenorrhoea. Mifepristone, an antiprogesterone is given orally 36–48h before vaginal insertion of a prostaglandin E1 analogue pessary; complete abortion occurs in 95% of patients.

In the second trimester, synthetic prostaglandin pessaries are placed in the posterior fornix every 3–4 h; incomplete abortion is not uncommon and surgical evacuation must be performed.

Complications

- Infection: screen for chlamydia preoperatively and/or give prophylactic antibiotics.
- Trauma: to cervix or uterus including perforation (cervical incompetence only usually occurs with repeated procedures).
- Haemorrhage: might be secondary to the above or the result of incomplete evacuation.

- How are contraceptive failure rates described?
- What are the contraindications to using the combined contraceptive pill?
- What are the non-contraceptive benefits of the combined contraceptive pill?
- Name the progestogen-only methods of contraception and describe their mechanism of action.
- Describe the mechanism of action of the levonorgestrel intrauterine system.
- What are the possible options for emergency contraception and how long after intercourse can they be used?
- Describe the possible options for sterilisation.

Further reading

Guillebaud J (2003) *Contraception: Your questions answered* (Churchill Livingstone, London)

Llewellyn-Jones, D (1999) *Fundementals of Obstetrics & Gynaecology* 7th edn (Mosby, London)

Shaw R W, Soutter W P, Stanton S L (1997) *Gynaecology* 3rd edn (Churchill Livingstone, London)

Amenorrhoea – primary and secondary

Delayed puberty
This is discussed in Chapter 19.

Precocious puberty
Precocious puberty is said to have occurred when sexual maturation takes place before the age of 9 years.

Aetiology
The possible aetiologies for precocious puberty are summarized in Fig. 32.1 and an algorithm for identifying the most common causes is shown in Fig. 32.2. Although it is important to exclude androgen-secreting tumours in the ovary and adrenal glands, most cases are constitutional.

Investigations
- Full history and physical examination.
- Full endocrine profile (oestradiol, FSH, LH, testosterone, sex hormone binding globulin (SHBG), androstenedione, dehydroepiandrosterone sulphate (DHEAS), 17-OH progesterone).
- Bone age studies.
- Imaging: ultrasound scanning of the gonads and adrenals should be performed as first line but CT or MRI are the gold-standard investigations for excluding tumours.

Management
- Endocrinological: the mainstay of endocrine support is suppression of oestrogen and androgen production by GnRH analogues to reverse the physical changes. This can either be given as a daily sniff or monthly depot preparation.
- Psychological support: this is vital, and counselling important, because the affected girl will see herself as being different from her friends.
- Surgical: if a tumour is discovered then this must be dealt with, usually surgically.

Hirsutism and virilism

Hirsutism – excess facial and body hair growth – can be either genetic (idiopathic) or due to increased androgen levels or sometimes both. Virilism occurs secondary to high circulating levels of androgens and is diagnosed when clitoral hypertrophy, breast atrophy, deepening of the voice and male-pattern balding occur either alone or together. Approximately 10% of healthy normal women can be said to have some degree of hirsutism without signs of virilism, however, virilism rarely occurs in the absence of hirsutism (except in the newborn). The causes of hirsutism and virilism are shown in Fig. 32.3.

- The mainstay of treatment for PCOS is weight loss.
- Although the most common cause of hirsutism in women is PCOS, it is vital to exclude an androgen-secreting tumour.
- The psychological effects of precocious and delayed puberty can be profound and should not be neglected.
- Virilism is never idiopathic whereas hirsutism can be.
- Rapid-onset hirsutism and virilism is suggestive of an androgen-producing tumour.

History
The timing of onset and the speed of progression of symptoms need to be elicited from the history. For instance, women with polycystic ovary syndrome (PCOS) typically have mild symptoms that have been present since menarche, whereas androgen-secreting tumours of the ovary characteristically produce high levels of androgens, which cause severe symptomatology over a short period of time. A

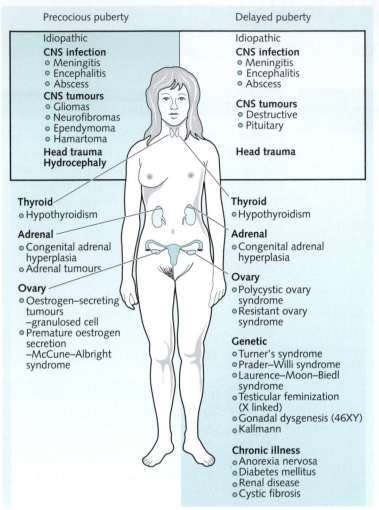

Precocious puberty

Idiopathic
CNS infection
- Meningitis
- Encephalitis
- Abscess
CNS tumours
- Gliomas
- Neurofibromas
- Ependymoma
- Hamartoma
Head trauma
Hydrocephaly

Thyroid
- Hypothyroidism

Adrenal
- Congenital adrenal hyperplasia
- Adrenal tumours

Ovary
- Oestrogen–secreting tumours
  –granulosed cell
- Premature oestrogen secretion
  –McCune–Albright syndrome

Delayed puberty

Idiopathic
CNS infection
- Meningitis
- Encephalitis
- Abscess

CNS tumours
- Destructive
- Pituitary

Head trauma

Thyroid
- Hypothyroidism

Adrenal
- Congenital adrenal hyperplasia

Ovary
- Polycystic ovary syndrome
- Resistant ovary syndrome

Genetic
- Turner's syndrome
- Prader–Willi syndrome
- Laurence–Moon–Biedl syndrome
- Testicular feminization (X linked)
- Gonadal dysgenesis (46XY)
- Kallmann

Chronic illness
- Anorexia nervosa
- Diabetes mellitus
- Renal disease
- Cystic fibrosis

Fig. 32.1 Causes of precocious puberty and delayed puberty.

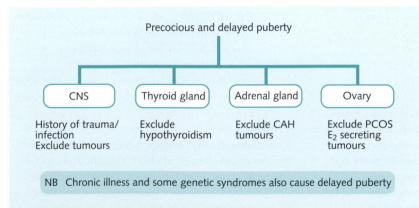

Precocious and delayed puberty

| CNS | Thyroid gland | Adrenal gland | Ovary |

History of trauma/ infection
Exclude tumours

Exclude hypothyroidism

Exclude CAH tumours

Exclude PCOS
E_2 secreting tumours

NB Chronic illness and some genetic syndromes also cause delayed puberty

Fig. 32.2 Algorithm for precocious and delayed puberty.

Fig. 32.3 Causes of hirsutism and virilism.

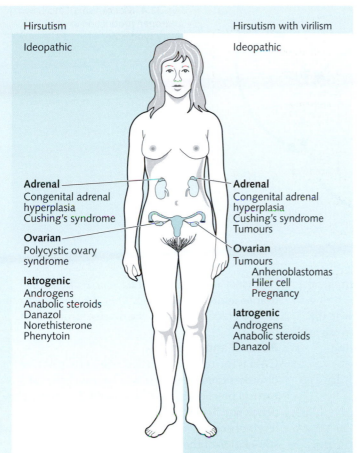

Hirsutism

Ideopathic

Adrenal
Congenital adrenal
hyperplasia
Cushing's syndrome

Ovarian
Polycystic ovary
syndrome

Iatrogenic
Androgens
Anabolic steroids
Danazol
Norethisterone
Phenytoin

Hirsutism with virilism

Ideopathic

Adrenal
Congenital adrenal
hyperplasia
Cushing's syndrome
Tumours

Ovarian
Tumours
   Anhenoblastomas
   Hiler cell
   Pregnancy

Iatrogenic
Androgens
Anabolic steroids
Danazol

detailed menstrual history is important because oligomenorrhoea (infrequent periods) is associated with PCOS and amenorrhoea is often associated with virilism. A family history of hirsutism is often present with idiopathic hirsutism and the menstrual history is usually normal.

PCOS typically presents with oligomenorrhoea and hirsutism from the time of menarche. There might be a history of subfertility secondary to chronic anovulation or a history of glucose intolerance. Although acne and seborrhoea occur relatively commonly, the androgen levels are not usually high enough to produce symptoms of virilism.

Congenital adrenal hyperplasia (CAH) usually presents in infancy with ambiguous genitalia but milder cases might not present until puberty and might have a history similar to women with PCOS.

Cushing's syndrome (excess cortisol) presents commonly with a gradual change in appearance associated with a host of other symptoms including central obesity, muscle wasting and weakness, hypertension and purple striae.

A careful drug history is imperative as not only do many of the hormonal therapies used in gynaecology have androgenic properties but there is an increase in the use of anabolic steroids even amongst women.

Examination

- Grading of hirsuties can be made objectively with detailed scoring systems but simple descriptive assessments are more practical. Signs of virilism should be looked for.
- Women with PCOS are often obese, although not always so. Acanthosis nigricans (pigmented raised patches found on the neck and skin flexures) is sometimes present in women with PCOS associated with insulin resistance.
- Severe CAH will have been diagnosed during childhood due to ambiguous external genitalia or salt-losing conditions. Women with milder, late-onset forms of CAH have little to distinguish them from those with PCOS, that is, obese, hirsute with some menstrual disorder.
- Women with Cushing's syndrome will have the

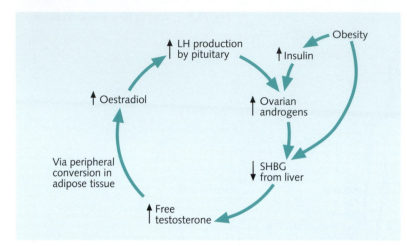

Fig. 32.4 Mechanism of increased androgen production in polycystic ovary syndrome.

typical appearance of central obesity, peripheral muscle wasting, hypertension and striae.

- Androgen-producing tumours cause little in the way of systemic upset apart from marked signs of virilism. They are usually too small to cause palpably enlarged ovaries.
- Women with idiopathic hirsutism usually have no abnormal findings on examination.

Aetiology

Hirsutism and virilism occur due to excess circulating endogenous or exogenous androgens. Endogenous production by the ovary is the most common source.

Ovarian androgens

PCOS is the most common cause of hirsutism (90%) and occurs in about 20% of women. Raised levels of circulating LH and sex steroids are characteristic of this syndrome and occur through different pathways (Fig. 32.4). Pituitary production of LH is raised in PCOS causing increased ovarian androgen production. This leads to a reduced production of SHBG by the liver and, as SHBG binds to circulating and androgens, increased free testerone levels. Androgens are converted to oestrogens in adipose tissue, raising oestradiol levels, which further stimulate pituitary production of LH. Obesity not only increases insulin levels, which stimulates further ovarian androgen production, but also reduces SHBG levels and increases the peripheral conversion of androgens to oestrogens.

Androgen-secreting tumours of the ovary are rare and include arrhenoblastomas and hilar cell tumours.

Pregnancy luteomas are a rare source of excess ovarian androgen secretion. They develop due to an exaggerated response by the ovarian stroma to hCG.

Adrenal androgens

CAH is the term used to describe a group of rare disorders caused by defects in hydroxylation of cortisol precursors, most commonly 21-hydroxylase deficiency. The net effect is increased circulating levels of cortisol precursors and androgens. Excessive stimulation of the adrenal cortex produces raised cortisol levels and is often associated with excess androgen production (Cushing's syndrome). Adenomas and adenocarcinoma of the adrenal gland produce high levels of androgens and are rare.

Exogenous androgens

Androgens and anabolic steroids will cause hirsutism and virilism, depending on the amount and length of time taken. Certain drugs prescribed for medical disorders have androgenic properties and, if taken in high enough doses and for long periods of time, can cause hirsutism (norethisterone, phenytoin) and virilism (danazol).

Investigation

Investigation is determined somewhat by the degree of symptoms (Fig. 32.5). Having excluded a history of exogenous androgens, if hirsutism is the only presenting complaint then PCOS is the likely cause accounting for 90% of cases. Diagnosis is made from the history, biochemical tests and ultrasound imaging of the ovaries. A rapid onset of symptoms, especially where virilism is present, would suggest high

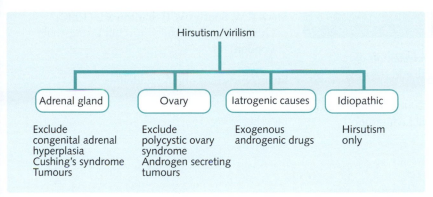

Fig. 32.5 Algorithm for hirsutism and virilism.

circulating levels of androgens secondary to more serious pathology. Testosterone levels more than twice the upper limit of normal suggest an ovarian or adrenal androgen-secreting tumour, which could be identified by imaging test such as ultrasound or CT scanning. Small tumours might be missed so a high level suspicion is needed. Investigations for CAH and Cushing's syndrome should be performed if symptoms and clinical signs suggest these diseases. Idiopathic hirsutism is a diagnosis made by excluding other pathology.

Complications

The main complication of hirsutism is psychosocial and this complaint should therefore be dealt with sympathetically. Some signs of virilism, such as deepening of the voice and cliteromegaly might be irreversible. Complications associated with PCOS include obesity, insulin resistance and glucose intolerance. Chronic anovulation affects fertility and can cause endometrial hyperplasia and adenocarcinoma as a result of the unopposed effect of oestrogens.

Treatment aims

Idiopathic hirsutism can be treated cosmetically using techniques such as bleaching or electrolysis. The effects of obesity in women with PCOS have been described above and encouraging weight loss in important in PCOS. Medical treatment of women with PCOS is most effective using a combination of ethinyloestradiol with an anti-androgen such as cyproterone acetate (Dianette™). Although improvement of hirsutism can take many months, the progestogentic effect of cyproterone acetate will protect the endometrium from the effects of unopposed oestrogen. Recent data suggest that PCOS might be driven by insulin resistance – as such, good results have been obtained by the use of the oral hypoglycaemic agent metformin.

Androgen-secreting ovarian and adrenal tumours should be surgically removed with preservation of the ovary in younger women.

Glucocorticoid and often mineralocorticoid replacement is the mainstay of treatment in CAH. Hirsutism and virilism should improve with therapy but it is sometimes necessary to perform surgical reconstructive procedures to the external genitalia.

Treating the cause of excess cortisol production in Cushing's syndrome should result in normal circulating levels of adrenal androgens.

Women with gynaecological conditions requiring treatment with drugs that have been androgenic properties should be forewarned of the potential virilizing side-effects. Immediate cessation should be advised. Phenytoin should not be stopped suddenly because this could precipitate status epilepticus.

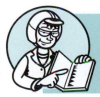

- What are the main causes of precocious puberty?
- Name four treatment options for women with PCOS.
- Does a normal ultrasound scan exclude polycystic ovarian syndrome?
- Is it possible for congenital adrenal hyperplasia to present in adult life and how?

Further reading

Llewellyn-Jones, D (1999) *Fundementals of Obstetrics & Gynaecology* 7th edn (Mosby, London)

McKay Hart, D & Norman, J (2000) *Gynaecology Illustrated* 5th edn (Churchill Livingstone, London)

Shaw R W, Soutter W P, Stanton S L (1997) *Gynaecology* 3rd edn (Churchill Livingstone, London)

http://www.rcog.org.uk/guidelines

33. Prenatal Diagnosis

Diagnosis of an ever-expanding number of conditions can now be made prior to birth. This allows for optimal preparation for the birth of an affected baby, including the place and mode of delivery (a tertiary centre rather than a district general hospital might be appropriate) and the involvement of neonatal or paediatric surgical teams, if necessary. The parents can be psychologically prepared for any intervention and can be put in touch with appropriate support groups. In some cases, once fully counselled, the parents might decide to terminate the pregnancy.

Prenatal diagnosis is not just about invasive procedures, which are detailed below. Ultrasound alone is used to diagnose many structural abnormalities, such as spina bifida and heart defects. Once structural anomalies have been diagnosed, the suspicion that the fetus might have an underlying chromosomal abnormality could arise and the parents would then be offered genetic testing.

Who has prenatal diagnosis?

- Women who have a family history of a disorder.
- Women who have had a previous pregnancy/baby affected by a disorder.
- Women whose babies are at increased risk of chromosomal disorders, as suggested by the maternal age alone, the result of serum screening ('double' or 'triple' test) or nuchal translucency scanning.
- Women who attend for a 'routine' ultrasound scan that reveals an abnormality.
- Women who have acquired an infection in pregnancy and there is any doubt as to whether the fetus is also infected.

Some of the most common conditions suitable for prenatal diagnosis are listed in Fig. 33.1.

Techniques for prenatal diagnosis

Ultrasound

Every ultrasound should be considered to be an opportunity for prenatal diagnosis.

Most centres advocate performing scans to examine the fetal anatomy in detail between 18 and 22 weeks. However, many women now have routine scans much earlier in pregnancy: dating scans take place at 7–12 weeks gestation and those for nuchal translucency at 10–14 weeks (Fig. 33.2); basic anatomy can be checked at this stage and some abnormalities will be apparent.

Amniocentesis

Amniocentesis has a 1% risk of miscarriage. Careful counselling prior to diagnostic procedures is vital; the risk of the baby being affected should always be weighed up against the risk of miscarriage caused by the procedure.

Transabdominal aspiration of amniotic fluid from around the fetus under continuous ultrasound guidance allows fetal cells (amniocytes) to be separated from the amniotic fluid and cultured to determine their genetic make-up (Fig. 33.3). Amniocytes can also be analysed for the absence of certain enzymes to diagnose the presence of fetal inborn errors of metabolism, or can be examined to diagnose infection such as toxoplasma.

Amniocentesis is performed from 15 weeks, ideally at around 16 weeks. Prior to this there are insufficient viable amniocytes within the fluid. Results of cell culture to determine karyotype or to

Conditions suitable for prenatal diagnosis	
Type of disorder/abnormality	**Description**
Chromosomal disorders	Trisomies, e.g. Down syndrome (trisomy 21), Edwards' syndrome (trisomy 18) and Patau's syndrome (trisomy 13)
	Triploidies
	Sex chromosome anomalies, e.g. Turner's syndrome (XO), Klinefelter's syndrome (XYY)
	X-linked disorders, e.g. Duchenne muscular dystrophy, haemophilia, fragile X
	Autosomal disorders, e.g. Huntington's disease, cystic fibrosis, thalassaemia, sickle-cell disease, Tay–Sachs disease, spinal muscular atrophy
Structural abnormalities	Neural tube defects, e.g. spina bifida or anencephaly
	Congenital heart defects
	Renal tract anomalies
	Skeletal dysplasias
Metabolic	Congenital adrenal hyperplasia
Fetal infection	Toxoplasma
	Rubella
	Parvovirus
	Listeria
Fetal anaemia	Fetal parvovirus infection
	Rhesus haemolytic disease

Fig. 33.1 Conditions suitable for prenatal diagnosis.

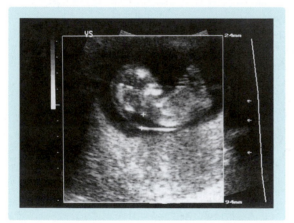

Fig. 33.2 Ultrasound scan showing increased nuchal thickness. Reproduced with kind permission from *High Risk Pregnancy* (2nd edn), published by WB Saunders.

look for specific gene anomalies can take around 2 weeks. With more expensive equipment the culture time can be reduced to 6 days but the UK national average is around 11 days. In around 1% of cases the cells will fail to culture.

Faster results – within 24–72 h – can be obtained by using fluorescent in situ hybridization (FISH) or polymerase chain reaction (PCR). These techniques give patients a 'preliminary' result, which is confirmed by culture, although many patients now make decisions regarding the future of the pregnancy on the basis of the preliminary result.

Because amniocentesis causes trauma to the uterus, with a risk of fetomaternal haemorrhage, anti-D is given to Rhesus negative women.

Chorionic villus sampling

 CVS can be performed earlier in pregnancy than amniocentesis so it gives the parents the option of earlier termination. However, it carries a higher risk of miscarriage of 2%.

Chorionic villus sampling (CVS) allows biopsy of chorionic villi under continuous ultrasound guidance to obtain a sample of cells that is examined to determine genetic make-up. It is performed from 11 weeks onwards and has a 2% risk of miscarriage. It can be performed transabdominally or transcervically (Fig. 33.4), depending on the preference of the operator. Some operators will always use the transcervical route with low-lying placentae. Like amniocentesis, it causes trauma to the uterus, so Anti-D is given to Rhesus negative women.

Results can be obtained more quickly from CVS samples, without resorting to FISH or PCR, because the mass of DNA obtained is greater than that from amniocentesis. 'Direct' CVS results – where a

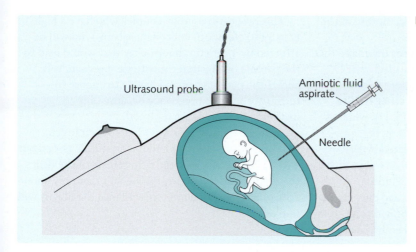

Fig. 33.3 Amniocentesis.

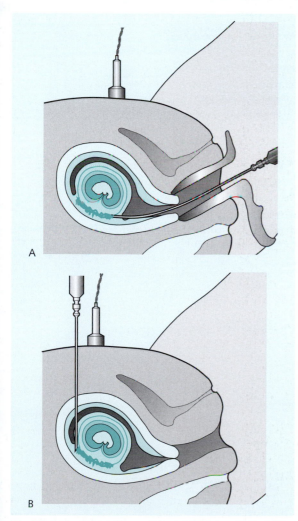

Fig. 33.4 Chorionic villus sampling. (A) Trans-cervical. (B) Transabdominal.

karyotype is determined without waiting for cell culture – are available within 3 days, although a complete result from culture is still considered the gold standard. However, FISH and PCR can still be used to reduce the result time to a minimum.

CVS has a false-positive rate of 1%, which is higher than amniocentesis due to the mosaicism of chorionic villi, which might show an abnormal karyotype when the fetus is normal. It also has a false negative rate of 0.1%, related to contamination with maternal cells.

Fetal blood sampling

Transabdominal needle aspiration of blood from the fetal hepatic vein or the umbilical cord (when the procedure is known as cordocentesis) under continuous ultrasound guidance. Conditions that can be diagnosed include:

- Chromosomal anomalies: if abnormalities are suspected later in pregnancy (because of ultrasound findings or early onset growth retardation) this method might be preferable to amniocentesis or CVS.
- Fetal anaemia.
- Fetal thrombocytopenia, e.g. where the mother has autoimmune thrombocytopenia.
- Fetal infection, using fetal IgM as a measure of immune response.

Fetal blood sampling can also be used for treatment of fetal conditions, for example to give transfusions, but this application is not considered in this chapter.

The complications include bleeding from the needling site (which can be fatal for the fetus), fetal bradycardia as a reaction to vasospasm of the umbilical artery, chorioamnionitis and rupture of the membranes.

Like the procedures above, it causes trauma to the uterus, so rhesus negative women are given anti-D.

Pre-implantation genetic diagnosis

Pre-implantation genetic diagnosis (PGD), which is only available at a few centres at present, is performed on eight-cell embryos created by IVF. One or two cells are removed and subjected to FISH or PCR to obtain a genetic diagnosis. Normal embryos are replaced into the uterus and develop normally, despite the 'insult' of having had cells removed at an early stage. Abnormal embryos are discarded.

This process is used by couples who have a high (25–50%) chance of conceiving a baby who will be affected by a genetic abnormality that would lead to the parents opting to terminate the pregnancy. It allows the parents to avoid having to choose to terminate a viable pregnancy because only unaffected embryos are replaced.

As it can only be performed on IVF embryos, PGD carries all the risks and uncertainties associated with IVF pregnancies – the side-effects of the drugs, the medical intervention and the fact that only about 25% of embryos that are replaced into the uterus will implant.

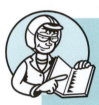

- What are the three main advantages of prenatal diagnosis?
- At what gestation is nuchal translucency scanning performed?
- What are the main differences between amniocentesis and CVS?
- Which technique is used to quantify fetal platelet levels?
- Why is anti-D given after the 'needling' tests described?

Further reading

Gonick & Wheelis *The Cartoon Guide to Genetics* (Harper & Row)
Miller AWF & Hanretty KP *Obstetrics Illustrated* (Churchill Livingstone, London)

Smith & Smith *Obstetric Ultrasound Made Easy* (Churchill Livingstone, London)

www.rcog.org.uk/guidelines
www.update-software.com/cochrane

34. Multiple Pregnancy

A multiple pregnancy is one in which two or more fetuses are present, that is, it is not a singleton pregnancy.

Multiple pregnancies are important to the obstetrician because they represent a high-risk pregnancy. The risk of all pregnancy complications is greater than in a singleton pregnancy, including preterm labour and IUGR. Perinatal mortality for a multiple pregnancy is about five times greater than that of a singleton.

- A multiple pegnancy is a high-risk pregnancy.
- Perinatal mortality rate is increased 4–5 times compared with a single fetus, mainly due to the risk of preterm labour.

Incidence of multiple pregnancy

The most common type of multiple pregnancy is a twin pregnancy, with an incidence of 1 in 80 pregnancies. The incidence of spontaneous triplets is 1 in 80^2 or 1 in 6400. The incidence of any multiple pregnancy increases with increasing maternal age. There has also been a rise over the last 2 decades, especially in Western countries, due to the increasing use of assisted conception techniques.

There is an ethnic variation in the frequency of multiple pregnancy (Fig. 34.1).

Diagnosis of multiple pregnancy

Nowadays, multiple pregnancies are normally diagnosed by routine dating ultrasound scan at 12–14 weeks gestation. The diagnosis should be excluded in a patient who presents with hyperemesis gravidarum. Clinical examination of the patient will reveal a large-for-dates uterus or the clinician will be able to palpate multiple fetal parts in later pregnancy (Fig. 34.2).

Aetiology of multiple pregnancy

Twins

The majority of twins (75%) are dizygotic, that is they arise from the fertilization (by two sperm) of two ova; monozygotic twins (25%) arise following the fertilization of a single ovum that then completely divides, so that each twin has the same genetic make-up.

However, rather than knowing the zygosity of a multiple pregnancy, the clinically important issue is the chorionicity of the pregnancy. This relates to the placentation of the pregnancy. If the placentae are separate, with separate amnions and chorions (dichorionic diamniotic twins), the blood supply to each fetus during the pregnancy is independent.

Conversely, if there are blood vessel anastomoses between the placentae (monochorionic diamniotic twins or monochorionic monoamniotic twins), then there is a risk of uneven distribution of blood. This results in discordant growth, with one twin showing signs of growth restriction and the other getting larger (see the section 'Twin-to-twin transfusion syndrome', p. 184). Thus diagnosing chorionicity determines the level of surveillance necessary in that particular pregnancy.

Dizygotic twins

Two ova from the same or different ovaries are released simultaneously and fertilized by two separate spermatozoa. Therefore, each fetus has its own chorion, amnion and placenta – dichorionic diamniotic placentation. If implantation occurs close together, the placentas can become fused. Subsequently, the twins can be of the same or different sexes and have different genetic constitutions, that is they have no more similarities than any other brother and sister.

The incidence of dizygotic twins varies widely between different populations, probably for

Ethnic variation in the frequency of twin pregnancies			
Country	Monozygotic	Dizygotic	Total
Nigeria	5.0	50	55
England and Wales	3.5	9.0	12.5
Japan	3.0	1.5	4.5

Fig. 34.1 Ethnic variation in the frequency of twin pregnancies shown as twinning rates per 1000 pregnancies.

Presentation of twin pregnancies at term	
Presentation	Percentage of pregnancies
Twin 1 cephalic/twin 2 cephalic	45
Twin 1 cephalic/twin 2 breech	37
Twin 1 breech/twin 2 breech	10
Other presentations including transverse	8

Fig. 34.2 Presentation of twin pregnancies at term.

multifactorial reasons such as genetic and nutritional factors. It also increases with increasing maternal age and increasing parity.

Monozygotic twins

A single ovum is fertilized by a single sperm and subsequently the zygote divides into two at various stages of embryonic development. This gives rise to different structural arrangements of the membranes (Fig. 34.3).

About two-thirds of monozygotic twins have monochorionic diamniotic placentation, that is a single blastocyst implants, developing a single chorion; the inner cell mass divides into two so that each embryo has its own amnion.

A third of monozygotic twins establish at an earlier stage than this, at the eight-cell stage, so that two separate blastocysts form and implant; such twins will thus have dichorionic diamniotic placentation.

The least common origin of monozygotic twins occurs by later splitting of the inner cell mass, before the appearance of the primitive streak, to produce a single amniotic cavity – monochorionic monoamniotic twins. Splitting even later than this causes conjoint twins to develop.

The incidence of monozygotic twins is constant around the world, at about 4 per 1000 births.

Triplets

Pregnancies of higher-order multiples (i.e. three or more fetuses) are less commonly formed by separate

ova. In the case of a triplet pregnancy, there are usually two ova' one of which splits as described above for monochorionic twins.

In such a pregnancy, and especially one of higher order, it is appropriate to counsel the parents about selective fetal reduction (see p. 186). The chorionicity of the pregnancy must be known to select the appropriate fetus. The procedure cannot be performed on a monochorionic twin because it shares placental circulation with its co-twin and therefore the drugs would affect both fetuses.

Diagnosis of chorionicity
Antenatally

Ultrasound assessment of the membrane dividing the amniotic sacs diagnoses the chorionicity; this is done before 16 weeks gestation. Figure 34.4 shows the thicker insertion of the membrane, known as the lambda sign, that is found in a dichorionic pregnancy and the thinner T sign of a monochorionic pregnancy. If there is no dividing membrane between the fetuses, then they share the placental blood flow and are monochorionic monoamniotic twins.

Fetal sex can also be assessed by ultrasound. If they are discordant, then the pregnancy must be dichorionic. Localization of the placental sites is also important. If the placentae can be seen completely separately, then again, the pregnancy must be dichorionic.

Postnatally

At this stage, chorionicity can be determined by:
- Macroscopic and microscopic examination of membranes.
- Analysis of red-blood-cell markers.
- DNA probes.

Complications of multiple pregnancy

A multiple pregnancy must be treated as a high-risk pregnancy. The majority of pregnancy-related

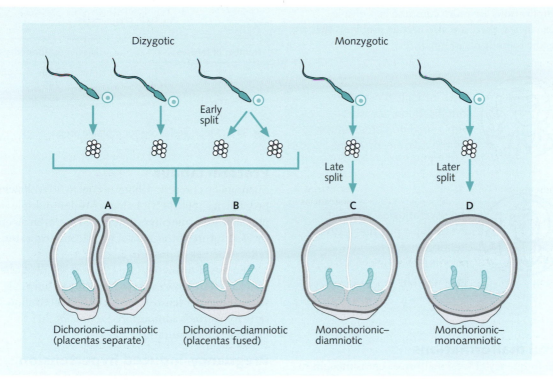

Fig. 34.3 Dizygotic and monozygotic twinning.

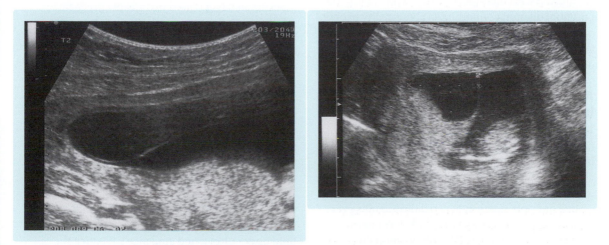

Fig. 34.4 Diagnosis of chorionicity. (A) The T sign is indicative of monochorionic diamniotic pregnancy. (B) The lambda sign is indicative of dichorionic diamniotic pregnancy.

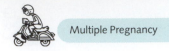

complications are more common in multiple pregnancies; there are also certain problems that are specific to multiple pregnancies.

The mother is at risk of any complication associated with a singleton pregnancy but the risks are increased.

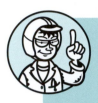

The psychological sequelae of a multiple pregnancy on the mother and her family, including existing children, should not be underestimated.

Multiple pregnancies	
Number of fetuses	Mean gestation (days)
1	280
2	245
3	231
4	203

Fig. 34.5 Mean gestations for multiple pregnancies.

Preterm labour

Spontaneous preterm labour occurs in 30% of twin pregnancies (Fig. 34.5). In higher-order multiple pregnancies, some physicians opt to put in an elective cervical suture at the start of the second trimester, to reduce the risk of preterm labour.

The use of tocolytics (see Chapter 38) might be considered to allow in utero transfer to a hospital with neonatal intensive care facilities and to allow time for steroids administered to the mother to improve lung maturation.

Pregnancy-induced hypertension

Hypertension is about three times more common in multiple pregnancies than in singleton pregnancies because of the larger size of the placental bed (see Chapter 35). It often develops earlier and is more severe.

Antepartum haemorrhage

The incidence of placental abruption and placenta praevia can be increased in multiple pregnancies.

Fetal malformations

The frequency of fetal malformations is thought to be almost double in a twin pregnancy compared with a singleton pregnancy, especially for monochorionic twins. In terms of screening for chromosomal anomalies (see Chapter 33), parents must be counselled about the possibility of a greater risk of pregnancy loss than in a singleton pregnancy with an invasive procedure. Separate sampling must be performed with dichorionic twins. There is also the potential dilemma of finding an abnormality in only one fetus; selective fetocide can result in the loss of the apparently normal fetus as well as the abnormal one.

Antenatal assessment of fetal well-being and growth

In a high-risk pregnancy, antenatal care should be more frequent, managed by a hospital consultant in a unit with facilities for regular ultrasound scans to check fetal growth and neonatal care facilities in case of preterm labour and delivery.

In a multiple pregnancy, serial ultrasounds every 2 to 4 weeks are necessary to exclude intrauterine growth restriction (IUGR). This is especially important in pregnancies with monochorionic placentation, which are at greater risk of discordant growth between the two fetuses and twin-to-twin transfusion syndrome (see below).

Twin-to-twin transfusion syndrome (TTTS)

This occurs in 5–15% of monochorionic twin pregnancies – blood is shunted across placental vascular anastomoses from twin to twin, such that the donor becomes anaemic and growth restricted, with oligohydramnios, and the recipient becomes plethoric with polyhydramnios. This syndrome usually occurs in the second trimester and results in fetal death in up to 80% of cases.

Treatment of this condition is still under discussion. Some centres have performed amniodrainage (i.e. taking off some of the excess fluid under ultrasound guidance to reduce the stretching of the uterus and therefore the risk of preterm labour). Other groups advocate laser treatment to the placental anastomoses to reduce the discordant blood flow between the fetuses.

With monochorionic placentation, fetal death of a twin in utero puts the surviving twin at risk of neurological damage and the mother at risk of developing DIC as thromboplastins are released into the circulation. The pregnancy can usually be managed conservatively until the surviving twin reaches a gestation with improved likelihood of survival; 80% of surviving twins can be delivered vaginally.

Intrapartum management of a twin pregnancy

Figure 34.6 provides a summary of the management of a vaginal delivery in a twin pregnancy.

Delivery of twin pregnancy

Delivery of multiple pregnancies should be managed in a unit with neonatal intensive care facilities. For a twin pregnancy, the mode of delivery depends on the presentation of the first twin; if it is anything other than cephalic, caesarean section is usually the method of choice. In the case of higher-order multiple pregnancies, delivery is almost always by caesarean section.

In a twin pregnancy, if the first twin presents as cephalic and there are no other complications then a vaginal delivery is usually planned. The onset of labour can be spontaneous or induced; induction might be advised for similar reasons to a singleton pregnancy (e.g. post dates) or for an indication more specific to a twin pregnancy, such as IUGR. The woman needs intravenous access and a sample of serum saved in the blood transfusion laboratory

because of the risk of post-partum haemorrhage (see below). An epidural block is often recommended to allow later manipulation of twin two (see below).

Both fetal heart rates should be monitored continuously, either both per abdomen or with a fetal scalp electrode on the first twin. If there is an abnormality in the heart rate pattern of twin one, fetal blood sampling might be appropriate (see Chapter 16). A problem with twin two should lead to immediate delivery by caesarean section. The reasons for augmentation of labour and for instrumental delivery of twin one are similar to those in a singleton pregnancy (see Chapter 41).

Once the first twin is delivered, the lie and presentation of the second twin must be determined by abdominal palpation and ultrasound. External cephalic version can be used to establish a longitudinal lie. Intravenous syntocinon might be necessary to maintain uterine contractions and the delivery of the second twin occurs either as a cephalic presentation or by breech extraction; again the reasons for instrumental delivery or caesarean section are similar to those of a singleton pregnancy.

Complications
Post-partum haemorrhage

Post-partum haemorrhage (PPH; see Chapter 42) is more likely with a multiple pregnancy than a singleton because of the larger placental site. Uterine atony due to the increased volume of the uterine contents – two fetuses, placentae, etc. – is a contributing factor. Active management of the third stage of labour is therefore appropriate; further treatment might include routine use of a post-partum syntocinon infusion.

Locked twins

This is a very rare complication of vaginal deliveries. The delivery proceeds with the first twin presenting as a breech but the aftercoming head of the first twin is prevented from entering the pelvis by the head of the cephalic-presenting second twin. If this is diagnosed in the first stage of labour, a caesarean section should be performed; during the second stage, general anaesthesia is necessary to allow manipulation.

The intrapartum management of twin pregnancy

- Neonatal unit intensive care facilities
- Allow vaginal delivery if normal pregnancy and twin 1 cephalic presentation
- IV access/full blood count/group and save
- Regional anaesthesia
- Continuous CTG monitoring ± fetal scalp electrode to twin 1
- IV syntocinon infusion to start after delivery of twin 1 to maintain contractions
- IV syntocinon infusion for third stage to reduce risk of PPH

Fig. 34.6 The intrapartum management of twin pregnancy.

Higher-order multiple pregnancies

In comparison to twin pregnancies, higher-order multiples are associated with a higher perinatal mortality rate and an increased incidence of the antenatal complications mentioned above. Fertility treatments have increased the numbers of high-order pregnancies and, in the case of IVF, guidelines in the UK now advise that a maximum of two embryos should be replaced (see Chapter 28).

Selective fetocide (fetal reduction)

Selective fetocide is a technique in which intracardial or pericardial potassium chloride is given to one or more fetuses in a high-order multiple pregnancy to improve the outcome of the remaining fetuses. Despite the procedure-related risk of miscarriage, the incidence of complications is low and improvements are seen in terms of reduction in rates of miscarriage and preterm labour. However, ethical dilemmas arise with respect to abortion in general, as well as possible miscarriage of the entire pregnancy.

- How is chorionicity diagnosed?
- Why is chorionicity important in the management of a twin pregnancy?
- What are the potential complications of a twin pregnancy?
- Discuss the intrapartum management of a twin pregnancy.
- What are the potential advantages and disadvantages of selective fetal reduction?

Further reading

Chamberlain,G & Steer, P (2001) *Turnbull's Obstetrics* 3rd edn

Enkin MW, Keirse MJNC et al (2000) *A guide to effective care in pregnancy and childbirth* 3rd edn

Nicolaides KH, Sebire NJ, Snijders JM *The 11-14 week scan*

Studd, J *Progress in Obstetrics and Gynaecology* 12

Ward RH, Whittle M (eds) (1995) *Multiple pregnancy* (RCOG Press, London)

35. Hypertension in Pregnancy

Hypertension can predate the pregnancy or might have been induced by the pregnancy. In some cases, hypertension is part of the syndrome of pre-eclampsia. Hypertensive disorders of pregnancy affect around 1 in 10 pregnancies.

> Due to the physiological changes seen in pregnancy, blood pressure falls in the first and second trimesters, reaching its lowest at around 23 weeks. From then on the blood pressure rises again until it has reached pre-pregnancy levels at term.

Non-proteinuric hypertension in pregnancy

Hypertension diagnosed prior to or early in pregnancy

This group includes known hypertensives and those whose hypertension is diagnosed in the first trimester, when the high blood pressure cannot be thought to be due to the pregnancy and was almost certainly present prior to pregnancy, but never measured. The risk factors for pre-existing hypertension are:

- Increasing maternal age.
- A family history.
- Medical disorders (e.g. diabetes, renal disease).
- Certain ethnic groups including those of Asian, Afro-Caribbean and South Pacific island origin.

Hypertension in a young woman not known to have any medical problems should be investigated to exclude the more unusual causes of hypertension: coarctation of the aorta, renal artery stenosis, Conn's syndrome, Cushing's syndrome and phaeochromocytoma.

Pregnancy-induced hypertension

Non-proteinuric hypertension that occurs in the second half of pregnancy can be thought of as a separate entity to essential hypertension and pre-eclampsia, but it is closely linked with both. Typically, it resolves within 6 weeks of delivery. The clinical sequelae are the same as those seen with essential hypertension and the management has the same aims.

Effects of non-proteinuric hypertension in pregnancy

The risks are threefold:

- Maternal health: above mean arterial pressures of 125 mmHg there is a risk of cerebral haemorrhage.
- Fetal health: pregnancies affected by essential hypertension are more susceptible to IUGR
- High risk of developing pre-eclampsia.

Management of essential hypertension and pregnancy-induced hypertension

Women known to be hypertensive prior to pregnancy should ideally receive preconception counselling, with advice about diet, weight and exercise to maximize control. If necessary, her antihypertensive medication can be changed to drugs that are considered safe in the first trimester. If hypertension is first diagnosed in early pregnancy an underlying cause should be sought (see Chapter 13).

As the risk of developing pre-eclampsia will be higher than for a normotensive woman, it is important that the patient knows the symptoms and signs to look out for, and to report them to her midwife or doctor. Some studies have shown value in Doppler scanning at 26 weeks gestation to look for changes in vessels that are said to predict pre-eclampsia. For this reason, some units arrange Doppler scans for all high-risk women. However, as there is no treatment to prevent the development of pre-eclampsia, predicting it might not be helpful.

Low-dose aspirin can reduce the risk of an 'at-risk' woman from developing severe pre-eclampsia early in pregnancy (before 32 weeks) but must be started at around 12 weeks gestation. Drug treatment that lowers blood pressure (see below) cannot prevent the development of pre-eclampsia but can reduce the risk of cerebral haemorrhage. Mother and fetus are closely observed with blood pressure and urinalysis checks and regular scans to monitor fetal growth.

Pre-eclampsia

The risk factors for developing pre-eclampsia are:
- Primiparous.
- Age > 35.
- Essential hypertension.
- Multiple pregnancy.
- Previous pregnancy affected by pre-eclampsia.
- Family history e.g. patient's mother or sister, with the strongest link being if the patient's sister had pre-eclampsia.

The recurrence rate of pre-eclampsia is around 10% but is higher if there is another medical problem contributing to the hypertension or if the next pregnancy is with a new partner.

Pathology

Pre-eclampsia is a multisystem disorder affecting different organs throughout the body. The underlying pathology relates to blood vessels and the chemicals that control them; women with pre-eclampsia have abnormal vessel responses to pregnancy. In normal pregnancy the peripheral resistance falls; in pre-eclampsia the drop in peripheral resistance is not as marked. Compared with a normal pregnancy the woman has increased sensitivity to pressor agents, reduced prostacyclin (a vasodilator) levels and increased thromboxane (a vasoconstrictor) levels. There is relative haemoconcentration due to less of the normal expansion in blood volume. The end-organ effects are shown in Fig. 35.1.

The symptoms and investigation of high blood pressure are detailed in Chapter 13.

The only cure for pre-eclampsia is delivery.

Management of pre-eclampsia

Treating high blood pressure in pre-eclampsia is important for the same reasons as with essential hypertension – to prevent intracerebral bleeds and to protect fetal health. However, treatment will not alter the course of the disease – the only treatment for pre-eclampsia is to end the pregnancy, that is, to deliver the baby. If the pregnancy has reached term and the cervix is favourable, induction of labour is sensible. If the cervix is not ripe and the pre-eclampsia is not severe, it may be better to monitor the condition until successful induction is more likely.

In labour, continuous monitoring is wise because the fetus will be more prone to distress and because treatment for high blood pressure can cause sudden hypotension, resulting in abruption and fetal compromise. If the mother has severe pre-eclampsia, fluid restriction should be exercised. Blood pressure can be controlled with intravenous hydralazine or labetalol, or intermittent doses of nifedipine.

When pre-eclampsia occurs preterm (before 37 weeks gestation), decisions about induction and delivery are more difficult. Bearing in mind the problems encountered by premature babies, it might be prudent to wait, monitor the condition of mother and baby, and try to achieve fetal maturity. In severe pre-eclampsia, however, the benefit of remaining in utero will not be great as compromised placental perfusion will result in little, if any, fetal growth.

Pre-eclampsia can be described as 'fulminating' – severe and of rapid onset. In these cases delivery is more likely to be by caesarean section, unless the woman is already in labour and is progressing rapidly. The classification of severity of pre-eclampsia depends on a combination of signs and symptoms (Fig. 35.2).

Complications of pre-eclampsia

The fetal and maternal effects of pre-eclampsia are reduced by careful control of the blood pressure and good fluid management but these measures will not necessarily prevent complications. These are:
- Eclampsia.
- Renal failure.
- Hepatic rupture.
- HELLP: haemolysis, elevated liver enzymes, and low platelets.
- Cerebral haemorrhage.
- DIC.

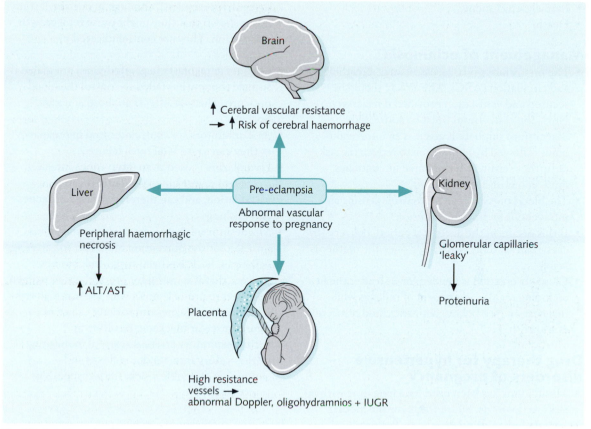

Fig. 35.1 End-organ effects of pre-eclampsia.

The criteria needed to diagnose severe pre-eclampsia

- BP ≥ 160/110 mmHg on two readings and proteinuria 2+ or more

or

- BP > 140/90 mmHg and proteinuria 2+ or more and at least one of:
  - oliguria: urine output < 400–500 mL in 24 h
  - visual disturbance/headache/right upper quadrant pain
  - platelets < 100, ALT > 50
  - creatinine > 100
  - three or more beats of clonus

Fig. 35.2 The criteria needed to diagnose severe pre-eclampsia.

- Pulmonary oedema.
- Increased perinatal mortality and morbidity due to increased preterm delivery, uteroplacental insufficiency and abruption (particularly in HELLP and severe PET).

Eclampsia

Eclampsia is defined as fitting secondary to pre-eclampsia. The appearance is the same as a grand mal epileptic seizure. It can occur in women who have previously been completely well through pregnancy, in whom there has been no suspicion of pre-eclampsia. Eclampsia affects 1 in 1600 pregnancies. Around 40% of eclamptic fits happen postnatally but usually within 48h of delivery. The mortality rate is between 0.5 and 5.5%. The differential diagnosis includes epilepsy, meningitis, cerebral thrombosis and intracerebral bleed.

Complications of eclampsia

As in severe pre-eclampsia, these are both fetal and maternal:

- Abruption (which can lead to fetal death and DIC).
- Pulmonary oedema.
- Cerebral haemorrhage.
- Liver rupture.

- Retinal detachment.
- Death.

Management of eclampsia

- The first priority is to assess airways, breathing and circulation (ABC). The airway should be secured and ventilation provided if necessary.
- Next, the convulsions must be addressed. Magnesium sulphate is given as an intravenous bolus followed by an infusion to reduce the risk of further seizures. If the initial fit continues, intravenous diazepam is used.
- The blood pressure can be controlled using an intravenous hydralazine infusion.
- If this occurs in the antenatal period, delivery (by caesarean section) is achieved once the mother is stable.
- Close observation is needed for 24h after the fit, including regular assessment of reflexes while on magnesium (see below) and strict fluid restriction of 85mL/h.

Drug therapy for hypertensive disorders of pregnancy

- Methyldopa has been used for a long time with no risks to the fetus. Side-effects for the mother include lethargy and diarrhoea. Postnatally, if antihypertensives are still required, methyldopa is no longer the drug of choice because depression is a possible side-effect.
- Beta-blockers such as labetalol are also used in tablet form and as an infusion (for rapid control of severe hypertension), although in one small study it was shown that they might cause fetal growth retardation. They are contraindicated in asthmatics.
- Calcium antagonists (e.g. nifedipine) are added if a single therapy has failed to control the blood pressure. The side-effects are headaches and flushing.
- ACE inhibitors are contraindicated in pregnancy as they can cause fetal renal failure.
- Hydralazine is used as an intravenous infusion to control severe blood pressure. It causes vasodilation, and can therefore cause headaches and flushing.
- Magnesium sulphate is used as an intravenous infusion for the prevention of further fits after an eclamptic fit. It has been suggested, but not proved, that it is useful for prophylaxis in women with severe pre-eclampsia who seem at high risk of eclampsia. Magnesium toxicity can cause neuromuscular blockade, resulting in cardiorespiratory arrest, so careful monitoring of respiratory rate, tendon reflexes and symptoms of double vision/slurred speech is important.

It is often necessary to continue antihypertensive medication postnatally. All the drugs listed above are safe in breastfeeding. If the woman is a known hypertensive on treatment she can return to her prepregnancy medication.

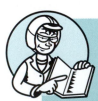

- How common is hypertension in pregnancy?
- At what level of blood pressure does the risk of cerebral haemorrhage become much higher?
- Why is ultrasound monitoring of the fetus important in pregnancies affected by hypertension?
- Which family of antihypertensive drugs are contraindicated in pregnancy?
- Can any measures be taken to reduce the risk of pre-eclampsia in subsequent pregnancies?

Further reading

Miller AWF & Hanretty KP *Obstetrics Illustrated* (Churchill Livingstone, London)
Nelson-Piercy, C *Handbook of Obstetric Medicine* (Isis Medical Media)

www.swot.org.uk
www.rcog.org.uk/guidelines
www.update-software.com/cochrane

36. Medical Disorders in Pregnancy

Anaemia

The lower limit of normal haemoglobin in pregnancy is 10.5 g/dL. The maximum increase possible in haemoglobin per week with iron tablets or injections is 0.8 g/dL.

Plasma expansion in pregnancy results in a physiological reduction in haemoglobin concentration. The body's handling of iron and folate changes (Fig. 36.1). However, due to the demands of the developing fetus and, in some cases, aggravated by pre-existing anaemia, women can become anaemic in pregnancy.

The symptoms of anaemia – fatigue, dizziness, fainting – are also common symptoms of pregnancy. Anaemia is proven by a full blood count looking at haemoglobin concentration and red cell indices.

It should not be assumed that anaemia is due to lack of iron. Renal clearance of folate doubles in pregnancy, making women prone to deficiency. Measuring serum iron, ferritin, folate and red cell folate will help to determine whether the anaemia is due to deficiency of iron, folate or both (Fig. 36. 2).

Many doctors believe that prevention is better than cure and that the disadvantages of the side-effects of iron and folate tablets are outweighed by the advantages that can be conferred by taking supplements routinely in pregnancy, thus avoiding the symptoms of anaemia and need for transfusions.

Iron absorption is aided by vitamin C (so washing down the tablets with orange juice helps) but impaired by caffeine (so tablets should not be taken with tea, coffee or cola).

Asthma

This affects at least 3% of women of childbearing age and can improve, deteriorate or stay the same during pregnancy. Peak flow and FEV_1 are unaffected by pregnancy, so remain the mainstay of monitoring asthma.

The main problem arises from women being worried to use their inhalers or to take oral steroids for fear of the possible harmful effect on the fetus. They can be entirely reassured, as the doses of drugs, and the types of drugs used are completely safe. The main danger to the fetus is if the woman suffers repeated severe attacks, so she should be encouraged to manage her asthma well.

Attacks in labour are very rare but the woman should bring her inhalers with her to the delivery ward. If she is on a high dose of oral steroids hydrocortisone, cover during labour will be needed.

Asthma attacks in labour are rare.

Breastfeeding while using inhalers or oral steroids is safe and might reduce the risk of the baby developing asthma in later life.

Diabetes

This section covers women with pre-existing diabetes, those with gestational diabetes, and the effect of these conditions on the fetus.

In normal pregnancy the woman becomes more resistant to her own body's insulin, partly due to the 'anti-insulin' hormones (human placental lactogen, glucagons and cortisol) secreted by the placenta. At the same time, glucose handling changes and the body loses its ability to regulate glucose levels smoothly, leading to lower fasting levels and higher postprandial levels than when not pregnant. These effects increase through the second and third trimesters.

The renal threshold for glucose also changes, so that most women will have glycosuria on urinalysis at some time in pregnancy. To cope with these changes, a pregnant woman will have doubled her insulin production by the end of pregnancy.

Pre-existing diabetes

The normal state explains some of the ways that pregnancy affects women with diabetes. The main points are that they:

- Need increased doses of insulin.
- Are more likely to experience 'hypos' (hypoglycaemic attacks).

'Anti-anaemia' changes	'Pro-anaemia' changes
↑ Production of red blood cells	↑ Plasma volumes i.e. haemodilution
↑ Iron absorption in gut	↓ Serum iron
↑ transferrin, so ↑ total iron-binding capacity	↓ Serum ferritin
	↑ Renal clearance of folate

Fig. 36.1 Anaemia in pregnancy.

- Might experience acceleration of the complications of diabetes (e.g. nephropathy, retinopathy).
- Can develop diabetic ketoacidosis if another factor 'tips them over' (e.g. hyperemesis, infection, administration of corticosteroids; see below).

Figure 36.3 shows the complications that can occur in pregnancy when there is pre-existing diabetes.

Management

Most of the complications listed above can be reduced by good control. Preconception and early pregnancy control can be assessed by measuring the HbA1c (glycosylated haemoglobin) level. The management of women with diabetes in pregnancy consists of:

- Joint care with midwives, obstetricians and diabetic physicians.
- Informing the woman: explaining to the woman why good control is so vital.
- Dietary advice: a low-sugar, low-fat, high-fibre diet will make it easier to keep glucose levels more stable; she is likely to need to snack in-between meals to protect against hypoglycaemia (but these can be healthy snacks!).
- Home blood glucose monitoring and clinic HbA1c monitoring.

Fig. 36.2 Determining anaemia deficiency.

Anaemia		
	Iron deficiency	**Folate deficiency**
Investigation results	Low haemoglobin Low mean cell volume Low serum iron Low serum ferritin	Low haemoglobin High mean cell volume Low serum folate Low red cell folate
Risk factors	Menorrhagia Multiple pregnancy Recent pregnancy Recent or current breastfeeding Iron-deficient diet	Anticonvulsant therapy Thalassaemia
Treatment	Iron tablets, solution or injections (blood transfusion)	Folate tablets
Side-effects	Constipation Indigestion Green/black stools	Few
Food sources	Liver Red meat Kidney beans, fresh vegetables Fortified cereals	Soy beans Walnuts Kidney beans, broccoli Fortified cereals

Pre-existing diabetes—complications of pregnancy	
Complication	**Comment**
Miscarriage	When control is poor
Fetal congenital abnormality	Related to control at the time of conception: can be as low as 5% or as high as 25%
Proteinuric hypertension	Especially if there is pre-existing hypertension or nephropathy
Macrosomia (baby > 4.5 kg)	Due to fetal exposure to high levels of insulin, which is a growth-promoting hormone
Shoulder dystocia	Due to macrosomia
Polyhydramnios	Due to fetal polyuria
Intrauterine death, stillbirth	
Candida and urinary tract infections	Due to glycosuria

Fig. 36.3 Pre-existing diabetes—complications of pregnancy.

- Increasing insulin doses as necessary, and converting women with non-insulin-dependent diabetes to insulin (tablets are contraindicated in pregnancy).
- Fundoscopy at regular intervals to assess for retinopathy.
- Anomaly screening: in the form of nuchal translucency scanning plus the detailed anomaly scan.
- Scans for growth and liquor.

It is particularly important to pay attention to sugar control at times when an additional stress has been placed on the body, for example at times of illness, infection or in labour, when a sliding scale is used for accurate control.

Corticosteroids, which might be given to the mother for the benefit of the baby when premature delivery is expected, are naturally diabetogenic and can cause high readings for a few days.

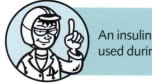 An insulin sliding scale is used during labour.

Although women with diabetes are more likely to have a caesarean section, this is because of the complications listed above rather than a recommended mode of delivery. The timing of delivery relates to the control of the diabetes – if control has been good the woman might be allowed to continue in pregnancy and to labour spontaneously, but if control has been poor induction of labour might be suggested to reduce the risk of intrauterine death and stillbirth after 37–38 weeks.

Postnatal considerations
The neonate is at risk of
- Hypoglycaemia.
- Respiratory distress.
- Jaundice.

Liaison with the paediatric team is sensible because the baby is likely to need some special care. Ongoing monitoring of the mother's glucose levels will be necessary, especially if she is breastfeeding, as her insulin requirements will take longer to return to prepregnancy levels.

Gestational diabetes
The incidence of this condition varies depending on the criteria used to diagnose it, but it is known to be far more prevalent in women of South East Asian, Mediterranean, and Afro-Caribbean origin. Other risk factors include:
- Past history of gestational diabetes.
- Previous macrosomic baby.
- Family history of diabetes.

It usually develops in the second or early third trimester; if diabetes is diagnosed earlier than this in pregnancy the suspicion should be raised that it was present but undiagnosed prior to pregnancy, and the management plans above should be applied.

Diabetes is diagnosed if a fasting blood glucose is greater than 7.8mmol/L or if a postprandial glucose is greater than 11.1mmol/L.

Diagnosis of gestational diabetes can be made:

- On screening: some units offer this to women with the risk factors listed above.
- As a result of maternal symptoms or signs: if the woman has recurrent infections, persistent glycosuria or feels 'large for dates' with macrosomia or polyhydramnios seen on scan.
- In retrospect, when HbA1c testing is done to investigate an intrauterine death/stillbirth or an unexpectedly macrosomic baby who was hypoglycaemic following delivery.

These pregnancies are not at increased risk of congenital abnormality but the risks of perinatal death and morbidity are higher than in non-diabetic pregnancies. The woman is also at increased risk of developing proteinuric hypertension.

All diabetic pregnancies are more at risk of stillbirth and neonatal morbidity and mortality, but pre-existing diabetics also have a higher risk of fetal abnormality, which gestational diabetics do not.

Management

The mainstay of management is dietary advice combined with home blood glucose monitoring. Insulin is needed if diet fails to control glucose levels. Fetal growth and liquor volume are monitored with regular scans and a joint approach should be taken to care, ideally involving a team of diabetic physician, obstetrician and midwife.

If on insulin, the woman is likely to need a sliding scale in labour, but this can be stopped when the third stage is complete. The neonate will be at risk of hypoglycaemia, so the paediatrician should be involved.

Women who develop gestational diabetes should be made aware that they are at high risk of developing

non-insulin dependant diabetes in the future and that their attitudes and actions regarding lifestyle, weight and diet can significantly affect this risk.

Epilepsy

Epilepsy affects 1 in 200 women of childbearing age. Pregnancy can exacerbate epilepsy but, equally, the frequency of seizures can decline. Seizures are particularly likely around the time of labour due to hyperventilation, dehydration and exhaustion. Seizures don't in themselves harm the baby but status epilepticus is dangerous for mother and fetus.

Complications

Women who have epilepsy should take higher than normal doses of folic acid before and throughout pregnancy – preconceptually and for the first 12 weeks of pregnancy to reduce the risk of neural tube defects and facial clefts, and later to counteract the anti-folate effects of anticonvulsants that make women with epilepsy more prone to folate-deficiency anaemia.

The main concern for pregnant women who are epileptic is that all drugs used to treat epilepsy are teratogenic; possible effects are shown in Fig. 36.4. The rate of abnormality is around 6% for women who are being treated for their epilepsy and 4% for women not receiving treatment, compared with 3% for non-epileptic women.

The discrepancy is accounted for by the inherent link between facial clefts and epilepsy that is

---

Fetal and neonatal complications of anticonvulsant therapy

- Cleft lip and palate
- Neural tube defects
- Congenital heart defects
- Haemorrhagic disease of the newborn

Fig. 36.4 Fetal and neonatal complications of anticonvulsant therapy.

independent of drug therapy. The teratogenic effect of the drugs used is cumulative (i.e. the risk of abnormality if the mother is on two drugs is > 12%) so monotherapy is the aim.

New anticonvulsants (e.g. lamotrigine and gabapentin) have shown encouragingly low levels of teratogenesis in animal studies but cannot be recommended for use in human pregnancy yet because there are no data as to their safety. Although no one anticonvulsant is particularly better than another, new patients are usually started on carbamazepine in pregnancy.

The woman should not have her usual drug changed unless it is one of the new drugs or phenobarbitone, which can lead to neonatal seizures and withdrawal. Control of seizures in pregnancy can deteriorate because drug levels change as a result of the difference in drug handling by the body. If seizures become frequent, drug levels should be monitored regularly, but the question of compliance should also be addressed – the patient might need further reassurance that it is safer for her baby that she takes her medication than that she run the risk of poor control.

Anticonvulsants affect hepatic handling of vitamin K, increasing the risk of haemorrhagic disease in the newborn, so women taking medication should receive vitamin K supplements from 36 weeks, and the baby should have vitamin K at birth.

Breastfeeding when on anticonvulsants is safe in the main. Occasionally, if the feed coincides with a peak in drug levels, the infant might become drowsy. All that is necessary is to change the time of feeding in relation to tablet taking.

Human immunodeficiency virus

Issues to be considered include the effect of pregnancy on the course of HIV infection, the risks of maternal HIV for the fetus and the screening of the antenatal population for HIV.

HIV is a disease of immunosuppression, and as pregnancy is a naturally immunosuppressed state it might be assumed to cause a deterioration in the condition of the woman affected. However, studies have not proven this to be the case. Women with HIV who become pregnant require specialized care and this is not just physical but also psychological and social.

Factors increasing the risk of vertical transmission of human immunodeficiency virus

- Advanced maternal disease, high viral load, low CD4 counts
- Procedures that risk fetal and maternal blood mixing:
  - amniocentesis / chorionic villous sampling
  - fetal blood sampling / fetal scalp electrodes in labour,
  - episiotomy
- Normal or instrumental vaginal delivery
- Breastfeeding

Fig. 36.5 Factors increasing the risk of vertical transmission of human immunodeficiency virus.

Complications

Women with HIV seem to have higher rates of miscarriage, premature labour and in utero growth restriction, but some of these might be accounted for by confounding variables such as smoking, poor nutritional status and general ill health. The main risk is of vertical transmission, that is of the baby becoming HIV positive, as neonatal and infant HIV infection carries a very poor prognosis. Transmission of the virus can occur antenatally or during labour (rates of around 30% without retroviral treatment and with vaginal delivery) or postnatally, through breastfeeding, which doubles the risk of transmission. Factors that increase the risk of vertical transmission are shown in Fig. 36.5.

Management

Women continuing in pregnancy should be monitored as usual, with regular blood tests for viral load and CD4 counts, but the physiological reduction in CD4 count must be taken into account. Treatment may be altered given the limited data available for the safety for the fetus of some of the newer combination regimens of antiretroviral and protease inhibitor drugs. Women at high risk of opportunistic infection such as pneumocystis and toxoplasma should be given prophylaxis.

The procedures that are known to increase the risk of vertical transmission are avoided if at all possible and women are offered elective caesarean section. Additional protection against vertical transmission may be gained by treating the mother with zidovudine (AZT), orally for the last month of pregnancy and intravenously around the time of delivery. The baby is given AZT syrup for the first 6 weeks of life.

Vertical transmission is reduced by giving antiretroviral therapy: orally to the mother in pregnancy, intravenously during delivery, then orally to the neonate.

Women in the developed world are advised not to breastfeed. In the developing world the risks of non-sterile bottlefeeding and the loss of the protection against common infant ailments afforded by breastfeeding might mean that breast is still best.

Screening

In the UK, the Department of Health has recommended that antenatal testing for HIV be part of routine care, offered to all women at booking. The identification of HIV infection has considerable implications for the management of the pregnancy and, since an agreement in the 1990s with the insurance industry, having had the test as part of antenatal screening does not alter premiums.

Most centres that have adopted the offer of testing to all women have had good take-up rates, and it is known that in some inner-city areas the incidence of HIV is as high as 0.5% in the booking population (although some of those women will already be aware of their diagnosis).

Liver disorders

Acute fatty liver

This is an extremely rare but potentially lethal liver condition of unknown aetiology. The incidence is approximately 1 in 10 000 pregnancies, and it carries mortality rates of 20–30% for the fetus and 10–20% for the mother. It is associated with obesity and with multiple pregnancy.

The woman presents with nausea, malaise and loss of appetite. She then develops severe vomiting and abdominal pain, jaundice and ascites. Fulminant liver failure can ensue, leading to renal failure, encephalopathy (with drowsiness and confusion) and clotting anomalies culminating in DIC.

Pathology specimens show fatty infiltration of hepatocytes, and the gold standard for diagnosis is liver biopsy, although this might be inadvisable given clotting problems. Ultrasound and MRI have been used as alternatives to visualize the fatty infiltration of the liver. Bloods show hypoglycaemia, extremely high transaminase (ALT and AST) levels, alkaline phosphatase raised to a lesser degree and a very high urate.

Management is to correct hypoglycaemia and clotting as far as possible and then to deliver the baby. Rapid reversal of the problem follows delivery.

Obstetric cholestasis

The unique symptom of obstetric cholestasis is itchy palms of the hands and soles of the feet.

This disorder is of unknown aetiology but there is a strong family history and it is postulated that there is autosomal dominant inheritance. Women present in the third trimester with severe pruritus that is worst on the palms of the hands and soles of the feet; on examination there is no rash. Direct questioning might reveal pale, fatty stools, dark urine and loss of appetite.

Investigation

Liver function tests show raised serum bile acids, raised transaminases (ALT and AST), mildly raised bilirubin and alkaline phosphatase raised even higher than is usually seen in pregnancy. Other causes for liver dysfunction should be investigated, including ultrasound scanning for gallstones and serology for hepatitis. The complications are shown in Fig. 36.6.

Complications of obstetric cholestasis	
Complication	**Comment**
Postpartum haemorrhage	Due to malabsorption of vitamin K
Intrauterine death	2–4%, with risk increasing with gestation
Premature labour	40% will deliver before 37 weeks
Fetal distress in labour	Meconium-stained liquor likely
Fetal and neonatal intracranial haemorrhage	Due to maternal malabsorption of vitamin K

Fig. 36.6 Complications of obstetric cholestasis.

Management

Management consists of:

- Reducing the itching: cholestyramine acts to reduce bile acids and can relieve itching but often causes vomiting and diarrhoea. Antihistamines work for some women, but have unwelcome sedative effects. Ursodeoxycholic acid (UDCA) lowers bile acids and reduces itching, but is not licensed for use in pregnancy, so is prescribed with caution.

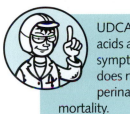

UDCA lowers serum bile acids and reduces symptoms of itching but does not reduce the perinatal morbidity and mortality.

- Reducing the risk of fetal and maternal haemorrhage: women are prescribed daily vitamin K tablets.
- Monitoring fetal well-being: unfortunately, the drugs listed above, which reduce bile acids, have not been shown to reduce the fetal risks of cholestasis. Regular CTG monitoring and growth scans are performed but probably do not make a difference in terms of preventing intrauterine death. The mother is warned to be aware of and to report any change or reduction in fetal movements.
- Delivery: once the fetus is considered sufficiently mature, that is, around 37 weeks. Obstetric cholestasis in itself is not an indication for elective caesarean section but because of the increased risk of fetal distress in labour there is a higher than average chance of the woman needing operative delivery.
- Counselling: regarding the risks to this pregnancy and to future pregnancies (there is a high recurrence rate). Women should also be warned to avoid the combined oral contraceptive pill because it can provoke similar liver dysfunction.

Multiple sclerosis

The typical female multiple sclerosis (MS) sufferer is of childbearing age but new presentation during pregnancy is unusual. The usual picture is of a relapsing and remitting course – often better in the third trimester but worse in the 6 months following delivery. The disease itself has no effect on the fetus or on pregnancy but if mobility is limited the risk of thrombosis should be considered and appropriate precautions (e.g. thromboembolic disease (TED) stockings) introduced; if there are pre-existing bladder problems, the risk of urinary tract infection will be higher.

The use of cannabis to relieve symptoms of MS is increasing. At present, the usual method of taking it is to smoke it mixed with tobacco. Women should be made aware that the risks to the baby are the same as for cigarette smoking.

Psychiatric disorders

Depression

Recognition of postnatal depression has received widespread attention in the media and in the medical literature. The subject of antenatal depression is less popular and yet, on closer questioning of women suffering from postnatal depression, many of them admit to symptoms of depression before the birth of their baby.

Society's view of pregnancy as something to be happy about and to be enjoyed can make it even harder for women to admit to depression or to ask for help. Women who suffered from depression prior to pregnancy might assume that drug treatments are contraindicated in pregnancy and that there is no point in them mentioning it to their carers.

Known risk factors for antenatal and postnatal depression include those common to all patients suffering from depression, and some that are specific to pregnancy (Fig. 36.7). The symptoms of depression are:

- Persistently low mood.
- Anhedonia.
- Loss of appetite.
- Insomnia or hypersomnia.
- Psychomotor agitation or retardation.
- Thoughts of self-harm.
- Anxiety (postnatally this might relate particularly to the baby, with worries of not being able to care for the baby or to love it enough).

Fig. 36.7 Risk factors for depression during and after pregnancy.

Postnatal depression affects around 1 in 10 women.

True postnatal depression, where symptoms are present for more than 2 weeks, affects around 1 in 10 women and should be distinguished from the 'baby blues', which lasts for a few days and is experienced by up to 70% of women. Once recognized, treatment should be started without delay as most antidepressants will not have an effect for 6 weeks. Good support is vital and hospitalization is sometimes necessary. In severe cases, electroconvulsive therapy (ECT) might be used.

Drug therapy

The older tricyclic antidepressants can cause drowsiness and antimuscarinic side-effects, such as dry mouth and constipation, but they have been used for years with no problems being seen for the fetus or, when breastfeeding, for the baby. However, depression outside pregnancy is often treated with selective serotonin reuptake inhibitors (SSRIs) such as sertraline (Lustral™), fluoxetine (Prozac™) and paroxetine (Seroxat™), so women will seek advice as to whether they should change their medication in pregnancy.

Sertraline has been shown to be potentially harmful to the fetus in animal studies but seems to be safe in breastfeeding. The other SSRIs show no evidence of teratogenicity in animal studies but the manufacturers advise that they are avoided in

pregnancy unless the benefit of their use outweighs the risk. Fluoxetine (Prozac™) shows high amounts in breast milk, so should be avoided, and the manufacturers of paroxetine (Seroxat™) advise that it is avoided unless the benefit outweighs the risk.

In conclusion, the choice of antidepressant treatment in pregnancy and during breastfeeding should be made on a case-by-case basis, actively involving the patient in the process and discussing the risks and benefits.

Puerperal psychosis

This disorder is seen most often in women who have a history of psychiatric illness (40% of women with bipolar disorder will develop a puerperal psychosis) but this is not always the case. It usually develops between 2 days and 3 weeks after the birth. The woman exhibits symptoms of mania, with accompanying delusional thoughts and visual or auditory hallucinations. The delusions and hallucinations might pertain to the baby and sometimes manifest as a desire to harm the baby, so a careful risk assessment must be made.

Admission to hospital is necessary – if possible to a specialized mother and baby unit. Treatment consists of antipsychotic medications. Breastfeeding should be avoided if at all possible while the mother is taking these because animal studies suggest possible adverse effects on the baby's developing nervous system. The risk of recurrence in future pregnancies is up to 50%.

Bipolar disorder

The main problem with this condition is that the drugs used as maintenance therapy (carbamazepine and lithium) are teratogenic. The risks associated with carbamazepine can be reduced to an extent by taking 5 mg of folic acid before conception and for the first 12 weeks of pregnancy, but detailed anomaly scanning is important. Lithium has a narrow therapeutic:toxic ratio and close monitoring of lithium levels is needed during pregnancy as dose requirements increase in the second and third trimesters, but they then come rapidly back to normal. High maternal levels at the time of delivery lead to the danger of toxicity in the neonate.

The most likely time for acute episodes of mania to occur is not during the pregnancy but in the puerperium. Close liaison between psychiatric and obstetric care providers will be very important. Breastfeeding while taking carbamazepine is safe but lithium is present in breast milk and can lead to toxicity in the infant. Acute episodes are treated with anti-psychotics (see below for their use in pregnancy and with breastfeeding).

Schizophrenia

Women who conceive when on the older antipsychotic drugs can be reassured that the risks to the baby from the medication are not high, although extrapyramidal side-effects are sometimes seen in the neonate. The manufacturers of other newer drugs advise their use only if the benefit outweighs the risk in pregnancy; others are to be avoided entirely if possible.

It is known that women with schizophrenia are more prone to preterm labour and that their babies have a higher than average risk of in utero growth retardation. All of these factors should be discussed carefully with the woman and careful liaison with her psychiatric carers is vital.

During the puerperium the woman is particularly vulnerable to exacerbations, so close support and observation is necessary during this time. Breastfeeding whilst on anti-psychotic medication is not advisable.

Drug and alcohol dependence

The misuse of drugs and alcohol is linked with poor obstetric outcome in many different ways. The keystone of obstetric care is to try to establish a link with the woman so that she will attend for antenatal appointments, but the involvement of drug liaison teams, paediatricians and social services may also be necessary.

Careful explanation of the risks for the fetus is necessary (see Chapter 45) and plans for a withdrawal programme should be drawn up if the woman agrees. Intravenous drug use should prompt discussion of screening for HIV and hepatitis B and C. Many centres have a named midwife with expertise in this area who will be a link between the hospital, social worker and the mother.

Thromboembolism

Pulmonary embolism (PE) is the most common pregnancy-related cause of death in the UK, so thromboembolism is to be taken extremely seriously

---

Factors increasing risk of thromboembolic disease related to pregnancy

- Obesity > 80 kg
- Age > 35
- Granmultiparity
- Past medical history of TED
- Prolonged bed rest
- Varicose veins, if severe
- Thrombophilia, e.g. protein C or S deficiency, antithrombin III deficiency, activated protein C resistance (the factor V Leiden mutation), antiphospholipid antibody syndrome

Fig. 36.8 Factors increasing risk of thromboembolic disease related to pregnancy.

in pregnancy. The underlying problem is that pregnancy is a hypercoaguable state, with increased levels of clotting factors and fibrinogen, decreased fibrinolysis and decreased levels of antithrombin; this state continues for at least 6 weeks postpartum. The added effects of venous pooling and increased abdominal pressure mean that pregnancy increases a woman's risk of a thromboembolic event by six times. Delivery by caesarean section raises the risk still further, by ten to twenty times, giving the risk of developing deep vein thrombosis (DVT) after an emergency caesarean section of 1–2%. The risk factors are summarized in Fig. 36.8.

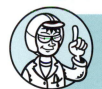

The increased risk of thromboembolism related to pregnancy continues for 6 weeks postpartum.

The diagnosis of thromboembolism on the basis of history and examination alone is more difficult in pregnancy. Signs and symptoms are less reliable. Leg oedema (which can be due to DVT) and breathlessness (which might be due to PE) are both common symptoms in pregnancy. The best advice is to have a high index of suspicion and to employ the investigations described below.

Cerebral vein thrombosis is very uncommon but is associated with high mortality; it usually occurs in the puerperium. Once again it can be difficult to make the diagnosis on clinical grounds; the picture is confused, with the woman suffering from fits (raising the suspicion of eclampsia), fever, vomiting and photophobia (suggesting meningitis).

Investigation

The diagnosis of DVT is best made using Doppler ultrasound unless the clot is above the inguinal ligament, in which case venography is the investigation of choice. The investigation of PE should include arterial blood gases, which show hypoxaemia and hypocapnia, ECG and chest X-ray.

The chest X-ray might be normal or might show an area of infarction or effusion. In non-pregnant patients a V/Q scan, showing ventilation and perfusion, or a spiral CT scan is performed to confirm the diagnosis. Although the dose of radiation is not contraindicated in pregnancy, it might be possible to reduce exposure by making the diagnosis on the basis of a perfusion scan alone. If, however, the original chest X-ray was abnormal, a ventilation scan will be necessary. The diagnosis of cerebral thrombosis is best made with MRI scanning.

Management

Pending the confirmation of the diagnosis of PE or DVT, the safest course of action is to anticoagulate. There is an ongoing discussion of the merits of intravenous heparin infusion compared with intermittent low molecular weight heparin (LMWH). LMWH is used extensively by physicians for treating DVT and PE but is still unproven for treatment in pregnancy. It is known that larger doses of intravenous heparin are needed in pregnancy to achieve the target of prolonging the activated partial thromboplastin time (APTT) by 1.5–2 times the control.

Treatment is continued for 1 week, after which prophylaxis against recurrence is started. Subcutaneous heparin or LMWH is used; warfarin is avoided because of its teratogenicity and the risk of maternal retroplacental bleeding and fetal intracerebral bleeds. Anticoagulation must be continued through labour and for 6 weeks postpartum.

Warfarin and heparin are both safe in breastfeeding, so some women might opt to switch to warfarin; the disadvantage is the frequent blood testing at first, but chronic treatment with heparin is not without its side-effects (see below).

Prophylaxis against thromboembolism in pregnancy

As is stated above, pregnancy itself is a major risk factor for thromboembolism. Some women have

Antithromboembolism prophylaxis in pregnancy	
Risk factor	**Prophylaxis**
Prosthetic heart valve	Warfarin through pregnancy and puerperium
Multiple deep vein thrombosis/pulmonary embolism in the past	Heparin through pregnancy and puerperium
Thrombophilia (proven or probable)	Heparin through pregnancy and puerperium
One previous deep vein thrombosis or pulmonary embolism	Aspirin through pregnancy, then heparin through labour and puerperium

Fig. 36.9 Antithromboembolism prophylaxis in pregnancy.

added risk factors and need the protection of prophylaxis. Women with a history of thromboembolism or a strong family history should be screened before pregnancy or in the first trimester. The duration and type of prophylaxis depends on the degree of the risk (Fig. 36.9).

Treatment with heparin for long periods of time results in bone demineralization, which can lead to vertebral fractures. As pregnancy and breastfeeding also cause demineralization, the rate of symptomatic osteoporosis in women on long-term therapy could be as high as 2%, although bone density does improve once therapy is stopped.

A rarer, but dangerous side-effect of heparin is thrombocytopaenia. The risks of these side-effects are thought to be lower with LMWH. Women on maintenance heparin have monthly platelet counts and clotting screens and, if therapy is for longer than 10 weeks in total, a dual-energy X-ray absorptiometry (DEXA) scan should be performed postnatally to assess bone loss. Low-dose aspirin is safe in pregnancy.

As operative delivery increases the risk of thromboembolism dramatically, prophylaxis is also given after caesarean section to some women, in the form of heparin and/or TED stockings.

Thyroid disorders

Hyperthyroidism

Hyperthyroidism affects 1 in 500 pregnant women. Most of them are hyperthyroid because they have Graves' disease, an autoimmune condition. Affected

Signs and symptoms of hyperthyroidism
• Lid lag • Tremor • Weight loss • Exophthalmos • Feeling hot • Racing heart • Palpitations • Vomiting • Goitre

Fig. 36.10 Signs and symptoms of hyperthyroidism.

Signs and symptoms of hypothyroidism
• Cold intolerance • Slowed pulse rate • Delayed relaxation of the tendon reflexes • Weight gain • Lethargy • Hair loss • Dry skin • Constipation • Carpal tunnel syndrome • Goitre

Fig. 36.11 Signs and symptoms of hypothyroidism.

women often have a family history. Some of the symptoms and signs are akin to those of pregnancy, but the first three listed in Fig. 36.10 should raise the suspicion of thyroid disease. Investigation reveals raised free T4 and low levels of thyroid stimulating hormone (TSH) in comparison with the normal range for that stage of pregnancy.

Like other autoimmune conditions, thyrotoxicosis often improves in pregnancy, but the deterioration in the puerperium might therefore be more marked. If untreated in pregnancy, thyrotoxicosis can predispose to miscarriage, IUGR, premature labour and increased perinatal morbidity, and the danger of thyroid storm. In 1–2%, thyroid antibodies cross the placenta and cause fetal and neonatal thyrotoxicosis. This is more likely to happen if control is poor in the third trimester, and carries a risk of 15% neonatal mortality if untreated.

Management

Treatment is with carbimazole or propylthiouracil. Both drugs cross the placenta and in high doses can result in fetal hypothyroidism. Efficacy of treatment is monitored with free T4 levels every other month. Women with Graves' disease should have serial ultrasound scanning looking for evidence of fetal thyrotoxicosis in the form of IUGR, goitre or fetal tachycardia. If the condition is diagnosed, increased doses of antithyroid drugs are administered to the mother. All neonates born to mothers with Graves' disease should have cord blood sent for thyroid function tests.

Antithyroid drugs are secreted in breast milk in small amounts, so the thyroid function of all breastfed babies should be monitored.

Hypothyroidism

Hypothyroidism is seen in about 1% of antenatal patients. New diagnosis in pregnancy is made more difficult by the fact that many of the symptoms are similar to those of normal pregnancy; the first three features shown in Fig. 36.11 are the most useful when trying to discriminate.

Fortunately, new diagnosis in pregnancy is unusual, and the management of hypothyroidism mainly consists of the care of women who are already on replacement therapy.

Most cases are due to autoimmune destruction of the thyroid – in this process the thyroid gland can atrophy or enlarge, forming a goitre. When a goitre is present the condition is known as Hashimoto's thyroiditis. Other cases are related to drug use (e.g. lithium, amiodarone) or to previous thyroidectomy. The diagnosis is confirmed by a low T4 level (normal ranges for different stages of pregnancy are used). TSH will be raised. A test for thyroid autoantibodies might be sent.

Untreated hypothyroidism leads to a higher risk of:
• Miscarriage.
• Fetal loss.
• Pre-eclampsia.
• IUGR.

It might also be related to lower intelligence in the child.

Well-controlled hypothyroidism does not affect maternal or fetal outcome except the rare cases of fetal and neonatal hypothyroidism, where TSH-receptor-blocking antibodies cross the placenta resulting in impaired neurological development.

Thyroxine replacement does not affect fetal thyroid function, and seldom needs adjustment during pregnancy if the dose was correct prior to pregnancy. Pregnant women receiving thyroxine replacement should have thyroid function checked once in each trimester, and, if the dose is altered, 4 weeks after any alteration.

Postpartum thyroiditis

It is estimated that this condition affects 5–11% of postpartum women. Those with a family history of hypothyroidism are particularly at risk. It is caused by an autoimmune thyroiditis, which results in an imbalance of thyroid hormones – the state resulting can be hypothyroid, hyperthyroid or a biphasic pattern of first hyperthyroidism and then hypothyroidism. Symptoms are often vague (e.g. fatigue, palpitations, lethargy, depression) and can be attributed (by the woman and her GP) to her recovery from childbirth and the demands of a new baby. It usually occurs around 12 weeks postpartum.

Investigation is first with biochemistry, to confirm thyroid malfunction. A radioactive iodine scan can be done to distinguish postpartum thyroiditis from Graves' disease.

Treatment is not always necessary; the condition is usually self-limiting and treatment will not speed recovery, although it will relieve troublesome symptoms. Overactive symptoms can be treated with β-blockers, underactive symptoms with thyroxine replacement. However, 3–4% of women will remain permanently hypothyroid, requiring replacement therapy, and around one-third will be euthyroid for a few years but then develop permanent hypothyroidism. Recurrence in future pregnancies is common.

Thyroid nodules

These are present in about 1% of women of childbearing age and are noteworthy because up to 30% might be malignant, so nodules must be investigated with fine needle aspiration or biopsy.

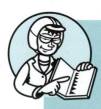

- What are the three common fetal structural abnormalities associated with anticonvulsant therapy?
- What is the main fetal concern in obstetric cholestasis?
- What should be done to reduce the thromboembolic risk of a woman with a thrombophilia in pregnancy?
- Why is good control of blood sugars so important for an insulin dependant diabetic woman who is trying to conceive?
- What three steps can be taken to reduce the risk of vertical transmission of HIV?
- When is a patient with bipolar affective disorder most likely to need psychiatric care related to pregnancy?
- If a woman is hypothyroid prior to pregnancy but is well controlled on treatment, what levels should be checked during pregnancy, and how often?

Further reading

Why Mothers Die, Report on Confidential Enquiries into Maternal Deaths in the United Kingdom, 1996–1999

Miller AWF & Hanretty KP *Obstetrics Illustrated* (Churchill Livingstone, London)

Nelson-Piercy, C *Handbook of Obstetric Medicine* (Isis Medical Media)

www.rcog.org.uk/guidelines (guideline: thromboembolic disease)

37. Antepartum Haemorrhage

Definition

An antepartum haemorrhage (APH) is defined as any vaginal bleeding that occurs after 24 weeks gestation and before the birth of the infant.

 Antepartum haemorrhge is an important cause of maternal and perinatal morbidity and mortality.

Incidence

The incidence of APH is 3%.

Aetiology

A summary is shown in Fig. 37.1. Placenta praevia combined with placental abruption accounts for about 50% of the causes of an APH. In both cases, the bleeding comes from maternal vessels that are exposed as the placenta separates from the decidua, that is, it is not fetal blood although fetal hypoxia can occur as a secondary process.

Placenta praevia

Definition

The placenta is wholly or partially attached to the lower uterine segment. The degree of attachment has traditionally been divided into four grades (Fig. 37.2) but, more recently, placenta praevia has been classified into two degrees, either minor – which encompasses grades I and II – or major – covering grades III and IV.

Incidence

Placenta praevia occurs in 0.4–0.8% of pregnancies; this figure has altered with routine use of ultrasound scanning. The incidence is increased with:

- Increasing maternal age.
- Increasing parity.
- Multiple pregnancy.
- Previous caesarean section.
- Presence of a succenturiate placental lobe.
- Smoking.

It is associated with a maternal mortality rate of about 0.03% in the developed world. The maternal and fetal morbidity is substantially higher in developing countries because of the complications of haemorrhage and prematurity.

History
Painless vaginal bleeding

Bleeding from a placenta praevia is usually unprovoked and occurs in the third trimester and in the absence of labour.

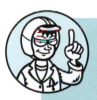 The presence of abdominal pain is the distinguishing clinical factor between placenta praevia and placental abruption.

Examination

General observations should always be performed, including maternal pulse and blood pressure. On abdominal palpation, the uterus is soft and non-tender. Because the placenta is low lying, it displaces the presenting part from the pelvis so that a cephalic presentation is not engaged, or there might be a malpresentation (see Chapter 46).

With a minor degree of bleeding, a speculum can be passed to exclude a lower genital tract cause for the APH. A digital examination should be avoided because it might provoke massive bleeding.

Diagnosis

As part of the routine 20-week ultrasound scan, the placental site is localized. If a low-lying placenta is

Aetiology of antepartum haemorrhage	
Source of haemorrhage	Type of haemorrhage
Uterine source	Placenta praevia
	Placental abruption
	Vasa praevia
	Circumvallate placenta
Lower genital tract source	Cervical ectropion
	Cervical polyp
	Cervical carcinoma
	Cervicitis
	Caginitis
	Vulval varicosities
Unknown origin (approx. 50%)	

Fig. 37.1 Aetiology of antepartum haemorrhage.

Ultrasound scan grading of placenta praevia		
Grade	Description	Degree of placenta praevia
I	Encroaches the lower segment	Minor
II	Reaches the internal os	Minor
III	Overlies the internal os in part	Major
IV	Centrally placed in the lower segment	Major

Fig. 37.2 Grading of placenta praevia determined by ultrasound scan.

noted then a follow-up scan in the third trimester is usually performed to make the diagnosis of placenta praevia. In the majority of patients, as the lower segment begins to form and the upper segment enlarges upwards, so the placenta appears to move up, away from the cervical os. A transvaginal scan is the diagnostic technique of choice due to its improved accuracy over the transabdominal mode.

Investigations
As well as an ultrasound scan, blood should be sent for haemoglobin count and group and save. AntiD is indicated if the patient is Rhesus negative. If the bleeding is heavy, cross-matching units for transfusion is indicated and a baseline clotting screen. Renal function tests might be necessary if the urine output is poor. A cardiotocograph should be done to check fetal well-being.

Management
Management depends first on assessing the severity of the bleeding and resuscitation of the patient if necessary (see Chapter 18). Immediate delivery by caesarean section might be appropriate if there is either maternal or fetal compromise.

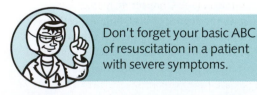
Don't forget your basic ABC of resuscitation in a patient with severe symptoms.

Expectant management depends on the gestation of the pregnancy and the placental site. If the

placenta remains at or over the cervical os, massive bleeding is likely to occur if the patient goes into labour and the cervix starts to dilate. Therefore, inpatient management is appropriate in the third trimester. Delivery by caesarean section is advised if the placenta is encroaching within 2 cm if the internal cervical os. If the head of the fetus becomes engaged (i.e. it passes below the leading edge of the placenta) then vaginal delivery may be possible.

Complications
Placenta praevia is associated with an increased risk of PPH (see Chapters 18 and 42). The lower uterine segment is less efficient at retraction following delivery of the placenta and thus less effective occlusion of the venous sinuses results in heavier blood loss.

Placenta accreta (see Chapter 42) is also a potential complication in up to 15% of patients with placenta praevia, especially those who have had a previous caesarean section. Whether this has been diagnosed preoperatively on ultrasound scan or not, preparations should be in place for potential PPH, for example, consultant obstetrician and anaesthetist input and counselling the patient.

Future pregnancy
Placenta praevia has a recurrence rate of 4–8%.

Placental abruption

Definition
The placental attachment to the uterus is disrupted by haemorrhage as blood dissects under the placenta, possibly extending into the amniotic sac or the uterine muscle.

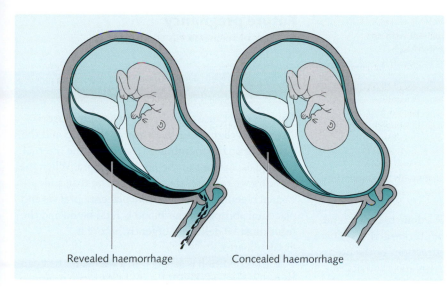

Fig. 37.3 Types of placental abruption.

Revealed haemorrhage   Concealed haemorrhage

Incidence

Placental abruption occurs in about 1% of pregnancies in the UK. In the majority of cases the cause is unknown but it is thought to be associated with:

- Maternal hypertension or pre-eclampsia.
- Abdominal trauma, e.g. assault, road traffic accident.
- Cigarette smoking.
- Lower socioeconomic group.
- External cephalic version.

History

Vaginal bleeding associated with abdominal pain

The patient can present at any stage of pregnancy with a history of bleeding and constant abdominal pain, which is usually unprovoked. This might be associated with uterine contractions.

As maternal blood escapes from the placental sinuses, it tracks down between the membranes and the uterus and escapes via the cervix; this is known as a revealed haemorrhage. Sometimes, the blood remains sealed within the uterine cavity such that the degree of shock is out of proportion to the vaginal loss; this is known as a concealed haemorrhage (Fig. 37.3).

Depending on the patient's previous antenatal history, she should be asked about symptoms of pre-eclampsia, including headache, blurred vision, nausea and epigastric pain (see Chapter 35).

Examination

The general maternal condition, including pulse and blood pressure, should be assessed. On abdominal palpation the uterus is typically tender. As bleeding extends into the uterine muscle, a tonic contraction can occur, making the uterus feel hard. Fetal parts are difficult to palpate. If the placental site is known (i.e. if placenta praevia has been excluded) a digital examination might be appropriate to diagnose the onset of labour.

Maternal hypertension and proteinuria must be excluded due to the association between abruption and pre-eclampsia. If present, liver tenderness, hyperreflexia and clonus should be excluded (see Chapter 35).

Investigations

Blood should be sent for haemoglobin count and group and save. AntiD is indicated if the patient is Rhesus negative. If the bleeding is heavy or if the patient is shocked, cross-matching units for transfusion is indicated and a baseline clotting screen.

Renal function tests might be necessary if the urine output is poor or in conjunction with liver function tests if pre-eclampsia is suspected. Urinalysis should be done to exclude proteinuria; if present, a 24-h urine protein level may be helpful to more accurately determine the degree of renal involvement (see Chapter 35).

Investigations for a patient with an antepartum haemorrhage
• Haemoglobin • Group and save/cross-match • Rhesus status • Renal function tests • Liver function tests • Cardiotocograph • Ultrasound scan

Fig. 37.4 Investigations for a patient with an antepartum haemorrhage.

A cardiotocograph should be done to check fetal well-being and also to monitor uterine activity. There might be palpable uterine contractions or the uterus might simply be irritable with irregular activity.

An ultrasound scan is of limited value since only a large retroplacental haemorrhage will be seen. The diagnosis of abruption is made on clinical grounds (Fig. 37.4).

Management

As for placenta praevia, management of a placental abruption must start with assessment of the severity of the symptoms. In a situation where the patient is clinically well and the fetus is not compromised, expectant management might allow the symptoms to resolve. However, in a more serious situation, active resuscitation of the patient could be necessary (see Chapter 18) with immediate delivery of the fetus as a life-saving procedure for the mother regardless of gestation.

Complications

- Accurate assessment of blood loss is necessary to assess the risks of developing disseminated intravascular coagulation and renal failure (see Chapter 18).
- Post-partum haemorrhage occurs in 25% of cases.
- Sheehan's syndrome as a result of PPH (pituitary necrosis secondary to hypovolaemic shock).

Future pregnancy

The risk of recurrence is about 6%.

Vasa praevia

This is a rare cause of antepartum haemorrhage. There is a velamentous insertion of the cord and the vessels lie on the membranes that cover the internal cervical os, in front of the presenting part. When the membranes rupture, the vessels can be torn and vaginal bleeding occurs. Unlike placenta praevia and placental abruption, this blood is fetal blood and the fetus must be delivered urgently before it exsanguinates.

If the condition is suspected, a Kleihauer test can be performed on the PV loss to test for the presence of fetal red blood cells.

Circumvallate placenta

This type of placenta develops secondary to outward proliferation of the chorionic villi into the decidua, beneath the ring of attachment of the amnion and chorion. This does not interfere with placental function, but it is associated with antepartum and intrapartum haemorrhage.

Unexplained antepartum haemorrhage

In up to 50% of cases of APH, no specific cause is found. The cervix should be visualized with a speculum examination and the date of the patient's last smear test checked. However, perinatal mortality with any type of APH is double that of a normal pregnancy, suggesting that placental function might be compromised. Therefore, it might be appropriate to consider delivery at term, by inducing labour.

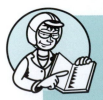

- What are the main causes of antepartum haemorrhage?
- How is the differential diagnosis made between placenta praevia and placental abruption?
- What investigations are appropriate for the patient who presents with an antepartum haemorrhage?
- What is the management of placental abruption?
- What are the main complications of placenta praevia?

Further reading

Chamberlain,G & Steer, P (2001) *Turnbull's Obstetrics* 3rd edn

Enkin MW, Keirse MJNC et al (2000) *A guide to effective care in pregnancy and childbirth* 3rd edn

RCOG (2001) *Placenta praevia: diagnosis and management* RCOG guideline no 27 (RCOG, London)

www.rcog.org.uk

38. Premature Labour

Premature labour is defined as labour occurring after 24 weeks and before 37 weeks gestation, so diagnosis depends upon the calculation of the estimated date of delivery. It is important to establish whether a labour is preterm for several reasons:

- Preterm labour is less predictable, and has more complications, than labour at term.
- There is an increased risk of fetal distress in labour.
- Neonatal problems are likely, so the paediatric team must be contacted

Prematurity is the single largest cause of neonatal mortality and long-term handicap in otherwise normal babies – premature babies have a 100-fold increased risk of dying than term babies.

- In most circumstances an effort can be made to stop the labour to administer corticosteroids to the mother, which will boost fetal lung surfactant production and therefore reduce neonatal respiratory distress.

Corticosteroids (e.g. betamethasone or dexamethasone) are given to the mother as two intramuscular injections 12 h apart. They have been shown to significantly reduce neonatal respiratory distress by stimulating fetal surfactant production and are recommended for any woman in threatened preterm labour between 24 and 36 weeks gestation. It is not known whether more than one course of steroids is beneficial but the effect is thought to decline over time.

Incidence

The incidence of preterm labour is currently around 6% in Europe, but this varies in different populations and the incidence is increasing. Risk factors for premature labour are shown in Fig. 38.1, with the most significant association being a history of a previous preterm labour.

The main causes of preterm delivery are shown in Fig. 38.2. Infection is thought to play a part in at least 20% of cases (see Fig. 38.3 for common pathogens implicated in preterm labour). Iatrogenic preterm delivery, accounting for one-third of preterm deliveries, occurs when obstetricians decide that delivery is necessary in the interests of fetal or maternal health, due, for example, to severe pre-eclampsia, or when scans have shown severe in utero growth retardation of the fetus.

Clinical evaluation and investigation of women in preterm labour

As preterm labour is often rapid and is almost always unexpected, some women will arrive in an advanced state of labour – in this case the mother should be assessed to make sure that she is stable (and not, for instance, shocked due to a large abruption), examined vaginally to check the dilatation of the cervix and fetal monitoring commenced. The paediatricians must be informed. As abnormal lie and presentation are far more common in preterm pregnancy, an ultrasound scan should be performed.

If the presentation is less acute a history should be taken and examination performed with the aim of finding out what the underlying cause of the threatened preterm labour is, and investigations arranged as appropriate. Any woman admitted with abdominal pain or discharge should have a speculum examination to allow inspection of the cervix (Fig. 38.4). Premature labour does not always present with obvious contractions and the cervix can undergo so-called 'silent' dilatation.

Cervical dilatation confirms labour but if the cervix

Characteristics of women more at risk of preterm labour

- Body mass index < 19
- Low social class
- Unsupported
- Afro-Caribbean ethnic group
- Extremes of reproductive age (under 20 and over 35)
- Domestic violence
- Smoking
- Previous preterm labour
- Bacterial vaginosis
- Chronic medical conditions

Fig. 38.1 Characteristics of women more at risk of preterm labour.

Causes of preterm delivery

- Infection, e.g. chorioamnionitis, maternal pyelonephritis/appendicitis
- Uteroplacental ischaemia, e.g. abruption
- Uterine overdistension, e.g. polyhydramnios, multiple pregnancy
- Cervical incompetence
- Fetal abnormality
- Iatrogenic

Fig. 38.2 Causes of preterm delivery.

Pathogens implicated in preterm labour

- Sexually transmitted: *Chlamydia*, *Trichomonas*, *Syphilis*, *Gonorrhoea*
- Enteric organisms: *Escherichia coli*, *Streptococcus faecalis*
- Bacterial vaginosis: *Gardnerella*, *Mycoplasma* and anaerobes
- Group B streptococcus (if a very heavy growth)

Fig. 38.3 Pathogens implicated in preterm labour.

Management checklist for patient presenting in threatened preterm labour

- Assess for signs of a precipitant of preterm labour, e.g. sepsis, polyhydramnios, abruption, severe pre-eclampsia, obstetric cholestasis. Take blood tests as appropriate. Perform urinalysis and send MSU
- Determine frequency and regularity of contractions. Monitor the fetal heart
- Perform a sterile speculum examination to examine the cervix. Take high vaginal and endocervical swabs. Start continuous electronic fetal monitoring (CTG) if there is cervical dilatation
- Ascertain fetal presentation (cephalic or breech)
- Give corticosteroids
- Give antibiotics if ruptured membranes or if obvious signs of sepsis
- Consider tocolysis
- Contact paediatricians and arrange transfer out if necessary and appropriate
- Discuss mode of delivery

Fig. 38.4 Management checklist for patient presenting in threatened preterm labour.

is closed in the presence of uterine contractions the diagnosis of 'threatened' preterm labour is made. Around half of women presenting with symptoms of threatened preterm labour are either not in labour or stop labouring spontaneously. If membranes have ruptured, delivery is far more likely.

The clinical picture alone does not allow us to predict accurately which women will settle spontaneously, so the management plan is formulated on the assumption that delivery will occur. Transvaginal scans to examine the length of the cervix have been used, where cervical shortening is a predictor of preterm delivery (Fig. 38.5). Evidence of fetal fibronectin in the mother's cervical secretions can be used; its absence has proved to be a reassurance that delivery is very unlikely but it is not a very sensitive test.

Liaison with the paediatric team is vital. Some hospitals do not have facilities for treating babies born under certain gestations and in these cases transfer to the nearest appropriate unit is made, preferably in utero, that is, transfer of the mother before she has delivered. If the mother is seriously unwell or if delivery is imminent, transfer of the baby can be arranged after delivery. Unless the mother is in advanced labour on arrival, there will be an opportunity for her and her partner to meet one of the paediatricians to find out what is likely to happen if her baby is born at an early gestation. They can be given a realistic outlook and warned about some of the problems that premature babies encounter. A tour of the neonatal intensive care unit could be arranged.

The main problems encountered by children surviving premature delivery are cerebral palsy, chronic lung disease, visual and hearing deficits and learning difficulties.

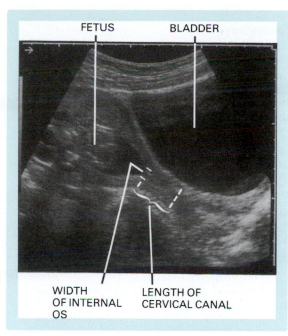

Fig. 38.5 Transvaginal scan of cervical canal. Reproduced with kind permission from *Obstetric Ultrasound: How, why and when*, published by Churchill Livingstone.

Treatment of women presenting in preterm labour

Although the mortality and morbidity of preterm infants has been reducing over the last decade, this cannot be ascribed to improved obstetric management, other than the increased administration of corticosteroids to the mother. Sadly, our attempts to stop preterm labour are unsatisfactory, being often ineffective and exposing women and their babies to drugs with significant side-effects. Part of the problem is our lack of knowledge about what triggers preterm labour.

Tocolysis

The different drugs used to try to stop contractions are shown in Fig. 38.6. Ethanol infusion is not included but it was used routinely until the 1970s. The common factor of all the drugs is that none has been shown to result in improved neonatal morbidity or mortality. Most have been shown to delay delivery for some time (24–48h), which gives the obstetricians the opportunity to administer corticosteroids and, if necessary, transfer to another hospital able to offer neonatal care. With all drugs, the side-effects on mother and fetus must be balanced against the benefit of prolonging the pregnancy. Tocolysis should not be used for all cases of preterm labour; instances when it might be inadvisable include:

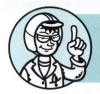 Ritodrine can cause pulmonary oedema, a potentially fatal side-effect.

- Maternal illness that would be helped by delivery, e.g. pre-eclampsia.
- Evidence of fetal distress.
- In the presence of chorioamnionitis.
- When there has been significant vaginal bleeding.
- Once the membranes have ruptured.

Antibiotic therapy

Antibiotics are given prophylactically if the membranes have ruptured before term (around a third of cases) to protect the fetus from ascending infection. If the membranes are intact the mother is screened for infection (vaginal and cervical swabs, blood cultures if pyrexial) and given antibiotics if there are signs of sepsis; prophylactic antibiotics are not indicated.

Cervical cerclage

When there is cervical incompetence resulting in cervical dilatation but the patient is not actively labouring, a suture can be placed in the cervix to attempt to reduce the prolapse of membranes that will otherwise ensue. Once the membranes prolapse into the vagina they weaken and their rupture is likely, followed by delivery or the development of infection. The MacDonald suture, which is inserted vaginally as high in the cervix as possible, is used most commonly (Fig. 38.7). Other options are the Shirodkar suture, which is inserted vaginally but involves the dissection of the bladder off the cervix, and a suture inserted into the cervix at laparotomy, which can be placed higher.

However, insertion of a suture can introduce infection or result in rupture of the membranes during the procedure.

Mode of delivery

The caesarean section rate might be presumed to be higher because of a higher incidence of low-lying

Drugs used to treat preterm labour

Beta-agonists, e.g. ritodrine, salbutamol, terbutaline
Most commonly used tocolytic in UK. Administered as IV infusion. Act on β-receptors in myometrium to cause relaxation. Common side-effects, occurring in up to 80% of mothers, include tachycardia, headache, tremor, nausea and vomiting, hyperglycaemia and hypokalaemia. Similar effects are seen in the fetus. The potentially fatal side-effects pulmonary oedema and myocardial ischaemia occur in around 5% of women

Calcium-channel blockers, e.g. nifedipine
Block calcium channels in the myometrium, interrupting contraction. Given orally. Their effectiveness has been questioned and they have the potential to alter uteroplacental blood flow, causing fetal compromise. Maternal side-effects are less common than with β-agonists but include headache, flushing and tremor

Oxytocin receptor antagonists, e.g. atosiban
This newly developed family of drugs has been proved to delay delivery but not to influence neonatal outcome. Atosiban seems to be well tolerated, with fewer side-effects than other drugs, but is expensive. Given as an intravenous infusion. Side-effects in the mother occur in around 8%, who experiences flushing and headache

Non-steroidal anti-inflammatory drugs (NSAIDs), e.g. indomethacin
NSAIDs are effective tocolytics, acting on the cyclo-oxygenase enzyme that catalyses production of prostaglandin vital for labour. They are cheap and easy to administer orally. Side-effects in the mother are mild, comprising gastrointestinal upset (nausea, heartburn) and headache. However they have potentially serious fetal side-effects, causing premature closure of the ductus arteriosus (which can result in pulmonary hypertension, tricuspid regurgitation and heart failure) and reducing renal function, leading to oligohydramnios. The neonatal complications necrotising enterocolitis (NEC) and intracerebral haemorrhage are also more common. The fetal effects are temporary and the neonatal effects are more common with prolonged administration of the drug, but the fetal morbidity that has been seen in the past has dissuaded clinicians from using NSAIDs

Magnesium sulphate
This competes at calcium channels in the myometrium. Given as IV infusion. Maternal side-effects are uncommon but potentially serious, occurring in around 5% and comprising blurred vision, loss of tendon reflexes and arrhythmias. Fetal and neonatal side-effects include reduced fetal heart rate variability, hypotonia and respiratory depression, and magnesium has been linked to increased perinatal mortality, so it is used with caution

Nitric oxide donors, e.g. glyceryl trinitrate (GTN) patches
Nitric oxide donors act on myometrium in vitro to cause relaxation. They have few side-effects for mother or fetus but their effectiveness in vivo has not been proven.

Fig. 38.6 Drugs used to treat preterm labour.

placenta, fetal distress and abnormal lie in prematurity, but there is also a trend to deliver all preterm babies by caesarean section, although there is no firm evidence to show that this is safer for the baby than vaginal delivery, especially when the presentation is cephalic. Caesarean section might have higher morbidity for the mother when performed at very early gestations because the lower segment is less well formed.

Management of future pregnancies

Any woman who has laboured prematurely is more at risk of doing so again in her next pregnancy. In many

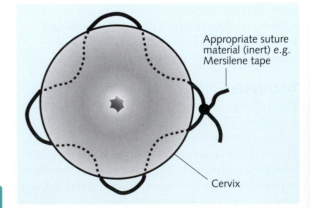

Fig. 38.7 The MacDonald suture.

cases there will be nothing that can be done to prevent this. Exceptions are when:

- Labour has been due to treatable, persistent infection, e.g. bacterial vaginosis.
- There is cervical incompetence.

Where infection has been proved it should be treated and the mother screened regularly for recurrence during subsequent pregnancies and treated as necessary.

Cervical incompetence can be treated by insertion of a cervical suture, either electively in early pregnancy (usually around 12 weeks after the high risk of early miscarriage has passed), or, if the cervix is monitored regularly in pregnancy with transvaginal scanning, when scan shows that the cervix is shortening.

The prescription of prophylactic tocolytics to women at increased risk of recurrent preterm labour is not helpful but some clinicians prescribe prophylactic corticosteroids at a point in the pregnancy before the last baby delivered.

- Between which weeks of pregnancy can labour be said to be premature?
- What is the greatest risk factor for premature labour?
- What is the purpose of antenatal steroid administration, and how are they given?
- What is the fibronectin test?
- What proportion of women presenting with symptoms of preterm labour will deliver on that occasion?

Further reading

Miller AWF & Hanretty KP *Obstetrics Illustrated* (Churchill Livingstone, London)
Smith & Smith *Obstetric Ultrasound Made Easy* (Churchill Livingstone, London)

www.swot.org.uk
www.rcog.org.uk/guidelines
www.update-software.com/cochrane

39. Malpresentation and Malpositions of the Occiput

Malpresentation

Any presentation other than a vertex presentation is a malpresentation. The vertex is the area between the parietal eminences and the anterior and posterior fontanelles. The most common malpresentation is the breech presentation but others include shoulder, brow and face presentations.

Malpresentation can occur by chance but it can also be caused by fetal or maternal conditions that prevent the vertex from presenting to the pelvis (Fig. 39.1). In all cases, management must include exclusion of important conditions such as fetal abnormality, pelvic masses and placenta praevia.

Breech presentation

Apart from the general causes of malpresentation, breech presentation is particularly associated with prematurity. The incidence of breech presentation increases with decreasing gestation:

- Term: 3%.
- 32 weeks: 15%.
- 28 weeks: 25%.

Classification of breech presentation

There are three types of breech presentation:
- Extended or frank breech.
- Flexed or complete breech.
- Footling breech.

Just over half of breech presentations are extended and the remainder are roughly equally divided between flexed and footling. With an extended breech, the hips are flexed and the knees extended with the feet situated adjacent to the fetal head. Flexed and footling breeches are flexed at both the hips and knees, but in the latter the feet present to the maternal pelvis not the breech (Fig. 39.2).

Diagnosis

The head can be felt as a hard lump at the uterine fundus by the examiner and the patient. Auscultation of the fetal heart at a higher level than is usual with a cephalic presentation might suggest a breech presentation, although this is not a reliable sign.

Vaginal examination can confirm the diagnosis, although if there is any doubt ultrasound examination is indicated, which will also determine the type of breech presentation.

Complications

There is an increased perinatal mortality and morbidity associated with vaginal breech delivery when compared with cephalic presentation of comparable birthweight and gestation. This is usually associated with difficulty in delivering the aftercoming head. The fetal trunk is softer than the head and can pass through a borderline pelvis, resulting in entrapment of the aftercoming head. Moulding of the fetal head as it passes through the pelvis can only occur after the body has delivered and in a relatively short period of time. Rapid compression and decompression of the head during delivery can produce intracranial injury. The presence of nuchal arms, that is when the fetal arms are extended posteriorly behind the head and sometimes crossed behind the head in the hollow of the neck, reduces the available space for delivering the aftercoming head. Unfortunately, no method of antenatal assessment – clinical, radiological or ultrasonic – will guarantee easy delivery of the aftercoming head.

Perinatal mortality

Four major causes account for the increased perinatal mortality associated with vaginal breech delivery. The relative importance of these depends on the gestational age of the fetus:

- Prematurity.
- Cord prolapse.
- Birth trauma.
- Congenital anomaly.

There has been a recent move towards more elective caesarean sections in breech presentation because of proven lower perinatal risks.

Cord prolapse can occur if the cervix is poorly applied to the presenting part and is most likely to occur with a footling breech (Fig. 39.3). Birth trauma is associated with difficulty in delivery of the aftercoming head or soft-tissue injury due to excessive traction to the fetus. The causes of death associated with birth trauma following vaginal breech delivery include:

- Intracranial haemorrhage/tentorial tear.
- Spinal cord injury.
- Soft tissue injury.
- Liver rupture.
- Adrenal haemorrhage.

Perinatal morbidity

Morbidity is also usually associated with difficulty in delivering the aftercoming head. Although the morbidity is distressing for all concerned with the delivery, the neonate usually makes a complete recovery. Typical injuries associated with vaginal breech delivery include nerve palsies, fractures and soft tissue injuries (Fig. 39.4).

Management

There are three management options for a breech presentation:

- External cephalic version (ECV).
- Planned vaginal breech delivery.
- Elective caesarean section.

Following the publication of a large, randomized, prospective trial in the *Lancet*, the tendency is now to deliver most breech presentation babies by caesarean section. This trial indicated a significantly

Causes of malpresentation	
Type of cause	**Description**
Maternal	Contraction of the pelvis
	Pelvic tumour
	Mullerian abnormality
	Multiparity
Fetoplacental	Placenta praevia
	Polyhydramnios
	Multiple pregnancy
	Fetal anomaly
	• hydrocephalus
	• extension of the fetal head by neck tumours
	• anencephaly
	• decreased fetal tone

Fig. 39.1 Causes of malpresentation.

Incidence of cord prolapse associated with fetal presentation	
Fetal presentation	**Incidence (%)**
Cephalic	0.5
Extended breech	1.0
Flexed breech	4.0
Footling breech	18.0

Fig. 39.3 Incidence of cord prolapse associated with fetal presentation.

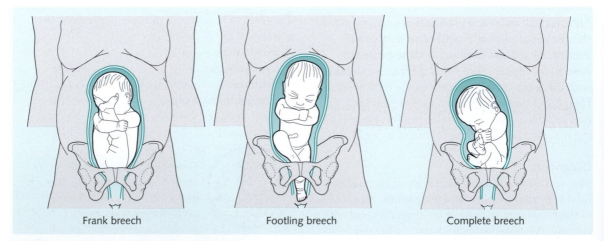

| Frank breech | Footling breech | Complete breech |

Fig. 39.2 Classification of breech presentation.

Fetal injuries associated with vaginal breech delivery	
Type of injury	Description
Nerve palsies	Brachial plexus palsy
	Facial nerve palsy
Fractures	Clavicle
	Upper limb
Soft tissue injury	

Fig. 39.4 Fetal injuries associated with vaginal breech delivery.

lower incidence of complications in term breech babies born by caesarean section than by the vaginal route.

External cephalic version
The fetus is turned to a cephalic presentation by manual manipulation through the maternal anterior abdominal wall. This is now usually performed at around 37 weeks gestation, by which time most breeches will have spontaneously turned. Contraindications to ECV include:

- Pelvic mass.
- Antepartum haemorrhage.
- Placenta praevia.
- Previous caesarean section or hysterotomy.
- Multiple pregnancy.
- Ruptured membranes.

ECV can be performed with the aid of tocolytics, to reduce uterine activity, and under ultrasound control. It should be performed on the labour ward because of the small risk of fetal distress requiring immediate caesarean section (< 1%). The fetus can be rolled forwards or backwards and version is successful in about half the cases. Extended breeches are more difficult to turn because the legs 'splint' the fetus. Rhesus negative women should be given anti-D immunoglobulin following attempted version because of the possibility of fetomaternal transfusion.

Antenatal assessment for vaginal breech delivery
Antenatal assessment for vaginal breech delivery includes assessment of:

- Fetal size.
- The maternal pelvis.

It is important to exclude a macrosomic fetus prior to vaginal breech delivery and this is best done by ultrasound estimated fetal weight (EFW). A fetus with an EFW of greater than 3.8 kg is probably best delivered by caesarean section. Ultrasound EFW at term is associated with an error of at least 10%. Measurement of the pelvic inlet and outlet is rarely performed now because of the inaccuracies and poor predictive value unless there is a significant past history of pelvic injury or rickets.

Management of labour with a breech presentation (Figs 39.5–39.14)
Delivery should be in an obstetric unit with an attendant paediatrician because vaginal breech delivery should be regarded as high risk. Management of the first stage of labour should be as for a vertex presentation, although some obstetricians do not advocate the use of syntocinon in the presence of secondary arrest preferring to perform a caesarean section. Continuous fetal heart rate monitoring is recommended. Exclusion of cord prolapse is mandatory when the membranes rupture or if the fetal heart rate pattern becomes abnormal. Epidural anaesthesia is recommended because of the increased level of manipulation during delivery. In only half of planned vaginal breech deliveries will vaginal delivery be successful because of the lower threshold to perform caesarean section.

During the second stage, the breech should be allowed to descend onto the pelvic floor before active pushing is commenced. If descent does not occur this could indicate disproportion or an unexpectedly large fetus, and caesarean section is indicated. Delivery in the lithotomy position allows access for the attendant to perform any necessary manipulation to the fetus. Routine episiotomy is recommended to further increase access and prevent delay due to the soft tissues. Two procedures are particularly valuable in the delivery of a breech presentation:

- Lovset's manoeuvre.
- The Mauriceau–Smellie–Veit manoeuvre.

Lovset's manoeuvre
Lovset's manoeuvre is used when the arms are extended. Grasping the fetal pelvis and upper thighs, gentle downwards traction is applied until the anterior shoulder lies behind the symphysis pubis and the inferior border of the scapula is visible. This allows the posterior shoulder to descend into the pelvic cavity. With the back uppermost, the fetal trunk is rotated through 180° to bring the posterior shoulder to an anterior position under the pubic arch. If the arm does not deliver spontaneously it is easily delivered using a finger. The posterior shoulder will now be situated in the sacral curve and, again with

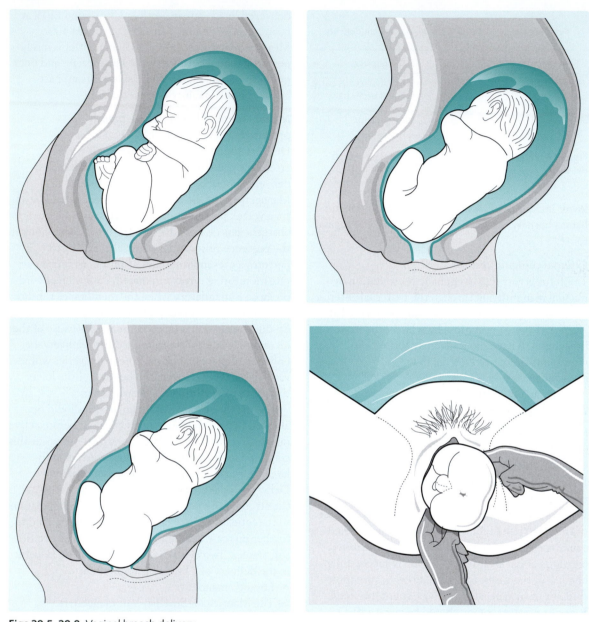

Figs 39.5–39.8 Vaginal breech delivery.

the back uppermost, the fetal trunk is rotated 180° in the opposite direction to bring the posterior shoulder anteriorly to lie under the pubic arch. The second arm will then deliver easily.

As soon as the trunk has been delivered, the fetal circulation will be compromised because the head will be compressing the cord at the level of the pelvic brim. Delivery of the head is therefore necessary in a matter of minutes to avoid asphyxia. The body of the fetus should be allowed to hang downwards while the head descends into the pelvis. The head usually enters the pelvis transversely and, during descent, undergoes rotation until the occiput lies beneath the pubic arch. If the head does not rotate and descend then the Mauriceau–Smellie–Veit manoeuvre can be used (often remembered as the 'smelly feet' manoeuvre by students!).

The Mauriceau–Smellie–Veit manoeuvre
This manoeuvre maintains flexion of the head as downwards traction is applied. With the body of the fetus lying on the attendant's lower arm, and with

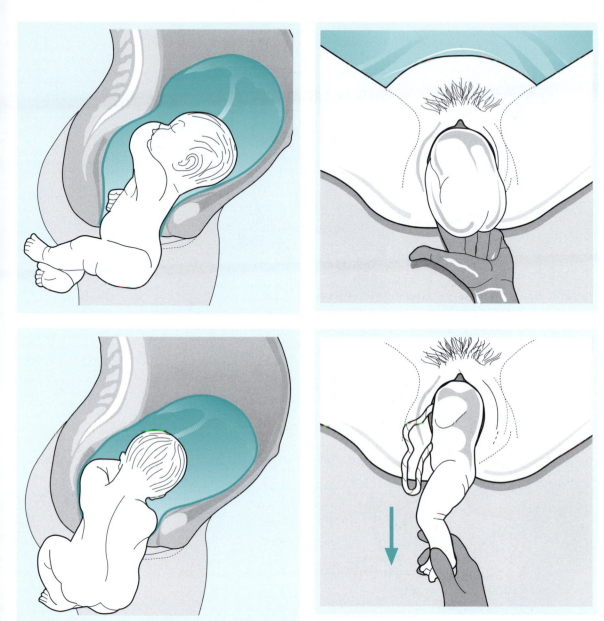

Figs 39.9–39.12 Vaginal breech delivery—cont'd.

the fingers of this arm in the vagina, the middle finger is used to apply pressure on the fetal jaw or gently inserted in the mouth to flex the fetal head. The index and middle finger of the other hand are placed over the fetal shoulders and used to apply downwards traction until the occiput lies under the pubic arch. The fetal legs are then grasped and elevated, extending the back and, by further gentle pressure on the fetal jaw, continuing flexion of the head allows delivery. Forceps can also be used to deliver the aftercoming head.

Elective caesarean section for breech presentation

The majority of breeches are now delivered by caesarean section, either emergency or elective. Some of the indications for elective caesarean section include:

- Footling breech.
- Maternal request.
- Ultrasound EFW > 3.8kg.
- Suboptimal pelvimetry.
- Failed ECV.
- Twins, where the first twin presents by the breech.

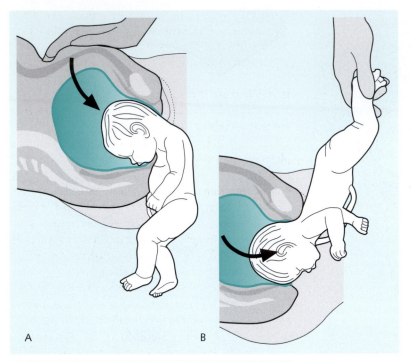

A   B

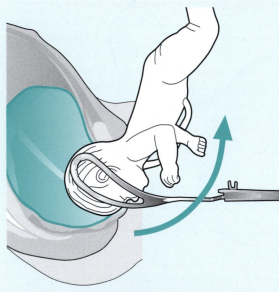

Figs 39.13–39.14 Vaginal breech delivery—cont'd.

- 'Breech plus another complication' (e.g. pregnancy-induced hypertension, previous caesarean section, diabetes mellitus).

As more and more breeches are delivered abdominally, gaining the required skills and experience needed for vaginal breech delivery is more difficult and it is likely that in the future we will see even fewer breeches delivered vaginally. Some would argue that this is not necessarily a retrograde step, particularly in light of the recent data.

Transverse lie and unstable lie

A transverse lie occurs when the long axis of the fetus lies transverse or oblique to the long axis of the uterus, usually with the shoulder presenting (Fig. 39.15). When the fetal lie is different at each palpation, the lie is said to be unstable.

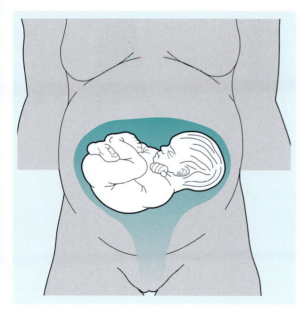

Fig. 39.15 Transverse lie.

The incidence of transverse lie diagnosed in labour with a single fetus is approximately 1 in 500 women but many more will have been identified and managed appropriately antenatally.

The causes of transverse lie include the general causes of malpresentation shown in Fig. 39.1 but there is particular association with:

- Multiparity, where the tone of the uterus and anterior abdominal wall is poor.
- Premature labour.
- The second twin.

The diagnosis of a transverse lie is usually made antenatally and the findings on abdominal palpation include the:

- Fetal head palpable laterally in the maternal abdomen.
- Fundal height being lower, and the uterus wider, than expected.

Vaginal examination, which should be avoided until placenta praevia has been excluded, will reveal an empty pelvis.

The most serious complication of a transverse lie is cord prolapse, and this is associated with spontaneous rupture of membranes, which can occur antenatally or in labour. As the shoulder usually presents, the arm can prolapse and, in an unsupervised situation, obstructed labour, infection

and uterine rupture can occur. Treatment depends on the situation at the time of diagnosis and is aimed at:

- Correcting the malpresentation.
- Avoiding serious complications.

If the diagnosis is made antenatally, exclusion of causes of malpresentation is important. Elective abdominal delivery at or approaching term is indicated in the presence of pelvic contraction, placenta praevia or a pelvic mass. In their absence, ECV can be attempted. If reversion to a malpresentation occurs, or an unstable lie is diagnosed, then admission to hospital from 37 weeks gestation is indicated when immediate delivery is possible if the membranes spontaneously rupture. At term, an unstable lie can be managed expectantly because spontaneous version to a cephalic presentation often occurs due to the increase in uterine activity. Transverse lie can be corrected by ECV followed by induction of labour. If the lie remains unstable then caesarean section is indicated.

If a transverse lie is diagnosed in early labour, ECV should be attempted only if the membranes are intact. If successful, ARM with the head in the pelvis can stabilize the lie by inducing uterine contractions. If version is not successful or the membranes have ruptured, caesarean section is indicated.

Following delivery of the first twin, if the second twin lies transversely the membranes must not be ruptured until external version to a longitudinal lie has been performed. When the presenting part has descended into the pelvis, ARM can be performed and vaginal delivery expected.

Face presentation

The incidence of face presentation is 1 in 300 labours and occurs when the head is fully extended (Fig. 39.16).

The causes of extension of the fetal head include congenital tumours of the neck but these are rare. Face presentation is more likely to occur when a normal fetus holds its head in an extended position. Historically, anencephaly is associated with face presentation but is now rare due to increased prenatal diagnosis and termination of pregnancy.

Diagnosis is usually made during vaginal examination in labour when the supraorbital ridges, the bridge of the nose and the alveolar margins in the mouth are palpable (Fig. 39.17). During labour, the face becomes oedematous and might be mistaken for a breech presentation.

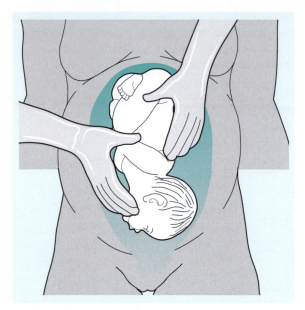

Fig. 39.16 Face presentation.

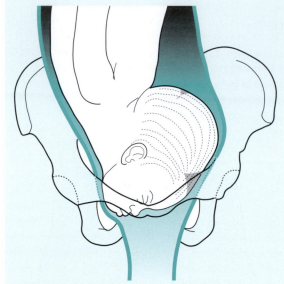

Fig. 39.18 Vaginal delivery of face presentation.

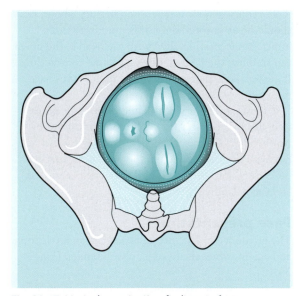

Fig. 39.17 Vaginal examination findings in face presentation.

Face presentation will deliver vaginally if it is mentoanterior but not if it is mentoposterior.

Management of a face presentation in labour is essentially the same as for a vertex presentation. Vaginal examination should be performed when the membranes rupture to exclude a cord prolapse. Mentoposterior positions rotate spontaneously to mentoanterior in 50% of cases, usually in the second stage of labour, and in those that do not a caesarean section is indicated. Caesarean section should also be performed when the fetal heart rate pattern is abnormal because a fetal blood sample for pH measurement should not be taken from the face. Traction forceps can be applied to a mentoanterior position to correct delay in the second stage.

The face is nearly always swollen and bruised following a face presentation and the parents should be warned about this. Care must be taken during vaginal examination because the fetal eyes can be damaged by trauma or antiseptic lotions.

Brow presentation

The incidence of brow presentation is approximately 1 in 500 labours and the causes are the same as for a face presentation.

Mechanism of labour

The chin (mentum) is the denominator and in 75% of cases the position is mentoanterior. The submentobregmatic diameter is 9.5 cm so vaginal delivery is possible. Vaginal delivery occurs by flexion of the head, which is possible only in the mentoanterior position (Fig. 39.18).

Brow presentation should be suspected on abdominal palpation when there is prominence of the head on the side of the back in the presence of an unengaged head. Vaginal examination reveals a high presenting part, a palpable forehead with orbital ridges in front and the anterior fontanelle behind.

Mechanism of labour

The membranes tend to rupture early in labour and there is an increased risk of cord prolapse. With a brow presentation, the mentovertical diameter – one of the longest diameters of the fetal head (13 cm) – presents. An average-sized fetus will not engage with a normal-sized pelvis and obstructed labour results. When the fetal head is small in relation to the maternal pelvis descent might occur, allowing flexion of the head as it hits the pelvic floor.

In the absence of disproportion, labour should be allowed to continue. Further extension might occur to a face presentation or flexion to a vertex position.

Malposition

The fetal head normally engages in an occipitotransverse position. With descent, the head rotates to an occipitoanterior position, presenting the narrowest diameter for delivery through the outlet. Any position that does not follow this pattern is regarded as a malposition; the two most important being:

• Occipitoposterior position.
• Deep transverse arrest.

Theoretically, brow and face presentations could be regarded as malpositions but they are more commonly regarded as malpresentations.

Occipitoposterior position

In approximately 20% of women in early labour the fetus will present with an occipitoposterior (OP) position.

Anthropoid and android pelves, which have an anteroposterior diameter equal to or greater than the transverse diameter, predispose to an OP position. An anterior placenta is said to be associated with OP position.

An OP position is the most common cause of an unengaged head at term in a primigravida. Abdominal palpation reveals:

• A prominent fundus.
• A lower abdomen that is flattened or concave.
• A fetal back that can be palpated posteriorly.
• Fetal limbs that can be palpated anteriorly.

In labour, vaginal examination will ascertain the position by identifying the sutures and fontanelles. If the anterior fontanelle is at all palpable vaginally then the head is deflexed. If only the posterior fontanelle can be palpated then the head is well flexed. The degree of flexion of the head is important in the mechanism of labour.

Mechanism of labour

If the occipitofrontal diameter (11.5 cm) presents to a borderline pelvis then engagement will not occur, resulting in an obstructed labour requiring caesarean section. If the pelvis is adequate and the fetus not macrosomic, the mechanism of labour with an OP position depends on the degree of flexion of the fetal head. When the head is well flexed, rotation to an anterior position usually occurs as the occiput hits the pelvic floor first and rotates forward. When the head is deflexed, a persistent OP position is usual, although delivery in an OP position ('face to pubes') is possible if the pelvis is large enough.

Face-to-pubes delivery of an OP position is possible but rotation and OA delivery is usually preferable because this allows better flexion of the head and therefore less perineal trauma.

The first stage of labour should be managed in the normal way. During the second stage, if the head rotates anteriorly normal delivery can be anticipated. An episiotomy is recommended if the fetus is delivered face to pubes because a wider diameter presents and increases the risk of severe perineal trauma. If rotation fails to occur spontaneously, this can be achieved using the following techniques:

• Manual rotation.
• Kielland's rotational forceps.
• Ventouse extraction with spontaneous rotation.

Excluding those women who require caesarean section for cephalopelvic disproportion, the outcome for an OP position in labour is as follows:

223

- 70% rotate and spontaneously deliver occipitoanterior.
- 10% fail to rotate and deliver OP (face to pubes).
- 20% need assistance with rotation (manual, ventouse extraction or rotational forceps).

Deep transverse arrest

Deep transverse arrest is said to have occurred when a poorly flexed head arrests in the transverse position at the level of the ischial spines.

Deep transverse arrest usually occurs when a transverse position fails to rotate to an anterior position. The head is neither flexed enough for the occiput nor extended enough for the brow to influence rotation. An android pelvis, where the side walls are convergent, can prevent descent of the head to the pelvic floor, where rotation normally occurs.

Diagnosis is by vaginal examination in the presence of failure to progress in the second stage of labour. The head is at the level of the ischial spines, the sagittal suture is in the transverse position and both anterior and posterior fontanelles are usually palpable.

Rotation is required and can be achieved either manually or by rotational forceps. The fetal head should not be rotated in the presence of fetal acidosis because intraventricular haemorrhage might be precipitated. Caesarean section is indicated in this situation.

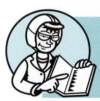

- What is the difference between a malposition and a malpresentation?
- What are the possible reasons for a malpresentation?
- What are the different types of breech presentation and what are their relative risks with regards to vaginal delivery.?

Further reading

Hannah et al (2000) 'Planned caesarean section versus planned vaginal birth for breech presentation at term: a randomized multicentre trial' 356 (9239): 1368-9, *Lancet*

40. Labour

Labour is divided into three stages:
- First stage: from the onset of established labour until the cervix is fully dilated.
- Second stage: from full dilatation until the fetus is born.
- Third stage: from the birth of the fetus until delivery of the placenta and membranes.

Onset of labour

Prior to the onset of labour, painless intermittent uterine tightenings, known as Braxton Hicks contractions, become increasingly frequent. As the presenting part becomes engaged, the fundus descends, reducing upper abdominal discomfort, and pressure in the pelvis increases. The signs and symptoms that define the actual onset of labour are:
- Painful regular contractions.
- A 'show' (passage of a mucoid plug from the cervix, often blood-stained).
- Rupture of the membranes.
- Cervical dilatation and effacement.

Labour is diagnosed when there are regular painful contractions in the presence of an effaced cervix, which is 3 cm or more dilated, with or without a show or ruptured membranes.

The exact cause of the onset of labour is not known. To some degree it might be mechanical, because preterm labour is seen more commonly in circumstances in which the uterus is overstretched, such as multiple pregnancies and polyhydramnios. Prostaglandins might play a role; they are thought to be present in the decidua and membranes in late pregnancy and are released if the cervix is digitally stretched at term to separate the membranes (a cervical sweep).

Progress in labour

Once the diagnosis of labour has been made, progress is assessed by monitoring:

- Uterine contractions.
- Dilatation of the cervix.
- Descent of the presenting part.

The rate of cervical dilatation is expected to be approx 1 cm/h in a nulliparous woman and approx 2 cm/h in a multiparous woman. A partogram is commonly used to chart the observations made in labour (Fig. 40.1) and to highlight slow progress, particularly a delay in cervical dilatation or failure of the presenting part to descend (see Chapter 15).

Progress is determined by the three factors:
- Passages.
- Passenger.
- Powers.

Passages
Bony pelvis
The pelvis is made up of four bones, the:
- Two innominate bones.
- Sacrum.
- Coccyx.

The passage that these bones make can be divided into inlet, cavity and outlet (Fig. 40.2). The pelvic inlet is bounded by the pubic crest, the iliopectineal line and the sacral promontory. It is oval in shape, with its longest diameter being transverse. The cavity of the pelvis is round in shape. The pelvic outlet is bounded by the lower border of the pubic symphysis, the ischial spines and the tip of the sacrum. Again the shape is oval, but with the larger diameter being anteroposterior (Fig. 40.3).

When a woman stands upright, the pelvis tilts forward. The inlet makes an angle of about 55° with the horizontal; this varies between individuals and different ethnic groups. The presenting part of the fetus must negotiate the axis of the birth canal with the change of direction occurring by rotation at the pelvic floor.

Soft tissues
The soft passages consist of:
- Uterus (upper and lower segments).
- Cervix.

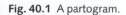

Fig. 40.1 A partogram.

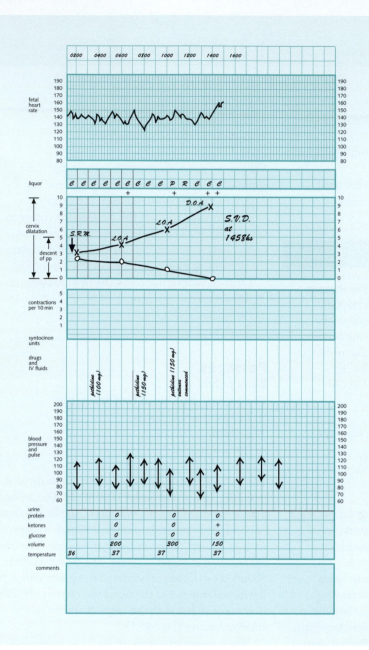

- Pelvic floor.
- Vagina.
- Perineum.

The upper uterine segment consists mainly of the fundus and is responsible for the propulsive contractions that deliver the fetus. The lower segment is the part of the uterus that lies between the uterovesical fold of the peritoneum and the cervix. It develops gradually during the third trimester, and then more rapidly during labour, incorporating the cervix, to allow the presenting part to descend.

The pelvic floor consists of the levator ani group of muscles, including pubococcygeus and iliococcygeus arising from the bony pelvis to form a muscular

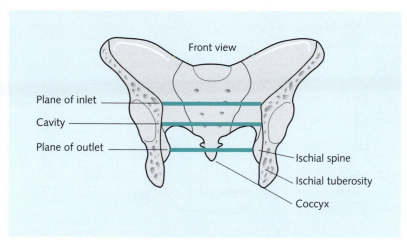

Fig. 40.2 The bony pelvis.

Front view

Plane of inlet

Cavity

Plane of outlet

Ischial spine

Ischial tuberosity

Coccyx

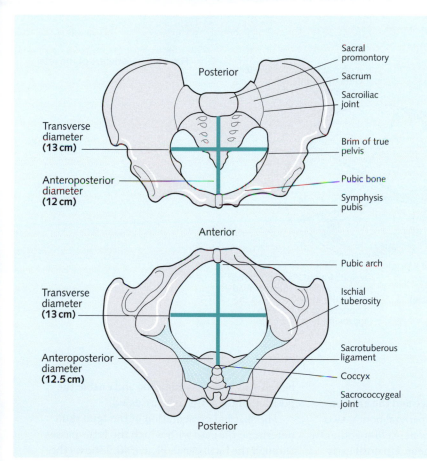

Fig. 40.3 The dimensions of the pelvic inlet and the pelvic outlet.

Posterior

Sacral promontory

Sacrum

Sacroiliac joint

Transverse diameter (13 cm)

Brim of true pelvis

Anteroposterior diameter (12 cm)

Pubic bone

Symphysis pubis

Anterior

Pubic arch

Transverse diameter (13 cm)

Ischial tuberosity

Anteroposterior diameter (12.5 cm)

Sacrotuberous ligament

Coccyx

Sacrococcygeal joint

Posterior

diaphragm along with the internal obturator muscle and piriformis muscle (see Chapter 27). As the presenting part of the fetus is pushed out of the uterus it passes into the vagina, which has become hypertrophied during pregnancy. It hits the pelvic floor, which acts like a gutter to direct it forwards and allow rotation. The perineum is distal to this and stretches as the head passes below the pubic arch and delivers.

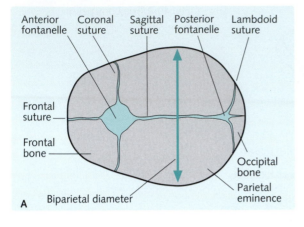

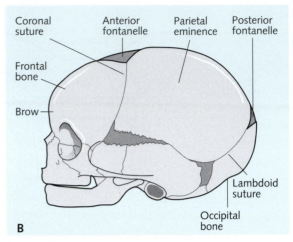

Fig. 40.4 The fetal skull from above (A) and from the side (B), showing the landmarks.

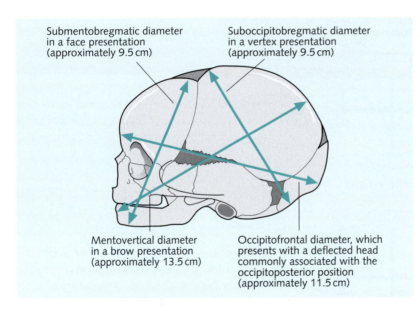

Submentobregmatic diameter in a face presentation (approximately 9.5 cm)

Suboccipitobregmatic diameter in a vertex presentation (approximately 9.5 cm)

Mentovertical diameter in a brow presentation (approximately 13.5 cm)

Occipitofrontal diameter, which presents with a deflected head commonly associated with the occipitoposterior position (approximately 11.5 cm)

Fig. 40.5 Diameters of the fetal skull.

Passenger

The fetal skull consists of the face and the cranium. The cranium is made up of two parietal bones, two frontal bones and the occipital bone, held together by a membrane that allows movement. Up until early childhood, these bones are not fused and so can overlap to allow the head to pass through the pelvis during labour; this overlapping of the bones is known as moulding.

Figure 40.4 shows the anatomy of the fetal skull, including the sutures between the bones, and the fontanelles. These are important landmarks that can

be felt on vaginal examination and enable the position of the fetus to be assessed.

The size and presentation of the fetal skull determine the ease with which the fetus passes through the birth canal. Figure 40.5 shows the diameters of the fetal skull; the one that presents during labour depends on the degree of flexion of the head, thus the suboccipitobregmatic diameter represents a flexed vertex presentation, giving the smallest diameter for delivery, along with the submentobregmatic diameter, which corresponds to a face presentation. The widest diameter is the

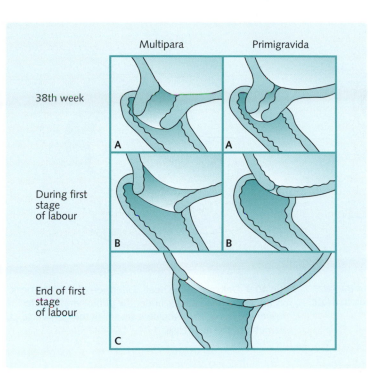

Multipara · Primigravida

38th week — A · A

During first stage of labour — B · B

End of first stage of labour — C

Fig. 40.6 Dilatation and effacement of the cervix in late pregnancy and labour.

mentovertical one, a brow presentation, which usually precludes vaginal delivery.

Power

The myometrial component of the uterus acts as the power to deliver the fetus. It consists of three layers, a:

- Thin outer longitudinal layer.
- Thin inner circular layer.
- Thick middle spiral layer.

From early pregnancy, the uterus contracts painlessly and intermittently (Braxton Hicks contractions). These contractions increase after the 36th week until the onset of labour. Each contraction starts from the junction of the fallopian tube and the uterus on one side, spreading down and across the uterus with its greatest intensity in the upper uterine segment.

During labour, the contractions are monitored for:

- Intensity.
- Frequency.
- Duration.

The resting tone of the uterus is about 6–12 mmHg; to be effective in labour this increases to an intensity of 40–60 mmHg. There should be three or four coordinated contractions every 10 min; each lasting 60–90 s.

In the second stage of labour, additional power comes from voluntary contraction of the diaphragm and the abdominal muscles as the mother pushes to assist delivery.

Mechanisms of normal delivery: action of the uterus

The myometrium acts like all muscle, that is, it contracts and relaxes, but it also has the ability to retract so that the fibres become progressively shorter. This effect is seen in the upper segment muscle: progressive retraction causes the lower segment to stretch and thin out, resulting in effacement and dilatation of the cervix (Fig. 40.6).

Delivery of the fetus

Active contractions of the uterus of increasing strength, frequency and duration cause passive movement of the fetus down the birth canal. At the beginning of labour, the lie, presentation and engagement of the fetus are assessed (see Chapter 46). As labour progresses (Fig. 40.7), the neck becomes fully flexed so that the

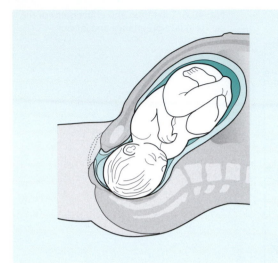

Fig. 40.7 Early labour. There has been flexion of the fetal head. The cervix is effaced but has not yet begun to dilate.

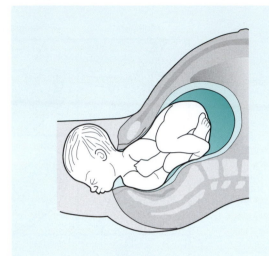

Fig. 40.9 Delivery of the head. Extension of the fetal neck occurs as the head passes under the pubic symphysis to deliver the head. The shoulders are still in the transverse diameter of the midpelvis.

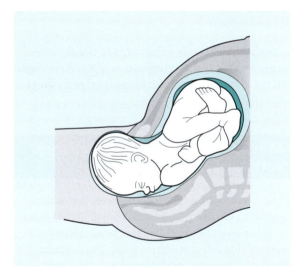

Fig. 40.8 The second stage of labour. The head has undergone internal rotation to bring the occiput into the anterior position. The cervix is fully dilated.

and the movement of extension pushes the head forward and delivers the occiput. Increasing extension round the pubic bone delivers the face (Fig. 40.9).

Delivery of the head brings the shoulders into the pelvic cavity, with the head oblique to the line of the shoulders. Restitution occurs: the head rotates to the natural position in relation to the shoulders (Fig. 40.10). Finally, in the process of external rotation, continuing descent and rotation of the shoulders brings their widest diameter (the bisacromial diameter) into the anteroposterior diameter of the pelvic outlet. This enables the anterior shoulder to pass under the pubis. Lateral flexion of the fetus delivers the posterior shoulder and the rest of the body follows (Fig. 40.11).

suboccipitobregmatic diameter is presenting (see above).

Descent occurs when the head is engaged, followed by internal rotation to bring the occiput into the anterior position when it reaches the pelvic floor. In the second stage of labour, the occiput descends below the symphysis pubis (Fig. 40.8)

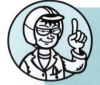

Mechanism of delivery of the fetus:
- Flexion.
- Internal rotation.
- Extension.
- External rotation (restitution).

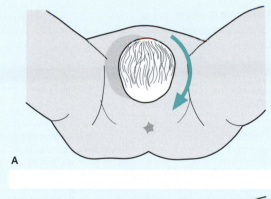

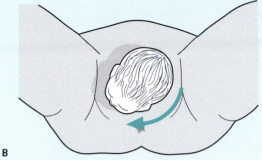

Fig. 40.10 External rotation (restitution). The head distends the perineum as it delivers in the occipitoanterior position and the external rotation occurs.

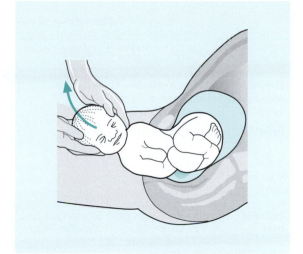

Fig. 40.11 Delivery of the shoulders. The anterior shoulder passes below the pubic symphysis, aided by downwards and backwards traction of the head from the midwife. The posterior shoulder delivers as the head is gently lifted upwards.

Management of the first stage of labour

When a patient presents in the first stage of labour, routine assessment includes:

- Mother: pulse, blood pressure, temperature, urinalysis, analgesia requirements.
- Fetus: presentation and engagement of the presenting part, fetal heart rate pattern (see Chapter 16).

- Contractions: frequency, duration, intensity.
- Vaginal examination: degree of cervical effacement, cervical dilatation, station of presenting part above ischial spines, position of presenting part, presence of caput or moulding.
- Liquor: clear/blood-stained, presence of meconium.

Maternal monitoring

The patient is encouraged to mobilize if possible and might be allowed to eat, depending on her risk of needing an operative procedure. There is delayed gastric emptying during pregnancy and labour and therefore a risk of inhalation of regurgitated acid stomach contents, causing Mendelson's syndrome if the patient is given a general anaesthetic.

The need for analgesia during labour varies markedly between different women, different ethnic groups and depending on their antenatal preparation. Non-pharmacological techniques include the use of psychoprophylaxis, hypnosis, massage and transcutaneous electrical nerve stimulation (TENS). The pharmacological methods are summarized in Fig. 40.12.

Fetal monitoring

Different degrees of fetal monitoring are appropriate, depending on the clinical picture. For

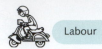

	Technique	Indication	Effectiveness	Duration of effect	Side-effects
Pharmacological methods of analgesia in labour					
Oxygen/ nitrous oxide	Inhalation of 50:50 mixture with onset of contraction	First stage	< 50% Takes 20–30 s for peak effect	Time of inhalation only	Does not relieve pain
Pethidine	Intramuscular injection 100–150 mg	First stage	<50% Takes 15–20 min for peak effect	Approximately 3 h	Nausea and vomiting – give with an antiemetic Respiratory depression in the neonate (this is easily reversed with intramuscular naloxone)
Pudendal block	Infiltration of right and left pudendal nerves (S2, S3 and S4) with 0.5% lidocaine	Second stage for operative delivery	Within 5 min	45–90 min	—
Perineal infiltration	Infiltration of perineum with 0.5% lidocaine at posterior fourchette	Second stage prior to episiotomy Third stage for suturing of perineal lacerations	Within 5 min	45–90 min	—
Epidural anaesthesia	Injection of 0.25% or 0.5% bupivicaine via a catheter into the epidural space (L3–4)	First or second stage Caesarean section	Complete pain relief in approximately 95% of women	Bolus injection every 3–4 h or continuous infusion	Transient hypotension – give intravenous fluid load Dural tap Risk of haemorrhage if abnormal maternal clotting Increased length of second stage because of reduced pelvic floor tone and loss of bearing-down reflex
Spinal anaesthesia	Injection of 0.5% bupivicaine into the subarachnoid space	Any operative delivery; manual removal of the placenta	Immediate effect	Single injection lasting 3–4 h	Respiratory depression

Fig. 40.12 Pharmacological methods of analgesia in labour.

example, in a high-risk pregnancy such as the presence of IUGR or if there is meconium-stained liquor, then continuous fetal monitoring is advisable (see Chapter 16). In a low-risk pregnancy, intermittent monitoring – either electronically or with a Pinard stethoscope – might be sufficient, approximately every 15 min during and after a contraction.

In some patients, abdominal monitoring can be difficult, for example, if the patient is obese, and so a fetal scalp electrode can be applied directly once the membranes are ruptured. If monitoring suggests that the fetal heart rate pattern is abnormal, it might be appropriate to measure the fetal pH by taking a blood sample from the fetal scalp (see Chapter 16).

Management of the second stage of labour

Once the cervix is fully dilated, the patient is encouraged to use voluntary effort to push with the contractions. If she has an epidural anaesthetic in situ she might be unaware of an urge to push, and so a further hour can be allowed for the presenting part to descend with the contractions alone.

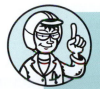

Descent of the presenting part is assessed by abdominal palpation (amount of head felt above the brim expressed in fifths—see below) and vaginal examination (descent in relation to level of ischial spines):
- 0/5   head not palpable
- 1/5   sinciput felt
- 2/5   head engaged
- 3/5   occiput felt
- 4/5   head just entering pelvic brim
- 5/5   head completely palpable above brim

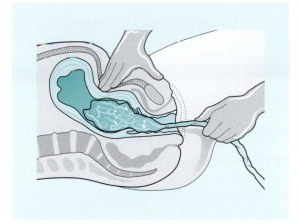

Fig. 40.13 Controlled cord traction to deliver the placenta.

Delivery of the infant is conducted as a sterile procedure, in the left lateral or dorsal position. As the head descends, the perineum distends and the anus dilates. Then the head crowns: the biparietal diameter has passed through the pelvis and there is no recession between contractions. The attendant applies pressure on the perineum to maintain flexion of the head and, once the occiput is free, encourages extension to allow delivery. The neck is felt to exclude the presence of the cord.

After external rotation, lateral flexion of the head towards the anus dislodges the anterior shoulder with the next contraction. Lifting the head in the opposite direction delivers the posterior shoulder. Holding the shoulders, the rest of the body is delivered either onto the bed or the mother's abdomen. Finally, the cord is divided and cut.

Management of the third stage of labour

Active management of the third stage has been shown to reduce the incidence of postpartum haemorrhage (see Chapter 42). Management involves:
- Using an oxytocic drug.
- Clamping and cutting the cord.
- Controlled cord traction.

In most units, syntometrine (5 units of oxytocin plus 0.5 mg of ergometrine) is given with delivery of the anterior shoulder; it takes about 2–3 min to act. As the placenta detaches from the uterine wall, it descends into the lower segment and the cut cord will appear to lengthen. There is slight bleeding and the fundus becomes hard. Brandt-Andrews' method of controlled cord traction is commonly used once the placenta has separated to reduce the incidence of uterine inversion (Fig. 40.13). The placenta and membranes must be checked to ensure that they are complete.

Finally, the vagina, labia and perineum are examined for lacerations. The uterine fundus is palpated to check that it is well contracted, approximately at the level of the umbilicus. The estimated blood loss should be recorded.

Induction of labour

Definition
Induction of labour is the artificial initiation of uterine contractions prior to spontaneous onset resulting in delivery of the baby.

Indications
The rate of induction varies widely between different units and even within different units. Figure 40.14 shows possible reasons for induction of labour, maternal or fetal. In the UK, the most common indication is prolonged pregnancy.

233

Indications for the induction of labour	
Type of indication	**Description**
Maternal	Severe pre-eclampsia
	Diabetes
	Social
Fetal	Prolonged pregnancy
	Intrauterine growth restriction
	Rhesus disease

Fig. 40.14 Indications for the induction of labour.

Amniotomy and oxytocin associated complications	
Treatment	**Complication**
Amniotomy	Cord prolapse
	Infection
	Bleeding from a vasa praevia
	Placental separation
	Failure to induce efficient contractions
	Amniotic fluid embolism
Oxytocin	Abnormal fetal heart rate pattern
	Hyperstimulation of the uterus
	Rupture of the uterus
	Water intoxication

Fig. 40.15 Complications associated with the use of amniotomy and oxytocin.

Methods

Prior to induction of labour, the favourability of the cervix should be assessed to give an indication of the likely success of the procedure. This is usually done by using the Bishop score (see Chapter 46); a higher score suggests a more favourable cervix.

With regards to the Bishop score to assess the cervix :
- Unfavourable cervix = hard, long, closed, not effaced (low Bishop score).
- Favourable cervix = soft, beginning to dilate and efface (high Bishop score).

Prostaglandins

Local application of a prostaglandin, usually prostaglandin E2, given as a vaginal gel, has been shown to ripen the cervix as part of the induction process and reduce the incidence of operative delivery when compared to use of oxytocin alone (see below). Used locally, the gastrointestinal side-effects are minimized. Strict guidelines have been produced to restrict the dose of prostaglandin given, to reduce the risk of uterine hyperstimulation.

Amniotomy

Artificial rupture of the membranes is thought to cause local secretion of endogenous prostaglandins and thus is performed using an amnihook. It might be part of the induction process, or accelerate slow progress in labour. It can also be done with an abnormal CTG to exclude meconium-staining of the liquor, or to apply a fetal scalp electrode.

Oxytocin

An intravenous infusion of synthetic oxytocin (syntocinon) is commonly used to induce labour, to stimulate contractions after amniotomy. The dose must be carefully titrated according to the strength and frequency of the uterine contractions, and continuous fetal monitoring is necessary. Uses of oxytocin include:
- To augment labour after spontaneous rupture of the membranes without the onset of contractions.
- In primary dysfunctional labour (see below).

Complications

Figure 40.15 lists the possible complications associated with the use of amniotomy and oxytocin.

Failure to progress in labour

As described above, progress in labour is related to the passages, the passenger (i.e. the baby) and the power.

The diagnosis of labour is made in the presence of regular contractions, with the cervix fully effaced and at least 3 cm dilated. There might also be a show or ruptured membranes.

Causes of abnormalities of the bony pelvis	
Type of cause	**Description**
Congenital	Osteogenesis imperfecta
	Ectopia vesicae
	Dislocation of the hip
Acquired	Kyphosis of the thoracic or lumbar spine
	Scoliosis of the spine
	Spondylolisthesis
	Pelvic fractures
	Rickets/osteomalacia
	Poliomyelitis in childhood

Fig. 40.16 Causes of abnormalities of the bony pelvis.

Failure to progress related to the bony pelvis
Abnormal bony shape

Antenatal X-ray pelvimetry and routine pelvic assessment by vaginal examination are no longer commonplace. However, certain points in a patient's history and examination can give clues to the likelihood of failure to progress in labour (Fig. 40.16).

Cephalopelvic disproportion

With cephalopelvic disporportion (CPD), the size of the pelvis is not in proportion to the fetus. It should be suspected antenatally if the head does not engage, particularly in a woman of short stature. Usually, a trial of labour is still appropriate but in some cases an elective caesarean section is planned.

During labour, CPD is diagnosed if the head remains high on abdominal palpation. This is confirmed on vaginal examination by the relationship of the head to the ischial spines (known as the station) and the presence of caput (swelling under the fetal scalp caused by reduction in venous return) and moulding.

Failure to progress related to the soft tissues of the pelvis
Uterus

A uterine malformation, such as the presence of a midline septum, might prevent the fetus from lying longitudinally, so that a malpresentation is responsible for failure to progress. This can also be caused by uterine fibroids, which often increase in size during pregnancy and might obstruct labour; a cervical fibroid might even necessitate caesarean section.

Cervix

Failure of the cervix to dilate during labour despite adequate uterine contractions may be secondary to cervical scarring causing cervical stenosis. This could be the result of cervical amputation or cone biopsy.

Vagina

Congenital anomalies of the vagina rarely cause problems with respect to labour and delivery, except for patients who have had reconstructive surgery. Other types of surgery, such as a colposuspension for urinary stress incontinence or repair of a vesicovaginal fistula, might indicate the need for an elective caesarean section at term, but more to prevent recurrent symptoms than because of possible slow progress in labour.

Vulva

Previous perineal tears or episiotomy should not present difficulties during delivery. More problematic is a female circumcision, which usually necessitates an elective episiotomy to prevent more severe tears and the risk of fistula formation.

Ovary

Ovarian cysts in pregnancy are usually incidental findings at routine ultrasound. They can present with abdominal pain during pregnancy, secondary to torsion or haemorrhage (see Chapter 12). Rarely, they cause slow progress in labour if they fail to rise up out of the pelvis as the uterus increases in size.

Failure to progress related to the passenger
Fetal size

The possibility of a large infant might be suggested by the patient's past medical history, for example, insulin-dependent diabetes or from the antenatal history, with development of gestational diabetes or hydrops fetalis secondary to rhesus isoimmunization or parvovirus infection (see Chapter 11).

Abdominal palpation is not particularly accurate as a method of diagnosing a large baby, although it should be suspected if the presenting part fails to engage in labour. Ultrasound is more accurate, provided that gestational age has been correctly estimated early in pregnancy. During labour, signs of cephalopelvic disproportion may indicate a large infant (see above).

Fetal abnormality

Routine ultrasound scanning is likely to diagnose abnormalities such as a congenital goitre or a lymphangioma. These extend the neck, resulting in a face presentation. Abdominal enlargement such as in the presence of ascites or an umbilical hernia may make delivery difficult.

Abnormalities of the fetal skull such as anencephaly should be suspected in labour if the head does not engage and the sutures feel widely spaced on vaginal examination.

Fetal malposition

Labour is more prolonged if the occiput is in the posterior or transverse (OP or OT) position. This can be determined abdominally by easy palpation of fetal parts and confirmed on vaginal examination by checking the positions of the sutures and fontanelles (see Chapter 46).

Fetal malpresentation

Malpresentation of the fetus is defined as a non-vertex presentation (see Chapter 39). This can be:

- Face.
- Brow.
- Breech.
- Shoulder.

Failure to progress related to the power

Uterine palpation monitors frequency, duration and intensity of the contractions. The cardiotocograph checks the frequency and duration but the recording of the intensity can be altered by position of the monitor on the abdomen and maternal obesity. In some centres, intrauterine pressure catheters are used to monitor contraction pressure. Inefficient uterine action can be diagnosed if labour is prolonged and the contractions are:

- Uncoordinated.
- Fewer than 3–4 in 10 min.
- Lasting less than 60 s.
- Less than 40 mmHg.

CPD and a malpresentation should be excluded. Then, careful use of oxytocic drugs, most commonly intravenous syntocinon infusion, can improve the contractions. Caution must be taken to avoid too frequent contractions because this can reduce the oxygen exchange in the placental bed and lead to fetal hypoxia. Continuous electronic monitoring is advisable.

Particular care is essential in a multiparous patient because the diagnosis of inefficient uterine action is much less common than in a primiparous patient. A fetal malposition, malpresentation or fetal size should be considered as the causes of the slow progress; inappropriate use of oxytocic drugs is more commonly associated with uterine rupture in this group.

- How do you diagnose labour?
- What maternal factors affect the progress of labour?
- What fetal factors affect the progress of labour?
- What comprises active management of the third stage of labour?
- What are the interventions in induction of labour, and their complications?

Further reading

Enkin MW, Keirse MJNC et al (2000) *A guide to effective care in pregnancy and childbirth* 3rd edn
NICE (2001) National evidence-based clinical guidelines *Electronic Fetal Monitoring* (NICE, London)

NICE (2001) National evidence-based clinical guidelines *Induction of Labour* (NICE, London)
RCOG Working Party Report (1999) *Childbirth: towards safer childbirth*
available online: www.rcog.org.uk

41. Operative Intervention in Obstetrics

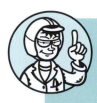

For all interventions in obstetrics, the following general principles apply:
- Make sure all documentation includes the time and date, and a legible signature.
- Clearly record the indication for the intervention, the abdominal and vaginal examination findings as appropriate and the operative findings including any complications.
- Obtain informed consent from the patient, either verbal or written, depending on the procedure.

Episiotomy

The purpose of an episiotomy is to increase the diameter of the vulval outlet by making an incision in the perineal body. The indications for this procedure are shown in Fig. 41.1. Since the 1980s, the routine episiotomy rate has been reduced dramatically because studies have demonstrated its association with increased blood loss, as well as long-term morbidity such as pain and dyspareunia.

To make them easier to remember, the indications for any intervention can be divided into maternal and fetal.

Two techniques are used for episiotomy (Fig. 41.2). Both should be performed with adequate analgesia, either an epidural or perineal infiltration with local anaesthetic, and should start in the midline at the posterior fourchette.

1. Mediolateral: widely used in the UK, this type of incision is more likely to protect the anal sphincter if the incision extends during delivery.

2. Midline: this technique is widely used in the USA and, although it is easier to repair and likely to result in less postpartum pain, it is more likely to involve the anal sphincter if it extends.

Repair of an episiotomy should be performed by an experienced operator. There should be adequate light and appropriate analgesia. A three-layer technique is usual with absorbable subcuticular sutures (Fig. 41.3):

- First layer – vaginal skin: identify the apex of the incision and suture in a continuous layer to the hymen to oppose the cut edges of the posterior fourchette.
- Second layer – perineal body: deep sutures to realign the muscles of the perineal body.
- Third layer – perineal skin: continuous or interrupted subcuticular sutures to close the skin.

At the end of the procedure, all needles and swabs should be checked. An examination of the vagina should be performed to ensure that the apex of the episiotomy is secure. Rectal examination should ensure that the rectal mucosa has not been broached by any deep sutures because this can result in fistula formation.

Perineal repair

Approximately 70% of mothers who deliver vaginally will sustain some degree of perineal trauma. This can be classified as:

- 1st degree: involves skin only.
- 2nd degree: involves skin and perineal muscle.
- 3rd degree: includes partial or complete rupture of the anal sphincter.
- 4th degree: as for 3rd degree but with the tear involving the anal mucosa.

The principles for repair are the same as for episiotomy. Some 1st-degree tears can be allowed to heal by secondary intention if they are not actively bleeding. It is very important to recognize and repair appropriately any damage to the anal sphincter or mucosa; failure to do so can result in long-term morbidity such as incontinence of flatus or faeces (this occurs in approximately 5% of women).

Ventouse delivery

Since the 1950s, when the vacuum extractor was invented in Sweden, it has increasingly been seen as the instrument of choice for assisted vaginal delivery. Metal cups were used initially, either anterior or posterior, and subsequently the silicone rubber ones

were developed; the former are more likely to be associated with vaginal trauma but might be more appropriate for delivery in certain situations such as the presence of excessive caput on the fetal head. Both types are available in different diameters depending on the gestation of the fetus. It is not an appropriate instrument at less than 34 weeks gestation.

Indications for ventouse

These are shown in Fig. 41.4.

Indications for episiotomy	
Type of indication	Description
Maternal	Female circumcision
	Consider if previous perineal reconstructive surgery
Fetal	Shoulder dystocia
	To precipitate delivery in cases of an abnormal CTG when the presenting part is on the perineum
	Consider in instrumental delivery
	Consider in breech delivery

Fig. 41.1 Indications for episiotomy.

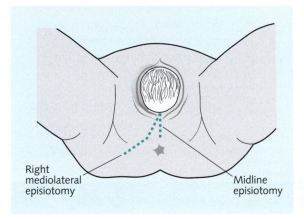

Fig. 41.2 Types of incision for episiotomy.

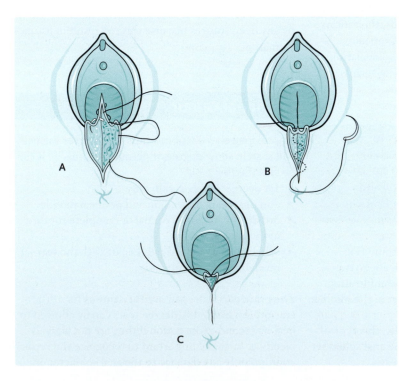

Fig. 41.3 Repair of an episiotomy. A. Suturing the vaginal wall. B. Suturing the perineal muscles. C. Tying the strands together – the knot disappears beneath the vaginal mucosa.

Indications for ventouse delivery	
Type of indication	Description
Maternal	Delay in 2nd stage due to maternal exhaustion
Fetal	Delay in 2nd stage due to fetal malposition (occipitoposterior or occipitotransverse position) Abnormal CTG

Fig. 41.4 Indications for ventouse delivery.

Criteria for instrumental vaginal delivery

1. Adequate analgesia: perineal infiltration/pudendal block/epidural anaesthesia (see Chapter 40)
2. Abdominal examination: estimation of fetal size – head either 1/5 or 0/5 palpable
3. Vaginal examination: cervix fully dilated – head either at or below the ischial spines, known fetal position, note presence of caput or moulding
4. Adequate maternal effort and regular contractions necessary for ventouse delivery
5. Empty bladder for forceps delivery

Fig. 41.5 Criteria for instrumental vaginal delivery.

Technique for ventouse

The criteria shown in Fig. 41.5 must be fulfilled. Instrumental delivery should not be attempted if the head is above the ischial spines because of the risks to the fetus – a caesarean section is indicated.

Both types of cup rely on the same technique. The cup is applied in the midline over the occiput avoiding the surrounding vaginal mucosa; the pressure in the connecting pump is raised to $-0.8\,\mathrm{kg/cm^2}$.

Traction with the maternal contractions and with maternal effort should be along the pelvic curve, that is, initially in a downwards direction and then changing the angle upwards as the head crowns. This action basically mimics the passage of the fetal head during a normal delivery, but uses the vacuum pump to increase traction and flexion.

The operator should judge whether an episiotomy is needed and the procedure should be complete within approximately 15 min of cup application. The CTG should monitor the fetal heart rate throughout and, in most units, it is standard practice for a paediatrician to be present. Complications are listed in Fig. 41.6.

Complications of instrumental delivery	
Type of complication	Description
Maternal	Genital tract trauma (cervical/vaginal/vulval) with risk of haemorrhage and/or infection
Fetal	Ventouse delivery is likely to cause a chignon (scalp oedema) or, less commonly, a cephalohaematoma (subperiosteal bleed) Forceps can cause bruising if not appropriately applied, or possibly facial nerve palsy or depression skull fracture

Fig. 41.6 Complications of instrumental delivery.

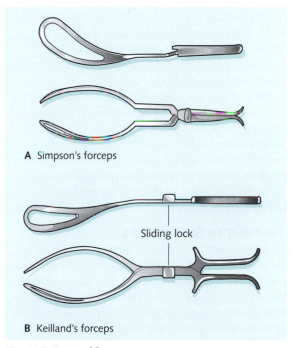

A Simpson's forceps

Sliding lock

B Keilland's forceps

Fig. 41.7 Types of forceps.

Forceps delivery

Over the last three or four centuries, forceps have been used for delivery. There are two main types of forceps (Fig.41.7):
- Non-rotational or traction forceps (Simpson's, Anderson's, Neville–Barnes or Wrigley's).
- Rotational forceps (Keilland's).

Indications for forceps rather than ventouse delivery	
Type of indication	**Description**
Maternal	Medical conditions complicating labour, e.g. cardiovascular disease
	Unconscious mother, i.e. conditions where the mother is unable to assist with pushing
Fetal	Gestation less than 34 weeks
	Face presentation
	Known or suspected fetal bleeding disorder
	After-coming head of a breech
	At caesarean section

Fig. 41.8 Indications for forceps rather than ventouse delivery.

Indications for forceps

These differ slightly from those for the ventouse, mainly because the ventouse requires maternal effort and adequate contractions (Fig. 41.8). Non-rotational forceps are suitable only for certain positions of the fetal head – direct occipitoanterior or direct occipitoposterior.

By contrast, the mode of action of the ventouse cup allows rotation to take place during traction and so it is suitable for a malposition (see Chapter 15). With a decline in the use of rotational forceps in some units due to fetal and maternal complications, it is essential to define the fetal position before attempting delivery, so that the appropriate instrument is chosen.

Technique for forceps

As for the ventouse, the necessary criteria must be fulfilled (see Fig. 41.5). The blades of non-rotational forceps are applied to the head, avoiding trauma to the vaginal walls. The direction of traction is similar to that of the ventouse, with episiotomy more likely to be performed when the head crowns than with the ventouse (Fig. 41.9).

Use of the rotational forceps involves a slightly different technique: the knobs on the blades must always point towards the occiput; asynclitism can be corrected using the sliding mechanism of the handles and then rotation achieved prior to traction in the manner described above.

Caesarean section

Caesarean section was first described by the ancient Egyptians. It was used increasingly throughout the twentieth century such that rates of 15–20% are now common in units in the UK. The lower segment procedure (lower segment caesarean section; LSCS) was introduced in the 1920s and has largely replaced the 'classical' midline uterine incision. Although the latter is sometimes indicated for preterm delivery with a poorly formed lower segment or for a preterm abnormal lie, it is associated with higher rates of haemorrhage and rupture in future pregnancies (up to 5% for midline operation, <1% for lower segment procedure).

Indications for LSCS

These are shown in Fig. 41.10.

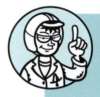

It is not appropriate to attempt an instrumental delivery if the fetal head is above the ischial spines. An LSCS should be performed.

Technique for LSCS

Under general or regional analgesia, depending on the indication for LSCS, a low transverse skin incision is made. The rectus sheath is divided and the uterovesical peritoneum is incised to allow the bladder to be reflected inferiorly. The lower uterine segment is incised transversely and the fetus is delivered manually.

Intravenous oxytocin is given by the anaesthetist and the placenta and membranes are removed. The angles of the uterine incision are secured to ensure haemostasis and then the uterus is closed with an absorbable suture, usually in two layers. The rectus sheath is secured to avoid incisional hernias and finally the skin is closed with either an absorbable or non-absorbable suture.

Complications of LSCS

Although LSCS has become an increasingly safe procedure, particularly with the introduction of regional anaesthesia, there is still significant morbidity associated with it:

- Haemorrhage: it is important to cross-match blood for certain patients, e.g. those with placenta praevia.
- Gastric aspiration: particularly with general anaesthetic (Mendelson's syndrome), this is reduced by routine use of antacids.

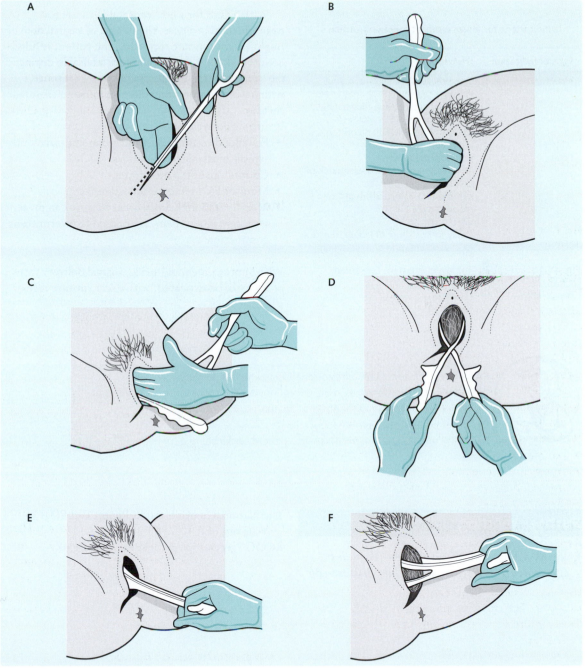

Fig. 41.9 Forceps delivery.

- Infection: reduced by routine use of prophylactic antibiotics.
- Thromboembolic disease: consider prophylaxis in all patients.
- Future pregnancy: subject to trial of scar (see below) or repeat operation with an increasing risk of complications.

Trial of scar

In patients who have had a pregnancy complicated by caesarean section, options for future deliveries should be discussed. In the case of a classical caesarean, the possibility of scar rupture is high (up to 5%) and thus repeat operation would be recommended.

Indications for lower segment caesarean section	
Type of indication	**Description**
Maternal	Two previous LSCSs
	Placenta praevia
	Maternal disease, e.g. fulminating pre-eclampsia
	Maternal request with no obstetric indication
Fetal	Breech presentation
	Twin pregnancy if the presentation of first twin is not cephalic
	Abnormal CTG or abnormal fetal blood sample
	Cord prolapse
	Delay in first stage of labour, e.g. due to malpresentation or malposition

Fig. 41.10 Indications for lower segment caesarean section.

With LSCS for a non-repeatable cause, for example cord prolapse, then a trial of vaginal delivery might be appropriate, providing the patient is fully counselled. Certain measures are advisable during labour to exclude the possibility of scar rupture, which would mean immediate recourse to caesarean section:

- Intravenous cannula.
- Full blood count (FBC) and group-and-save sample available in laboratory.
- Continuous CTG monitoring.
- Monitor PV loss to exclude bleeding.
- Monitor abdominal pain: scar rupture can present with continuous pain, as opposed to intermittent contractions.

With appropriate monitoring, vaginal delivery rates of 75% can be expected, with a scar rupture rate of <1%.

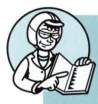

- What criteria must be fulfilled for an instrumental delivery?
- What are the differences in the indications for ventouse compared with forceps?
- What is the technique for repair of an episiotomy?
- What complications are associated with LSCS?
- What precautions are necessary in a patient undergoing a trial of scar?

Further reading

Enkin MW, Keirse MJNC et al (2000) *A guide to effective care in pregnancy and childbirth* 3rd edn

The National Sentinel Audit Report Oct 2001 (rcog.org.uk)

RCOG "green top" guidelines (rcog.org.uk)

42. Complications of the Third Stage of Labour and the Pueperium

Postpartum haemorrhage

Definition
Postpartum haemorrhage (PPH) is defined as vaginal bleeding of more than 500 mL. It can be either primary or secondary:
- Primary: occurring within 24 h of delivery.
- Secondary: occurring after the first 24 h and within 6 weeks of delivery.

Primary PPH

Incidence of primary PPH
The incidence of primary PPH in the developed world is about 5% of deliveries, in contrast to developing countries where it can occur in 28% of deliveries and is still a major cause of maternal mortality.

Aetiology of primary PPH
The main causes of primary PPH are shown in Fig. 42.1.

Uterine atony
The most common cause of PPH is uterine atony, when there is a failure of contraction and retraction of the uterus after the infant has been delivered. Risk factors include:
- Multiple pregnancy.
- Grand multiparity.
- Polyhydramnios.
- Fibroid uterus.
- Prolonged labour.
- Previous PPH.
- APH, especially placenta praevia or abruption.

In the case of a twin pregnancy, for example, there is overdistension of the uterus, which might reduce its ability to contract effectively, as well as a larger placental site, which can bleed. Fibroids can also restrict efficient contraction of the uterus, depending on their position. APH secondary to placental abruption impairs the normal function of the uterine muscle because of damage caused by bleeding into the myometrium. The lower segment of the uterus does not contract after delivery and so a patient with placenta praevia is at risk of haemorrhage from the placental bed.

Genital tract trauma
A PPH can occur after any type of delivery but is more common in certain circumstances. For example, a difficult forceps delivery might cause cervical lacerations as well as needing an episiotomy for delivery. At caesarean section, delivery of a deeply engaged presenting part or a large infant might cause extension of the uterine incision and result in heavy bleeding.

Prevention
In the first instance, prevention of primary PPH involves treatment of anaemia during pregnancy and identifying patients who might be at risk. These women might be obvious antenatally, such as the patient with a known inherited coagulation factor deficiency or one who has had a previous PPH. Equally, PPH might be anticipated during labour, for example the patient who has a prolonged labour ending with a difficult instrumental delivery of a large baby.

Active management of the third stage of labour is routine in most obstetric units, with the patient's consent. It involves:
- Use of an oxytocic drug.
- Controlled cord traction to deliver the placenta (Brandt–Andrews method).
- Clamping and cutting the umbilical cord.

Prophylactic use of oxytocics in particular is known to reduce the incidence of PPH by 30–40%. Syntometrine is most commonly used in the UK (5 units of syntocinon and 0.5 mg ergometrine). If the patient has hypertension, syntocinon is given alone.

Management
History, examination and investigation of the patient who has a PPH is described in Chapter 17. Treatment must start with basic resuscitation (ABC) depending on the patient's condition and the extent

Causes of primary postpartum haemorrhage	
Cause	**Frequency (%)**
Uterine atony	Approximately 90%
Genital tract trauma	Approximately 7%
• Retained placenta/placenta accreta	
• Coagulation disorders	
• Uterine inversion	
• Uterine rupture	

Fig. 42.1 Causes of primary postpartum haemorrhage.

Treatment of primary postpartum haemorrhage secondary to uterine atony
• IV access/cross-match blood
• Rub-up uterine contractions by massaging the uterine fundus
• Give IV oxytocin or ergometrine
• Start oxytocic infusion
• Give intramuscular or intramyometrial prostaglandin
• Consider surgical options or uterine artery embolization

Fig. 42.2 Treatment of primary postpartum haemorrhage secondary to uterine atony.

of the bleeding. It is important to get an accurate estimation of the blood loss; it is frequently underestimated. Intravenous access must be established. Blood is sent for haemoglobin, platelets, clotting and cross-matching. In cases of massive obstetric haemorrhage, generally classified as ≥2000 mL, a multidisciplinary approach to management is very important, involving liaison between the obstetrician, the anaesthetist and the haematologist.

Multidisciplinary management is important with:
- **Haematologists** in cases of massive PPH.
- **Microbiologists** in cases of sepsis of uncertain origin that does not respond to regular treatment.
- **Psychiatrists** in cases of postnatal mental illness.

All these disorders are associated with maternal mortality.

Retained or incomplete placenta

The cause of the bleeding must be identified so that appropriate management can be instigated. If the placenta is still in situ, delivery should be attempted by controlled cord traction. Once delivered, the placenta must be examined to ensure that the cotyledons and the membranes are complete. If the placenta is still retained, manual removal is necessary under regional analgesia. This is usually performed with antibiotic cover and with further doses of oxytocics.

Examination of the patient under anaesthetic allows exploration of the uterus if the placenta is thought to be incomplete. It also enables suturing

of genital tract trauma such as cervical or vaginal lacerations once uterine atony is excluded as the cause of the PPH.

Uterine atony

With uterine atony, the uterus is palpated and a contraction rubbed up by massaging the uterus abdominally. Further oxytocic drugs are given, commonly intravenous syntocinon, initially as a single dose, then proceeding to an intravenous infusion. Prostaglandin may be beneficial. This is commonly given in the form of carboprost ($PGF_{2\alpha}$) injected intramuscularly or intramyometrially (also known as hemabate™).

In severe cases, surgery is necessary and even life-saving. This includes bilateral uterine artery ligation or bilateral internal iliac artery ligation. A B-Lynch compression suture can be performed to avoid hysterectomy and this preserves future fertility. However, prompt recourse to hysterectomy is essential to reduce maternal morbidity and mortality. This management is summarized in Fig. 42.2.

Complications
Sheehan's syndrome

Severe PPH can lead to avascular necrosis of the pituitary gland, resulting in hypopituitarism. This can present as secondary amenorrhoea or failure of lactation.

Placenta accreta

With routine active management of the third stage of labour, the placenta is usually delivered within minutes of the infant. If the patient is not bleeding, up to an hour can be left before undertaking manual removal under anaesthesia. Rarely, the placenta is found to be morbidly adherent to the uterine wall, known as a placenta accreta. This condition is associated with paucity of underlying decidua:

- Placenta praevia.
- Uterine scar such as previous caesarean section.
- Multiparity.

 The potential morbidity and mortality associated with PPH are so significant that earlier rather delayed recourse to hysterectomy is important.

If the patient is not bleeding, conservative management includes observation and antibiotics. However, more commonly, the patient has significant bleeding and surgery is necessary, including hysterectomy.

Uterine inversion

This rare complication of labour can be complete, when the uterine fundus passes through the cervix, or incomplete, when the fundus is still above the cervix. It can occur spontaneously, for example in association with a fundal placental site or a unicornuate uterus, or be the result of mismanagement of the third stage.

The more serious presentation is of severe lower abdominal pain followed by collapse and haemorrhage. The pain is secondary to tension on the infundibulopelvic ligaments. Treatment involves resuscitation of the patient, replacement of the uterus, either manually or hydrostatically, and oxytocic infusion.

Uterine rupture

This is seen very rarely in the UK, except in association with a previous caesarean section. The incidence has fallen dramatically with the introduction of the lower segment procedure (<1%), as opposed to the classical vertical incision of the uterus (up to 5%). Spontaneous rupture is much less common, seen in a patient of high parity, associated with the use of syntocinon to augment labour, and has a high maternal and fetal mortality.

Uterine rupture can present with an abnormal CTG in labour (see Chapter 16), or with continuous abdominal pain and vaginal bleeding. Diagnosis is made at laparotomy and the treatment is surgical, either repair of the rupture or hysterectomy.

Secondary PPH

This can be caused by:

- Retained products of conception.
- Endometritis.
- Molar pregnancy or choriocarcinoma.

Chapter 17 gives the relevant points in the history, examination and investigations for the disorder, which most commonly presents with persistent vaginal bleeding.

Lactation

There are two main hormonal influences on breast tissue during pregnancy:

- Oestrogen increases the number and the size of the ducts.
- Progesterone increases the number of alveoli.

Colostrum, which is rich in antibodies, is secreted in late pregnancy and production increases after delivery. The level of oestrogen falls in the first 48 h after delivery so that prolactin can act on the alveoli and initiate lactation.

Suckling stimulates two reflexes:

1. the anterior part of the pituitary gland releases prolactin into the bloodstream, which induces the alveoli to secrete milk.
2. the posterior part of the pituitary gland releases oxytocin into the bloodstream, which causes contraction of the myoepithelial cells surrounding the alveoli so that the milk is ejected.

Postnatal infection

Definition
Also known as puerperal infection, this is defined as a maternal temperature of ≥38°C maintained for 24 h.

Incidence

Infection remains a major cause of maternal mortality (see Chapter 43). However, with improved hygiene and the use of antibiotics, the incidence has fallen to 1–3%.

 Maternal sepsis is still one of the top five causes of maternal mortality and so must be investigated thoroughly and treated promptly.

Sites of infection

- Uterus.
- Abdominal incision.
- Perineum.
- Chest.
- Urinary tract.
- Breast.

History

The site of infection might be obvious from the patient's history. Dysuria and urine frequency would suggest a urinary tract infection. If there is also loin pain then there might be an ascending infection to the kidneys causing pyelonephritis. If the patient has a productive cough and complains of feeling breathless, then she is likely to have a chest infection. This is typically a postoperative complication, seen in the patient who has had a caesarean section.

A uterine infection is also more common after an operative intervention, such as a caesarean section or a manual removal of placenta. It typically presents with lower abdominal pain, sometimes with unpleasant-smelling vaginal discharge. Retained products of conception must be excluded. It is now routine practice to give prophylactic antibiotics at the time of a caesarean section. As well as protecting against a uterine infection, this also reduces the risk of a wound infection.

Infection in the perineum can also present with vaginal discharge, as well as localized discomfort. There is usually a history of a vaginal tear or an episiotomy. Acute mastitis, or infection of the breast, typically presents at the end of the first week after birth, as organisms that colonize the baby affect the breast. Infection presents with pain in one or both breast associated with fever.

Examination

Check for pyrexia and tachycardia, which will be present with infection. Then examine the patient from head-to-toe, as suggested in Fig. 42.3.

Investigations

A white blood cell count will be raised and a C-reactive protein level will also be high. Blood cultures are indicated if the temperature is ≥38°C.

Other investigations depend on the system that seems to be involved:

- High vaginal swab for uterine infection.
- Perineal swab.
- Wound swab for caesarean section patient.
- Mid-stream urine sample.
- Sputum sample.

Management

The antibiotic of choice will depend on local protocol but usually involves a broad-spectrum antibiotic and anaerobic cover with metronidazole for 5 to 7 days. Flucloxacillin might be more appropriate for mastitis or for a wound infection because the usual pathogen is a staphylococcus.

Postnatal mental illness

Incidence

Postnatal depression is one of the most common medical diseases of pregnancy, with 10% of women fulfilling the criteria for a depressive disorder. Psychosis is much rarer, affecting 0.2% of births.

These disorders should be distinguished from the 'baby blues', which affects up to 70% of women, with a peak incidence on day 4 to 5. Tearfulness, anxiety and irritability normally settle with reassurance and support from family and friends.

History

Chapter 36 lists the risk factors for postnatal depression and some of these should be sought at the time of the antenatal booking, as recommended in the triennial report into maternal death (see Chapter 43). Puerperal psychosis in particular has associated risks: previous psychotic illness gives the woman a 1:2 chance of postnatal disease and a family history a 1:4 chance.

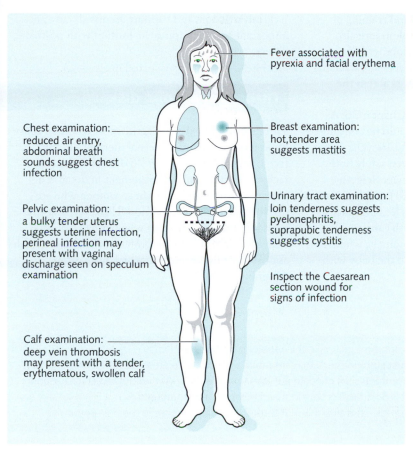

Fig. 42.3 Examination of the patient with a postnatal pyrexia.

Fever associated with pyrexia and facial erythema

Chest examination: reduced air entry, abdominal breath sounds suggest chest infection

Breast examination: hot, tender area suggests mastitis

Pelvic examination: a bulky tender uterus suggests uterine infection, perineal infection may present with vaginal discharge seen on speculum examination

Urinary tract examination: loin tenderness suggests pyelonephritis, suprapubic tenderness suggests cystitis

Inspect the Caesarean section wound for signs of infection

Calf examination: deep vein thrombosis may present with a tender, erythematous, swollen calf

 Prediction from the antenatal history is one of the main factors in the early management of postnatal mental illness.

The common symptoms of postnatal depression and puerperal psychosis are shown in Figs 42.4 and 42.5, respectively. The peak time of onset for postnatal depression is 4 to 6 weeks postpartum, whereas the onset of psychosis is usually very sudden.

Management
- Prevention.
- Pharmocological.
- Psychological/social.

The mainstay of management is prevention, which has improved recently as media interest increases

Symptoms of postnatal depression

- Anxiety
- Low mood
- Tiredness
- Irritability
- Feelings of inadequacy
- Ambivalence towards the baby
- Reduced or absent libido

Fig. 42.4 Symptoms of postnatal depression.

Symptoms of puerperal psychosis

- Insomnia or early morning wakening
- Lability of mood
- Overactivity
- Disorientation
- Lack of insight
- Hallucinations
- Persecutory beliefs

Fig. 42.5 Symptoms of puerperal psychosis.

public awareness. Early diagnosis and training of professionals to recognize the problems are also vital and have resulted in the development of the Edinburgh Postnatal Depression Scale, which is used successfully by health visitors across the UK.

Drug treatment is described in Chapter 36. As with any drug in pregnancy, use should be considered if its benefits outweigh its risks. The Tricyclic Antidepressants (TCAs) can be given safely both antenatally and postnatally. The newer Selective Serotonin Reuptake Inhibitor (SSRI) antidepressants are probably safe, although there is less evidence at this stage. Lithium is associated with cardiac anomalies, particularly Ebstein's anomaly, when used antenatally. It might also be toxic to the baby with breastfeeding. ECT is safe.

Health visitors and support groups all have an important role in helping the mother with postnatal illness.

Thromboembolic disease

Thromboembolic disease is the most common cause of pregnancy-related maternal mortality in the UK (see Chapter 43). Chapter 36 describes the risk factors, diagnosis and management in detail. Of particular importance are those women who are delivered by caesarean section. However, it is vital not to forget that a woman who has had a normal delivery might still have significant risk factors, such as obesity or hypertension, which necessitate thromboprophylaxis.

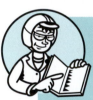

- What are the important factors in the aetiology of primary PPH?
- What are the first steps in the management of a patient who presents with a primary PPH?
- What are the common sites of postnatal infection, and how you would investigate them?
- How prevalent is postnatal depression, and how can it be managed?
- What is the diagnosis and treatment of thromboembolic disease in the puerperium?

Further reading

Chamberlain,G & Steer, P (2001) *Turnbull's Obstetrics* 3rd edn
Enkin MW, Keirse MJNC et al (2000) *A guide to effective care in pregnancy and childbirth* 3rd edn
Confidential Enquiry into Maternal Deaths 1997-1999
www.doh.gov.uk/cmo/mdeaths

Thromboembolic disease in pregnancy and the puerperium
RCOG Clinical Green Top Guideline
www.rcog.org.uk

43. Maternal Death

Maternal mortality is defined as death of the mother during pregnancy, labour and within 42 days of delivery or abortion, but recently deaths up to 1 year have been studied. Maternal deaths are divided into four categories: direct, indirect, coincidental (which used to be called fortuitous) and late (Fig. 43.1).

The maternal mortality rate for the United Kingdom in the 1997-1999 triennia was approximately 1 in 10,000 maternities (only Direct and Indirect maternal deaths are included in this statistic).

Confidential Enquiries into Maternal Deaths

Since 1952, a triennial report of the Confidential Enquiries into Maternal Deaths (CEMD) has been published. Recently titled *Why mothers die*, it examines deaths in England, Wales, Scotland and Northern Ireland. The CEMD aims are to:

- Assess the main causes of death.
- Examine the trends, comparing rates of death to those in previous reports.
- Identify avoidable deaths and look at substandard care.
- Make recommendations about improving clinical care.
- Suggest areas for future research.

At a local level, hospitals can use the report to develop guidelines for the management of complications of pregnancy, and to review the care that their patients receive.

Figure 43.2 shows the maternal mortality rate since 1952. The fall in maternal mortality is thought to be due to a combination of improved obstetric and midwifery care and an improvement in the standards of living. The increasing rates seen in the last two reports are due to a change in the way that figures are collected; before 1994 the CEMD relied upon clinicians reporting deaths, so inevitably the data was incomplete. The last two triennial reports include deaths that were discovered by analysis of a death certificate database at the Office of National Statistics.

Causes of maternal death

Figure 43.3 shows the main causes of maternal death in 1997–9. The case studies below are drawn from the most recent confidential enquiry document.

Direct maternal deaths

Thromboembolism is the commonest cause of direct maternal deaths.

Thromboembolic disease

Thromboembolic disease is the most common cause of direct maternal death, accounting for more than one-third of deaths. Great effort has been made in recent years to improve prophylaxis for women at increased risk of thromboembolism in pregnancy, particularly those undergoing caesarean delivery, and national guidelines exist recommending heparin and Thromboembolic (TED) stockings as appropriate. However, all pregnant women are at risk (see Chapter 36) and women are still dying, often after the problem has been put down to muscle strain, as illustrated in the case study below.

Case study: thromboembolic disease

An overweight woman aged over 30 with a strong family history of thromboembolic disease developed thrombophlebitis and was admitted to A&E at 8 weeks gestation with chest pain. Although the woman's GP had suggested a diagnosis of pulmonary embolism (PE), the medical registrar thought that chest X-ray and anticoagulation were contraindicated and the woman went home with a diagnosis of 'musculoskeletal pain'. Two days later she was readmitted and a V/Q scan was arranged to exclude PE; she died of PE before the scan was done.

Hypertensive disorders

Deaths from hypertensive disorders, including pre-eclampsia and eclampsia, are decreasing. The largest single cause of death of women in this group is intracranial haemorrhage, a complication of uncontrolled hypertension reflecting a failure to treat high blood pressure effectively. The need for monitoring to continue after delivery is vital, as illustrated in the following case study.

Case study: hypertension in pregnancy

A woman complained to her GP of abdominal pain. Her period was late and a pregnancy test was positive. An appointment for a scan was arranged but abdominal pain with diarrhoea recurred before the date of the scan and the woman was taken to hospital by ambulance. In transit she was noted to be pale, sweaty and hypotensive. She then had a cardiac arrest with prolonged asystole. She was resuscitated and taken to the operating theatre where laparotomy was performed. A ruptured tubal pregnancy was discovered. Unfortunately, major cerebral damage had resulted from prolonged asystole, and she died in the intensive care unit.

Haemorrhage

Haemorrhage-related deaths are also decreasing. Recommendations made by the CEMD emphasize the fact that the speed with which haemorrhage becomes life-threatening means that any woman at

---

Definitions of the classes of maternal death

- Direct: resulting from obstetric complications
- Indirect: previous existing disease, or disease arising in pregnancy, aggravated by the physiological effect of pregnancy (includes all asthma, cardiac disease, epilepsy and suicide)
- Coincidental: unrelated cause, occurring in pregnancy or puerperium
- Late: >42 days, <12 months after termination/miscarriage/delivery

Fig. 43.1 Definitions of the classes of maternal death.

Causes of maternal death 1997–9

Category	Cause	Rate per million maternities
Direct	Thromboembolic disease	16.5
	Early pregnancy	8
	Hypertensive disorders	7.1
	Sepsis	6.6
	Amniotic fluid embolism	3.8
	Haemorrhage	3.3
Indirect	Indirect	16.5
	Psychiatric	7.1
	Cancer-related	5.1
Coincidental		10.8
Late		50.3

Fig. 43.3 Causes of maternal death, 1997–9.

Fig. 43.2 Death rates from 1952 to the present.

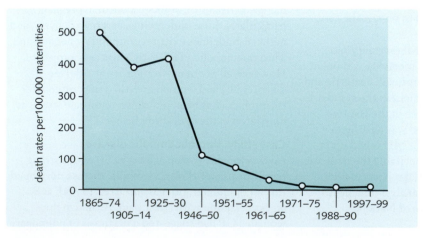

increased risk should be identified antenatally and advised to deliver in a hospital with a blood-bank on site (see the following case study). Placenta praevia poses a major risk, so consultant obstetricians and anaesthetists should be in charge of caesarean sections performed for this reason.

Case study: haemorrhage

A woman with a multiple pregnancy had a booking blood pressure of 90/60 mmHg. She was admitted to hospital during the pregnancy with pre-eclampsia and was subsequently delivered by caesarean section. Immediately prior to delivery her blood pressure was 140/80 mmHg and she had 3+ proteinuria. There was inadequate monitoring of her blood pressure after delivery and 8 h postnatally the reading was 260/140 mmHg. She developed neurological symptoms and was transferred to intensive care, where she died of a cerebral haemorrhage.

Sepsis

Deaths from septic abortion following illegal termination of pregnancy were, sadly, not uncommon before the Abortion Act of 1967. Sepsis declined as a major cause of maternal death thereafter but has recently been increasing again. Deaths seen in 1997–9 included those after miscarriage, after late intrauterine death and following prolonged rupture of membranes, with septicaemia associated with DIC.

Amniotic fluid embolism

Amniotic fluid embolism remains a significant cause of death but, frustratingly, we still do not have any clear ideas of how to prevent or to treat this condition.

Ectopic pregnancy

Of the direct deaths associated with early pregnancy in 1997–9, most were due to ectopic pregnancy, with the main problem being a failure to suspect the possibility of ectopic pregnancy in the first place. Presentation might be atypical with, for example, gastrointestinal symptoms confusing the issue, but the diagnosis must be suspected in any woman who is unwell and has a positive pregnancy test (see Chapter 7).

Indirect maternal deaths

Central nervous system (CNS) disorders, cardiac disease and psychiatric disease are the main categories in this section.

CNS disorders

Cerebral haemorrhage and epilepsy are the most common cause of CNS deaths. Close monitoring of epilepsy in pregnancy is important because anticonvulsant levels can change and women often feel ambivalent about continuing treatment due to the fetal side-effects (see Chapter 36).

Cardiac disease

Heart disease is now as common as thromboembolism as a cause of maternal death. About 30% is due to congenital disease, including pulmonary hypertension, and 15% to ischaemic heart disease. The remainder is due to other acquired heart disease. Rheumatic heart disease is uncommon in the UK and when seen is usually in new immigrants.

Psychiatric disorders

Psychiatric disease is known to have caused or to have contributed to 12% of maternal deaths, 10% of which were due to suicide. Suicide often occurred later than 42 days after delivery, so is also counted as a 'late' death and was often not reported as a maternal death. Alcohol and drug misuse is also covered in this category. The 1997–9 triennial report particularly emphasizes the high risk of recurrence of serious psychiatric illness postnatally (see the case study below) and warns health professionals to be aware of this (see Chapter 36). The lack of specialist mental health teams and mother-and-baby units makes it more difficult to treat these women optimally.

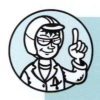

If all categories of maternal death are considered i.e. indirect, coincidental and late, mental illness is the leading cause of maternal death.

Case study: postpartum psychosis

A woman died in a road traffic accident when absconding from an inpatient psychiatric unit where she was being treated for postpartum psychosis. She had previously suffered from postpartum psychosis following the birth of a child some years earlier. There was no mention in her antenatal notes of her previous psychiatric history and she had midwifery-led care and a home delivery. Shortly after this she became psychotic and required inpatient admission, during which time she expressed suicidal intentions.

Coincidental deaths

This section includes many different causes of death but of particular concern are those due to domestic violence. Women suffering domestic violence are more likely to book late, to be poor attenders at antenatal clinic and to have poor obstetric histories. Ideally, all women at the booking visit should be asked, directly but sensitively, about violence. A pregnant woman should be seen at least once on her own during pregnancy and relatives should not be used as interpreters.

About 30% of domestic violence starts in pregnancy.

Risk factors for maternal death

Maternal mortality increases with increasing maternal age and parity. Other factors include multiple pregnancy and IVF treatment, non-white ethnic origin, late booking and lower social class.

Women from the most deprived social class are 20 times more likely to die of direct or indirect causes than women in social classes 1 and 2.

Substandard care was identified in 60% of cases of direct maternal deaths studied in the 1997–9 report. The main causes were summarized as:

- Lack of communication and teamwork.
- Failure to appreciate the severity of illness.
- Suboptimal treatment.
- Wrong diagnosis.
- Failure of juniors/GPs to refer-on to senior staff in hospital.
- Failure of consultants to attend, or inappropriate delegation of responsibility.
- Lack of clear policies for prevention and management of serious conditions.
- Failure to seek advice from other specialties when appropriate.

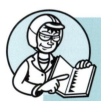

- How often is the report of the Confidential Enquiries into Maternal Deaths published?
- What is the most common direct cause of maternal death?
- What is the longest period of time that can elapse between end of pregnancy and death for the case to be studied by the Enquiry?
- In what proportion of the cases studied in the last enquiry was substandard care identified?
- What is the main direct cause of death in early pregnancy?

Further reading

Why Mothers Die, Report on Confidential Enquiries into Maternal Deaths in the United Kingdom, 1996–1999

Nelson-Piercy, C *Handbook of Obstetric Medicine* (Isis Medical Media)

www.rcog.org.uk/guidelines

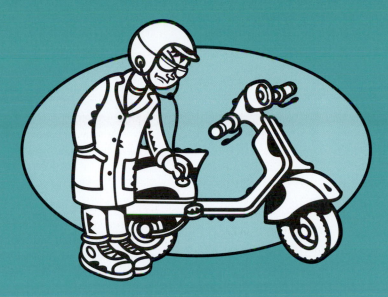

HISTORY AND EXAMINATION

44. Taking a History

The history plays a vital role in obstetrics and gynaecology, often giving pointers to a diagnosis that is not always evident from examination and investigation of the patient. Many women are embarrassed by having to discuss their gynaecological problems, especially to someone who is often younger than they are, so it is important to overcome this by developing a confident, friendly and relaxed atmosphere. Always introduce and present yourself in an acceptable manner, be courteous and friendly without being overfamiliar, and always pay attention.

Patient details

It is surprising how often patient details are omitted from a history. Always record the following:
1. Name, date of birth, age and address (sticky labels with this information are usually available).
2. Marital status, ethnic group and occupation.
3. The date, time and place of the consultation.
4. Source of referral, e.g. GP referral, self-admitted to A&E, labour ward.

It is useful to get into the habit of writing certain details in the top right hand corner of the clerking sheet, for example:

- Age.
- Parity.
- Date of LMP.
- Date of last smear.

Presenting complaint

The presenting complaint documented in the referral letter or the casualty card does not always correlate to what the patient perceives as the main problem. Some patients have already been labelled with a diagnosis before you get to see them. It is therefore vital to ask the patient what she sees as her primary complaint and document this – preferably in her own words. If there are multiple symptoms, document each one and do so in order of severity.

During the examination, investigations and treatment never lose track of the presenting complaint; management plans are not always appropriate. Conversely, the presenting complaint might be a cover for a different problem that the patient has difficulty discussing. Always ask if there is anything else bothering the patient that she wishes to discuss.

History of presenting complaint

Details of the history of the presenting complaint should be ascertained. For instance:
- How long has the complaint been present or a problem? For example, a woman might complain that she has always had heavy periods but they have only been a problem for the last 2 years.
- Was the onset of symptoms sudden or gradual? For example severe hirsutism of rapid onset is likely to be due to an androgen-producing tumour.
- Was the onset associated with a previous obstetric or gynaecological event? For example, stress incontinence and childbirth.
- Are there any relieving or exacerbating factors? For example symptoms of prolapse are often worse on standing and better on lying down.
- Are there any associated symptoms? For example the painful periods of endometriosis is sometimes associated with frequent bowel action.

If pain is the presenting complaint then the following characteristics should be discussed and noted:
- Site: is the pain pelvic or abdominal? For example ovarian pain can be felt quite high in the abdomen.
- Severity: how severe is the pain and to what extent does it disrupt every day life? For example the cyclical pain of endometriosis might necessitate regular time off work.
- Onset: sudden or gradual? For example. the pain from a torted ovarian cyst is usually of very sudden onset.

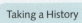

- Character: is the pain sharp/knife-like, dull, heavy/dragging, colicky, stretching or twisting? Many adjectives have been used to describe pain or discomfort of gynaecological origin. For example women with uterine prolapse might describe a pulling or a dragging pain/sensation, dysmenorrhoea might be likened to labour pain.
- Duration: is the pain constant, intermittent, frequency if intermittent? The pain of a degenerating fibroid in pregnancy will be constant whereas the pain of threatened premature labour will be intermittent and frequent.
- Radiation: does the pain radiate? For example endometriosis pain might radiate to the back or into the upper thighs.
- Relieving/exacerbating features: does anything make the pain better or worse and this should include self-prescribed analgesia? For example endometriosis symptoms are usually cyclical and associated with menstruation.
- Associated symptoms, for example symptoms of peritonitis or advanced malignancy.

Past gynaecological history

Menstrual history

The following characteristics of menstruation and the menstrual cycle should be noted:
- Age at menarche.
- Last menstrual period (LMP).
- Menstrual cycle: usually denoted as 5/28, where the numerator is the length of the period in days and the denominator is the length of the cycle in days. If period and cycle length are variable the shortest and longest are noted, e.g. 3–10/14–56.
- Menstrual flow: whether light, normal or heavy. If heavy, the presence of clots, flooding, night time soiling and the number of sanitary pads/towels used should be noted.
- Menstrual pain: is the pain mild, moderate or severe? Has it been present since menarche or is of recent onset. Is the pain worse before or during the period?
- Associated symptoms: for example bowel or bladder dysfunction, nausea.
- Other bleeding: intermenstrual bleeding (IMB), postcoital bleeding (PCB), pre- or postmenstrual spotting.
- Age at menopause.

Sexual activity and contraception

Is the patient sexually active or in a relationship. Does the patient suffer from dyspareunia and if so is it superficial or deep? Is she or her partner using contraception and if so what? If she is on the pill, was it prescribed for contraceptive purposes or menstrual disorder?

Cervical screening

Has the patient undergone regular cervical screening? When was the last smear taken? Have there ever been abnormal smears?

Vaginal discharge

Is vaginal discharge present and if so is it normal or abnormal? If abnormal, what is the colour and consistency and is it irritant? Was the onset associated with a change in sexual partner? Is there a history of sexually transmitted disease?

Past obstetric history

The parity and gravidity should be noted. Parity denotes the number of livebirths or stillbirths after 24 weeks gestation and gravidity the number of pregnancies. Use of the terms 'parity' and 'gravidity' can become very complicated, especially with a history of multiple pregnancies. A more straightforward way of documenting previous pregnancies is to document the number of:
- Children.
- Miscarriages.
- Terminations.

Document the details of each pregnancy:
- The number of children with age and birth weight. Note any complications of pregnancy, labour and the puerperium.
- The number of miscarriages, their gestation and complications if any.
- The number of terminations of pregnancy, their gestation, method and indication and complications if any.

Past medical history

This should include previous surgery, for example sterilization.

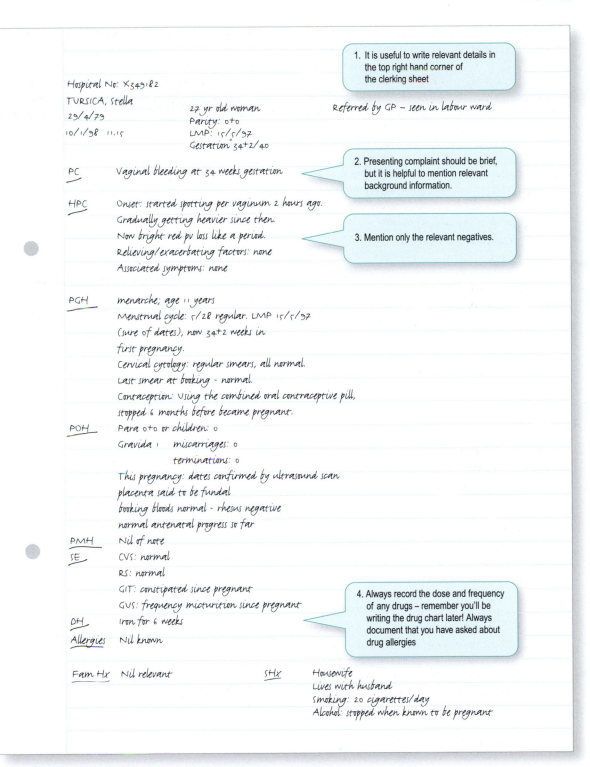

Hospital No: X349182

TURSICA, Stella
29/4/79
10/1/98 11.15

27 yr old woman
Parity: 0+0
LMP: 15/5/97
Gestation 34+2/40

Referred by GP – seen in labour ward

1. It is useful to write relevant details in the top right hand corner of the clerking sheet

PC   Vaginal bleeding at 34 weeks gestation

2. Presenting complaint should be brief, but it is helpful to mention relevant background information.

HPC   Onset: started spotting per vaginum 2 hours ago.
        Gradually getting heavier since then.
        Now bright red pv loss like a period.
        Relieving/exacerbating factors: none
        Associated symptoms: none

3. Mention only the relevant negatives.

PGH   menarche; age 11 years
        Menstrual cycle: 5/28 regular. LMP 15/5/97
        (sure of dates), now 34+2 weeks in
        first pregnancy.
        Cervical cytology: regular smears, all normal.
        Last smear at booking - normal.
        Contraception: using the combined oral contraceptive pill,
        stopped 6 months before became pregnant.

POH   Para 0+0 or children: 0
        Gravida 1   miscarriages: 0
                    terminations: 0
        This pregnancy: dates confirmed by ultrasound scan
        placenta said to be fundal
        booking bloods normal - rhesus negative
        normal antenatal progress so far

PMH   Nil of note
SE   CVS: normal
        RS: normal
        GIT: constipated since pregnant
        GUS: frequency micturition since pregnant
OH   Iron for 6 weeks
Allergies Nil known

4. Always record the dose and frequency of any drugs – remember you'll be writing the drug chart later! Always document that you have asked about drug allergies

Fam Hx Nil relevant   SHx   Housewife
                                     Lives with husband
                                     Smoking: 20 cigarettes/day
                                     Alcohol: stopped when known to be pregnant

Fig. 44.1 Clerking.

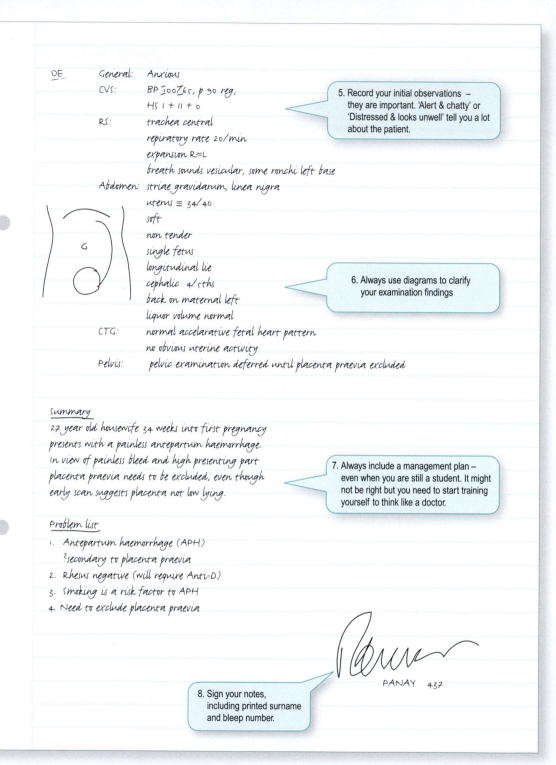

OE General: Anxious

CVS: BP 100/65, p 90 reg,
      HS I + II + o

> 5. Record your initial observations –
> they are important. 'Alert & chatty' or
> 'Distressed & looks unwell' tell you a lot
> about the patient.

RS: trachea central
     repiratory rate 20/min
     expansion R=L
     breath sounds vesicular, some ronchi left base

Abdomen: striae gravidarum, linea nigra
          uterus ≡ 34/40
          soft
          non tender
          single fetus
          longitudinal lie
          cephalic 4/5ths
          back on maternal left
          liquor volume normal

> 6. Always use diagrams to clarify
> your examination findings

CTG: normal accelerative fetal heart pattern
      no obvious uterine activity

Pelvis: pelvic examination deferred until placenta praevia excluded

Summary

27 year old housewife 34 weeks into first pregnancy
presents with a painless antepartum haemorrhage.
In view of painless bleed and high presenting part
placenta praevia needs to be excluded, even though
early scan suggests placenta not low lying.

> 7. Always include a management plan –
> even when you are still a student. It might
> not be right but you need to start training
> yourself to think like a doctor.

Problem list

1. Antepartum haemorrhage (APH)
   ?secondary to placenta praevia
2. Rhesus negative (will require Anti-D)
3. Smoking is a risk factor to APH
4. Need to exclude placenta praevia

PANAY 437

> 8. Sign your notes,
> including printed surname
> and bleep number.

Fig. 44.1 cont'd.

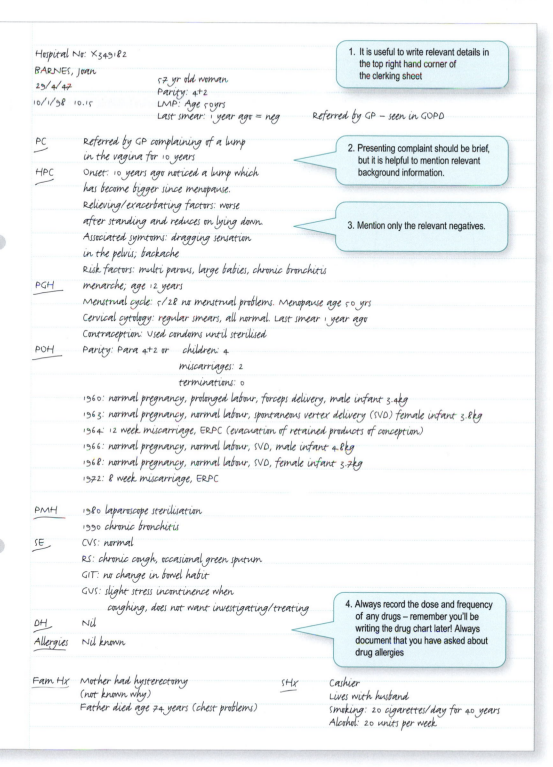

Hospital No: X349182

BARNES, Joan
29/4/47   57 yr old woman
10/1/98 10.15   Parity: 4+2
                 LMP: Age 50yrs
                 Last smear: 1 year ago = neg   Referred by GP — seen in GOPD

> 1. It is useful to write relevant details in the top right hand corner of the clerking sheet

PC   Referred by GP complaining of a lump
      in the vagina for 10 years

> 2. Presenting complaint should be brief, but it is helpful to mention relevant background information.

HPC   Onset: 10 years ago noticed a lump which
      has become bigger since menopause.
      Relieving/exacerbating factors: worse
      after standing and reduces on lying down.
      Associated symtoms: dragging sensation
      in the pelvis; backache
      Risk factors: multi parous, large babies, chronic bronchitis

> 3. Mention only the relevant negatives.

PGH   menarche; age 12 years
      Menstrual cycle: 5/28 no menstrual problems. Menopause age 50 yrs
      Cervical cytology: regular smears, all normal. Last smear 1 year ago
      Contraception: Used condoms until sterilised

POH   Parity: Para 4+2 or   children: 4
                            miscarriages: 2
                            terminations: 0
      1960: normal pregnancy, prolonged labour, forceps delivery, male infant 3.4kg
      1963: normal pregnancy, normal labour, spontaneous vertex delivery (SVD) female infant 3.8kg
      1964: 12 week miscarriage, ERPC (evacuation of retained products of conception)
      1966: normal pregnancy, normal labour, SVD, male infant 4.8kg
      1968: normal pregnancy, normal labour, SVD, female infant 3.7kg
      1972: 8 week miscarriage, ERPC

PMH   1980 laparoscope sterilisation
      1990 chronic bronchitis

SE   CVS: normal
      RS: chronic cough, occasional green sputum
      GIT: no change in bowel habit
      GUS: slight stress incontinence when
           coughing, does not want investigating/treating

DH   Nil
Allergies Nil known

> 4. Always record the dose and frequency of any drugs – remember you'll be writing the drug chart later! Always document that you have asked about drug allergies

Fam Hx Mother had hysterectomy   SHx   Cashier
        (not known why)   Lives with husband
        Father died age 74 years (chest problems)   Smoking: 20 cigarettes/day for 40 years
                                               Alcohol: 20 units per week

Fig. 44.2 Clerking.

OE

General:	Well, overweight
CVS:	BP 140/90, pulse 80 reg,
	heart sounds normal,
	no cardiac murmurs

> 5. Record your initial observations – they are important. 'Alert & chatty' or 'Distressed & looks unwell' tell you a lot about the patient.

RS: trachea central
        respiratory rate 20/min
        expansion R=L
        breath sounds vesicular, some ronchi left base

Abdomen: laparoscopy scar
         soft
         non tender
         no masses
         normal bowel sounds
         rectal examination not done

> 6. Always use diagrams to clarify your examination findings

Vulva: normal
cervix sitting at antroitus
Bimanual: uterus 6 weeks size, mobile,
          non tender, smooth outline
Speculum: cervix excoriated
moderate cystocoele
moderate rectocoele

Summary

57 year old multiparous woman complaining of symptoms of prolapse. Pelvic examination reveals 2nd degree prolapse of uterus associated with moderate pelvic floor prolapse.

> 7. Always include a management plan – even when you are still a student. It might not be right but you need to start training yourself to think like a doctor.

Problem list

1. Uterine and pelvic floor prolapse
2. Associated stress incontinence
3. Obesity and chronic bronchitis are exacerbating factors
4. Heavy smoker, moderate alcohol

PANAY   437

> 8. Sign your notes, including printed surname and bleep number.

Fig. 44.2 cont'd.

Systems enquiry

A brief systems enquiry should be made with especial reference to the:
- Gastrointestinal tract: change in bowel habit, especially with menstruation.
- Genitourinary system: urinary frequency, nocturia, dysuria, incontinence.

Drug history

A careful drug history should be taken and should include hormonal contraception and HRT, which are often overlooked by the patient.

Family history

Enquire as to a family history of ovarian, uterine and breast disease.

Social history

Occupation, smoking habits and alcohol consumption should be noted. If surgery is contemplated, what is the support network at home?

Allergies

Document all known allergies.

45. Antenatal Booking and Ongoing Care

Fundamental to the planning of antenatal care is the identification, at the booking visit, of factors that reveal the woman to be at risk of complications during her pregnancy, labour and postpartum period (Fig. 45.1).

The history

History of the current pregnancy

First, ascertain the gestation of the present pregnancy. Ask for the date of the first day of the LMP and whether it was a normal period. Also check the usual cycle length and whether her periods are regular or irregular. Ask if she was on the oral contraceptive pill when she conceived (the baby will not suffer any ill effects but the date of her LMP cannot be relied upon for estimation of gestation). Find out if she has had any problems so far, and if she has had any admissions or scans.

Naegele's rule for calculation of the estimated date of delivery (assumes a 28-day cycle): add 7 to the first day of the LMP for the due day, and take 3 from the month of the LMP for the due month. For example, an LMP of 1 March gives a due date of 8 December.

Past obstetric history

Past obstetric history records the outcome of all past pregnancies (Fig. 45.2). For pregnancies less than 24 weeks, document whether she had a miscarriage or a termination, and at what gestation. If the termination was for fetal abnormality this should be noted. For pregnancies lasting longer than 24 weeks, record:

- Mode of delivery, and reason for caesarean/instrumental delivery.
- Gestation at delivery.

- Whether onset of labour was spontaneous or induced.
- Weight and sex of baby.
- Any significant antenatal problems.
- Problems experienced by the baby in the neonatal period.

Past gynaecological history

The date of the last smear is recorded. If there have been abnormal smears in the past, the outcome of these, and treatment performed, must be noted. Most CIN in the UK is treated by LLETZ, which does not result in obstetric complications. Cone biopsy, which is used to treat a minority of cases, can result in significant cervical damage, resulting in cervical incompetence or stenosis (see Chapter 23).

Past medical history

Any admissions to hospital, operations or ongoing medical conditions should be documented. Particular attention should be paid to psychiatric history – not all psychiatric illness following childbirth is 'simple' postnatal depression. Conditions that are likely to cause obstetric complications, or to worsen in pregnancy and the puerperium, include insulin-dependent diabetes, thromboembolism, thyroid disease, recurrent UTIs (urinary tract infections), depression, cardiac disease, anorexia nervosa, epilepsy, genital herpes infection and (especially if the mother decides to discontinue her treatment) asthma (see Chapter 36).

Social history

This might need to be particularly sensitively elicited, and it might be appropriate to wait until the woman is alone before questioning. The key points to cover include:

- Smoking.
- Drug and alcohol use, documenting types of drug and amount used.
- Domestic violence: all women should be asked about this as a matter of routine (see Chapter 43).
- Support and social circumstances.

Factors in history and examination that make a pregnancy high risk		
History	**Risk factors**	**Associated problems**
Age	<18 years	Hypertensive disorders
		IUGR
	>38 years	Fetal chromosomal abnormality
		IUGR
		Stillbirth after 40 weeks
		Hypertensive disorders
Weight at booking	<45 kg	IUGR
	>100 kg	Hypertensive disorders
		Impaired glucose tolerance
		Shoulder dystocia
		Thromboembolism
Past obstetric history	Primaparous	Pre-eclampsia
	Granmultiparous (>4)	Anaemia
		IUGR
		Malpresentation
		Unstable lie
		Postpartum haemorrhage
	Previous manual removal of placenta	Recurrence of retained placenta
		Placenta praevia
		Postpartum haemorrhage
	Previous caesarean section	Placenta praevia
	Previous baby >4 kg	Shoulder dystocia
	Previous baby affected by medical or chromosomal abnormality	Recurrence: consider referral to paediatrician, fetal medicine unit and/or geneticist
Past medical history	Hypertension	Hypertensive disorders
	Insulin-dependent diabetes	Miscarriage
		Stillbirth
		Congenital anomaly
		Macrosomia
		Shoulder dystocia
		Neonatal hypoglycaemia
	Epilepsy	Cardiac abnormalities
		Palate abnormalities
		Neural tube defects
		Haemorrhage disease of the newborn
		Labile drug levels
	Thromboembolism	Deep vein thrombosis/pulmonary embolism in pregnancy and puerperium
	Thyroid disease	Maternal thyroid 'storm'
		Neonatal hypo-/hyperthyroidism
	Recurrent urinary tract infections	UTIs in pregnancy, leading to premature labour or IUGR
	Psychiatric disorders	Acute exacerbation in the postnatal period
	Anorexia nervosa	IUGR
Past gynaecological history	Cone biopsy	Cervical incompetence and midtrimester miscarriage
Family history	Genital herpes	Neonatal herpes encephalitis if lesions present at delivery
Social history	Diabetes	Impaired glucose tolerance
	Domestic violence	Physical injury
		Depression and suicide
		Premature labour
		IUGR
	Cigarettes and cannabis	IUGR
		Neonatal respiratory distress
		Cot death
		Childhood asthma and ear infections

Fig. 45.1 Factors in history and examination that make a pregnancy high risk.

History	Risk factors	Associated problems
Social history—cont'd	Alcohol: > 4 units/day > 8 units/day Cocaine	Fetal alcohol syndrome Cardiac defects Abruption IUGR Premature labour Microcephaly Cot death
	Amphetamines	Palate abnormalities Cardiac abnormalities IUGR
	Ecstasy (MDMA) Barbiturates Smoked heroin	Musculoskeletal and cardiac abnormalities Neonatal withdrawal Miscarriage Stillbirth IUGR Neonatal withdrawal
	Injected heroin Methadone	Hepatitis B and C, HIV Neonatal withdrawal
Present pregnancy	Assisted conception	Multiple pregnancy Premature IUGR
	Recurrent antepartum haemorrhage Multiple pregnancy	IUGR Miscarriage Chromosomal abnormality Hyperemesis Premature labour Anaemia IUGR Postpartum haemorrhage
	Fibroids	Postpartum haemorrhage Unstable lie or obstructed labour if in the lower segment of the uterus

Fig. 45.1 cont'd.

Fig. 45.2 Past obstetric histories.

Past obstetric histories

Shorthand for the number and type of pregnancies includes talking of 'primips' to denote women who have not had a >24-week pregnancy before, and 'multips' who have. 'Gravidity' means the number of pregnancies of any gestation, whereas 'parity' is the number of deliveries (by vaginal or operative route). An obstetric history can be abbreviated as shown in the examples below:

Lynne is currently 22 weeks into this pregnancy and in the past has had two normal deliveries, one miscarriage at 8 weeks and a termination at 8 weeks. She is therefore Para 2 Gravida 5, or Para 2 + 2.

Hayley is booking at 12 weeks. She had a caesarean section last year and a stillbirth at 37 weeks 10 years ago. She is Para 2 Gravida 3, or Para 2 + 0 – the shorthand does not take into account the outcome of her first pregnancy.

Sonia is now 15 weeks. Her last pregnancy was twins, who were delivered – vaginally – prematurely at 25 weeks. Twins count as one delivery, so she is Para 1 Gravida 2, or Para 1 + 0.

Michelle is late to book, at 30 weeks. She has had one previous pregnancy, an ectopic that was detected at 7 weeks and was treated medically. She is Para 0 Gravida 2, or Para 0 + 1.

Family history

A family history of diabetes should prompt screening for gestational diabetes at 28 weeks gestation. Other conditions that have a strong familial element and can affect the pregnancy include thromboembolism, pre-eclampsia and obstetric cholestasis.

Examination

Examination should include:
- Weight and height, to calculate BMI.
- Blood pressure.
- Urinalysis.
- Uterine size (abdominally) and auscultation of fetal heart if > 12 weeks.

Listening to the heart and lungs and performing breast and pelvic examinations are part of the booking visit in some centres.

Booking investigations

These are summarized in Fig. 45.3.

Full blood count

An FBC is performed at booking and again, later in pregnancy, to detect anaemia (for treatment of anaemia, see Chapter 36). This will also detect a low platelet count – idiopathic thrombocytopaenia. If mild to moderate (platelets $50–100 \times 10^9$/L) this poses little risk to the mother, but platelet levels must be monitored regularly. If severe, the woman might require intravenous immunoglobulin (Ig). The risk of the fetus having thrombocytopaenia is around 1 in 10, and is not predicted by the severity of the mother's condition.

Booking investigations
• Full blood count
• Blood group and antibody screen
• Syphilis, rubella, hepatitis and HIV serology
• Haemoglobin electrophoresis
• Midstream urine
• Ultrasound scan for dating

Fig. 45.3 Booking investigations.

Haemoglobin electrophoresis

Haemoglobinopathies can result in a mistaken diagnosis of anaemia – carriers of the genes for sickle cell and thalassaemia have a 'normal' haemoglobin that is lower than average. Diagnosis of haemoglobinopathy avoids unnecessary iron supplementation and allows identification of fetuses at risk of major thalassaemia or sickle-cell disease. All women whose racial background predisposes them to haemoglobinopathy should be offered screening and if the local population contains more than 15% of people of these races screening should be universal.

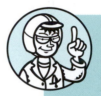

Sickle-cell trait affects 1 in 10 people of AfroCaribbean origin and 1 in 100 people originating from Cyprus and the Indian subcontinent. Alpha-thalassaemia trait affects 1 in 15 people of Chinese origin and 1 in 50 people of Cypriot origin. Beta-thalassaemia trait affects 1 in 7 people of Cypriot origin, 1 in 30 of Chinese origin and 1 in 50 of AfroCaribbean origin.

Blood group

If the woman is Rhesus negative (dd) and her fetus is Rhesus positive (DD or Dd) she might form anti-D antibodies in the event of fetal and maternal blood mixing. As these can cross the placenta and attack the fetal blood cells, fetal anaemia due to haemolysis can result. Giving therapeutic anti-D, which does not cross the placenta, after any incident where mixing of the fetal and maternal circulations is likely is known to reduce the mother's risk of developing her own anti-D, and reduces the risk of fetal haemolytic disease (Fig. 45.4). Prophylactic anti-D can also be administered, routinely, at 28 and 34 weeks gestation.

Antibody screen

This is performed at booking and on at least one other occasion later in pregnancy, usually around 34 weeks. Antibodies can occur in all women, not just those who are Rhesus negative. A rising antibody titre raises worries of fetal anaemia, prompting ultrasound scans looking for signs of this, and, if indicated, fetal blood sampling.

Events after which anti-D is given
• Delivery
• External cephalic version
• Termination of pregnancy
• Manual removal of placenta
• Bleeding in pregnancy after 12 weeks gestation
• Ectopic pregnancy
• Abdominal trauma in the third trimester
• Amniocentesis/CVS
• Evacuation of retained products of conception
• Abruption

Fig. 45.4 Events after which anti-D is given.

Rubella antibodies

Rubella acquired in pregnancy can have serious consequences, so the test is done to see if a woman has immunity. If IgG is present she has had the infection or has been vaccinated in the past. Exposure in the pregnancy should still be investigated if she develops symptoms but the risk of reinfection is extremely low. If she is not immune, she can be advised to avoid any contact with the infection and a vaccination can be given after the baby is born so that she will be protected in future pregnancies. As the vaccine is live it cannot be given during pregnancy.

Syphilis antibodies

Happily, syphilis is rare but because fetal infection can have devastating consequences and is easily treated by giving the mother penicillin, a case remains for screening in pregnancy.

Hepatitis antibodies

Detection of hepatitis B or C has implications for fetal health and for the long-term health of the woman and her partner. Hepatitis B can be transmitted to the fetus in utero, via transplacental haemorrhage, or at the time of delivery (vertical transmission). If infected, the baby will have a 90% chance of developing chronic hepatitis, with the possible sequelae of cirrhosis and primary hepatocellular carcinoma. Identifying a woman who is positive for hepatitis B antenatally allows the paediatric team the chance to try to prevent the baby from infection by administering vaccine neonatally. It also allows the woman to be monitored by the medical team; her partner and any other children can be screened.

HIV antibodies

All women should be encouraged to have HIV screening. Diagnosis of HIV in pregnancy can improve the outcome for the unborn child, the mother, her partner and any other children (see Chapter 36). As this is now part of routine booking, there should be no stigma attached, and no penalty imposed by insurance companies.

Urinalysis

The urine is dipped for protein, blood, and glucose and can also be analysed for leucocytes and nitrites.

Proteinuria

If protein is detected on dipstix the first question should be whether the sample was contaminated with vaginal discharge and, if so, to ask for a repeat sample. If protein persists, it must be investigated. Leucocytes and nitrites would add to the suspicion of a UTI, which can be excluded by sending an MSU; do not be reassured by lack of symptoms as pregnant women are often unaffected by 'cystitis'. If this is negative and proteinuria persists, the possibility of renal disease or (later in pregnancy) pre-eclampsia should be considered (see Chapter 35). The first step is to obtain a 24-h urine collection to quantify the protein. Total protein excretion increases in pregnancy, so proteinuria should not be diagnosed until more than 0.3g is excreted in 24h.

Glycosuria

Finding glucose on dipstix is very common in pregnancy. In some cases it is due to impaired glucose tolerance or gestational diabetes but in others a glucose tolerance test will not reveal this diagnosis. In the past it was thought that these women's glycosuria could be explained by an altered renal threshold for glucose, but physiological studies have not proved this. Instead, we must recognize that in some women glycosuria is normal in pregnancy.

Haematuria

Contamination with vaginal blood must be excluded. An MSU should be sent to look for infection. If this is negative consider a renal ultrasound for evidence of stones or renal disease.

Screening and prenatal diagnosis

Assessing the risk that the fetus is affected by some chromosomal abnormalities can be done using a blood test that looks at proteins in the maternal blood or by using ultrasound, which measures the thickness of the fat pad in the nuchal fold of the fetal neck. Both types of test can give false-positive and false-negative results and are only risk assessments rather than diagnostic tests, but the result can help parents to decide if they want more invasive tests, for example amniocentesis.

 Nuchal thickness is measured on ultrasound scan between 11 and 14 weeks gestation. Serum screening is performed between 15 and 20 weeks gestation.

Women who opt for diagnostic testing in the form of amniocentesis or chorionic villus sampling might be doing so for a variety of reasons (see Chapter 33). It is now recognized that ultrasound scanning at 18–20 weeks is the best method of screening for neural tube defects (e.g. spina bifida).

Planning antenatal care

Most women in the UK currently have 'shared care', where they are booked to deliver in hospital under the care of a consultant obstetrician but the majority of their antenatal care is provided by the GP and/or midwife in the community. The frequency of hospital visits will be determined by their assessment as low or high risk at booking. Some women will not need hospital care at all, booking with the GP or midwife and arranging to deliver in hospital under their care or at home. Midwife-led 'home-from-home' birth centres are another option. A minority of women, who are particularly high-risk, will have all of their visits with the consultant team in hospital.

A plan for the woman's care should be made at her booking visit after any risk factors affecting the pregnancy have been identified (see Fig. 45.1). The number of visits needed varies from woman to woman; most antenatal visits follow the pattern: booking (around 12 weeks), followed by visits at 20, 28, 34, 38 weeks and then weekly until delivery. If there is cause for concern at any time this schedule will change to include extra visits, which may be in the community or at the hospital.

Education at booking

The booking visit is an opportunity for the woman to ask questions regarding her antenatal care and delivery, and for the midwife or doctor to ensure that advice about the following is given:

- Folic acid: taking folate supplements before conception and in the first trimester of pregnancy reduces the risk of fetal neural tube defects.
- Diet: certain foods are not advisable in pregnancy (Fig. 45.5).
- Exercise: it is safe to continue exercising in pregnancy but sensible to modify the exercise routines as the pregnancy advances and to bear in mind that it is far easier to strain muscles because of increased progesterone levels.
- Seatbelts: it is illegal to go without a seatbelt and pregnancy is not an exemption. The belt should be worn above and below, not across, the 'bump'.
- Smoking: smoking increases the risk of fetal and neonatal problems; it is also associated with cot death and childhood illnesses.
- Toxoplasma: infection is acquired from contact with cat faeces, which can contaminate soil, so pregnant women are advised to wash fruit and salad carefully, not to handle cat litter and to wear gloves if gardening. Animals can ingest infected soil, which can pass through the food chain unless meat is cooked through thoroughly, so women are advised against eating uncooked or 'rare' meat in pregnancy.

Dietary advice in pregnancy	
Food to avoid	Risk
Soft cheese Unpasteurized milk and cheese Uncooked fish, e.g. sushi, smoked fish Chill-cook meals	Listeria: fetal infection can lead to miscarriage or stillbirth
Unwashed salad/fruit/vegetables Raw and rare meat Unpasteurized milk	Toxoplasma: fetal infection can lead to miscarriage, stillbirth or long-term disability
Shellfish Uncooked egg	Can cause food poisoning, which can precipitate premature labour

Fig. 45.5 Dietary advice in pregnancy.

Antenatal visits after booking

At each visit following booking these points are covered:

- General health and well-being.
- Fetal movements.
- Urinalysis.
- Blood pressure.
- Abdominal palpation for fetal growth, lie and presentation.
- Auscultation of the fetal heart.

Any worries or symptoms can be discussed. The so-called 'minor' symptoms of pregnancy can cause major upset, yet some are simply treated. Common problems and suitable advice/treatment are shown in Fig. 45.6.

'Minor' symptoms of pregnancy

- Nausea: eating little and often, acupuncture and anti-emetics. If severe vomiting develops admission will be needed
- Constipation: increase fruit in diet, drink plenty of water, and regular aperients as necessary
- Headache: often due to dehydration but paracetamol is safe in pregnancy
- Pain due to ligament stretch and symphysis pubis separation: helped by regular paracetamol and physiotherapy
- Piles (haemorrhoids): soothing cream available, ice packs an alternative
- Reflux (heartburn): avoid spicy foods, sleep in a more upright position, use liquid antacid preparations, sometimes use H_2-blockers, e.g. ranitidine

Fig. 45.6 'Minor' symptoms of pregnancy – appropriate advice and treatment.

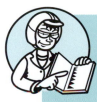

- What information will help you to estimate the gestation of pregnancy?
- Mrs Jones is booking in her fourth pregnancy. She has had two babies and a miscarriage. What is her gravidity and parity?
- Why screen for hepatitis and HIV in pregnancy?
- Which foodstuffs can transmit toxoplasma?
- What are the three main substances tested for at urinalysis?

46. Examination

General examination

General examination of the patient is extremely important and is often overlooked. Ensure that the patient is comfortable and not unduly exposed. Obstetric patients should not be examined flat on their backs because of the risk of postural supine hypotensive syndrome. The following general assessment should be made quickly:

- The patient's general well-being.
- The cardiovascular system, including pulse, blood pressure, cardiac murmurs and clinical signs of anaemia; oedema can affect the hands, the periorbital region, the legs and the sacral region.
- The respiratory system.

The urine should be tested for the presence of sugar and protein.

A chaperone should always be used when performing a gynaecological examination.

Abdominal examination

Inspection
Inspection of the abdomen is an important part of the abdominal examination.

Surgical scars
Surgical scars are often overlooked because of successful attempts to produce cosmetically pleasing scars. Transverse suprapubic and laparoscopy scars are commonly missed unless specifically looked for. Always check the umbilicus and pubic hairline for hidden scars. Multiple small scars might be present following minimal access surgical procedures.

Abdominal masses
Inspection for abdominal masses is important, although they might not be evident on inspection alone because of an increased BMI. The size and shape of the abdomen should be noted.

Stigmata of pregnancy
Striae gravidarum (stretch marks) caused by pregnancy hormones that stimulate the splitting of the dermis and can occur relatively early in pregnancy. New striae appear red and sometimes inflamed and can be sore and itchy, old striae from previous pregnancies are pale and silvery. They usually appear on the lower abdomen, upper thighs, buttocks and breasts.

Increased skin pigmentation can occur in pregnancy and results in the linear nigra – midline pigmentation from the xiphisternum to the symphysis pubis. Other areas that can undergo pigmentation in pregnancy include the nipples, the vulva, the umbilicus and recent abdominal scars.

Palpation
Before palpating the abdomen always enquire for areas of tenderness and palpate these areas last. Using the palm of the hand, gently palpate the four quadrants of the abdomen to elicit tenderness, guarding and rebound.

On discovering an abdominal mass, the size, shape, position, mobility and consistency should be assessed. If a mass is discovered you should first ascertain whether it is arising from the pelvis. If you cannot palpate the lower aspect of the mass it is probably arising from the pelvis. Pelvic tumours can generally be moved from side to side but not up and down. Percussion can help outline the borders of a mass in an obese patient. Auscultation of the abdomen is important to assess bowel sounds and in an obstetric patient the fetal heart should be auscultated using a pinard or a sonicaid.

Obstetric palpation
Uterine size
Uterine size is assessed by palpation and is a skill that is acquired through experience. A rough guide to the uterine size can be made from assessment of the fundal height in relation to the topography of the abdomen, for example the symphysis pubis, umbilicus and xiphisternum (Fig. 46.1). The fundus of the uterus should not be palpable abdominally until 12 weeks gestation. By 36 weeks the fundus

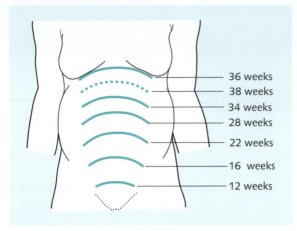

Fig. 46.1 Fundal height in relation to abdominal landmarks.

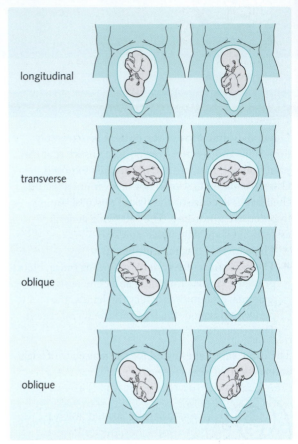

Fig. 46.2 The fetal lie. The relationship of the long axis of the fetus to the long axis of the uterus.

should be almost at the level of the xiphisternum, following which it drops as the fetal head engages into the maternal pelvis.

When palpating the uterine fundus, always start at the xiphisternum and work towards the umbilicus using the medial border of the hand or the fingertips. Percussing the fundus can be useful in obese women. Measuring the distance from the fundus to the symphysis pubis in centimetres (the symphysis–fundal height) is a more objective method of assessing fundal height than using topography alone but is not a replacement for careful palpation. The symphysis–fundal height measurement ± 3 cm should equal the number of weeks amenorrhoea after 24 weeks gestation. Similarly, after 28 weeks gestation the abdominal girth measured in inches at the level of the umbilicus should equal the number of weeks amenorrhoea, although this is less reliable and not routinely peformed

Number of fetuses

The number of fetuses present can be calculated by assessing the number of fetal poles present. 'Fetal pole' is the term used to denote the head or the breech. In a singleton pregnancy, two poles should be palpable unless the presenting part is deeply engaged in the pelvis. In multiple pregnancies, the number of poles present *minus one* should be palpable. For example, four poles are present in a twin pregnancy and only three should be palpable as one is usually tucked away out of reach. In a triplet pregnancy, six poles are present and five should be palpable, and so on. This requires a high level of skill in abdominal

palpation but don't worry, the patient will usually tell you how many fetuses are present!

Fetal lie

This is the relationship between the long axis of the fetus and the long axis of the uterus. This can be longitudinal, transverse or oblique (Fig. 46.2).

Fetal presentation

This is the part of the fetus that presents to the mother's pelvis. If the head is situated over the pelvis this is termed a 'cephalic presentation'. Three different types of cephalic presentation can occur, depending on the degree of flexion of the head on the fetal spine:

- A well flexed head will present by the vertex (the area bordered by the parietal bones and the anterior and posterior fontanelles).
- A partly extended head will present by the brow.
- A fully extended head will present by the face.

In a breech presentation the buttocks occupy the lower segment, and in an oblique lie the shoulder generally presents (Fig. 46.3). Any presentation other than a vertex presentation is called a malpresentation.

Engagement

The fetal head is said to be engaged when the widest diameter of the head (the biparietal diameter) has passed through the pelvic brim. Abdominal palpation of the head is assessed in fifths and is measured by palpating the angle between the head and the symphysis pubis (Fig. 46.4). When three or more fifths of the head are palpable abdominally the head is not engaged. When two or fewer fifths of the head are palpable the head is clinically engaged.

Position

The position of the presenting part is defined as the relationship of the denominator of the presenting part to the maternal pelvis. The denominator changes according to the presenting part, the occiput in a cephalic presentation, the mentum (chin) in a face presentation and the sacrum in a breech presentation. An idea of the position can be gained at abdominal palpation by determining the position of the fetal back. If the back lies:

- On the maternal left, the position is likely to be left occipitolateral.
- On the maternal right, the position is likely to be right occipitolateral.
- More posteriorly (i.e. towards the mother's spine), the position is likely to be left or right occipitoposterior.
- Anteriorly, the position is likely to be left or right occipitoanterior (Fig. 46.5).

The position of the presenting part can be assessed accurately only by vaginal examination, because the head might not lie in the same axis as the fetal trunk.

Attitude

This term is no longer commonly used. It describes the relationship of the fetal parts to the fetus itself. For instance, when the head, back and limbs of the fetus are flexed, as in the classic 'fetal position', the fetus has a flexed attitude; conversely it can be said to have an extended attitude.

Liquor volume

Clinical assessment of liquor volume is not as accurate as objective assessment using ultrasound. However, subjective assessment can alert the examiner to the possibility of reduced or increased liquor volume and instigation of the necessary investigations. Reduced liquor volume might be suggested when the uterus is small for dates with easily palpable fetal parts producing an irregular firm outline to the uterus. Increased liquor volume causes a large-for-dates uterus that is smooth and rounded and in which the fetal parts are almost impossible to distinguish. If suspected, an ultrasound scan should be ordered to assess objective measurements such as depth of deepest pool or amniotic fluid index.

Difficulty palpating fetal parts

Many students worry that they will not be able to ascertain all the above information during an obstetric abdominal palpation. This is not always possible even in the most experienced hands but it is important to understand why this might be so. Figure 46.6 shows some situations when palpation of the fetal parts might prove difficult.

Pelvic examination
Gynaecological pelvic examination

There are three important steps when performing a pelvic examination:

1. External inspection of the vulva.
2. Internal inspection of the vagina and cervix via a speculum.
3. Bimanual examination of the pelvis.

The most common position for carrying out a pelvic examination is the dorsal position with the woman lying on her back with her knees flexed. Make sure that the patient is as comfortable as possible and not too exposed.

During a gynaecological examination the pelvic examination should always be preceded by inspection of the external genitals, and vaginal walls.

External examination of the vulva

The presence of abnormal discharge on the vulva should be noted, as should the anatomy of the

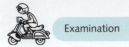

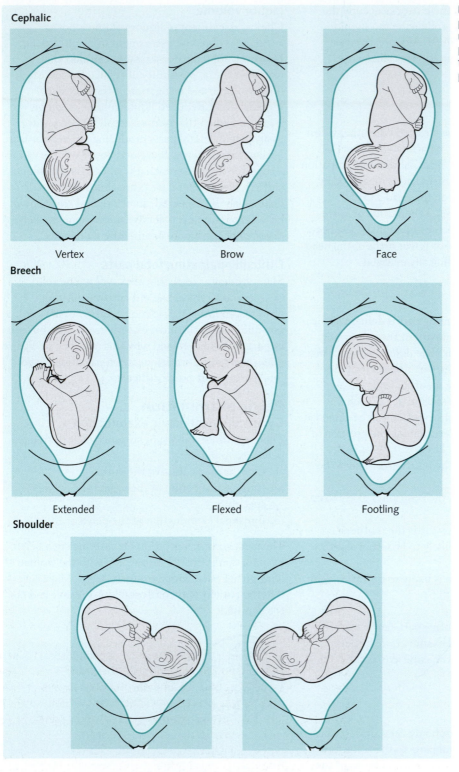

Cephalic

Vertex

Brow

Face

Breech

Extended

Flexed

Footling

Shoulder

Fig. 46.3 The fetal presentation. The relationship of the presenting part of the fetus to the maternal pelvis.

Fig. 46.4 Engagement of the fetal head.

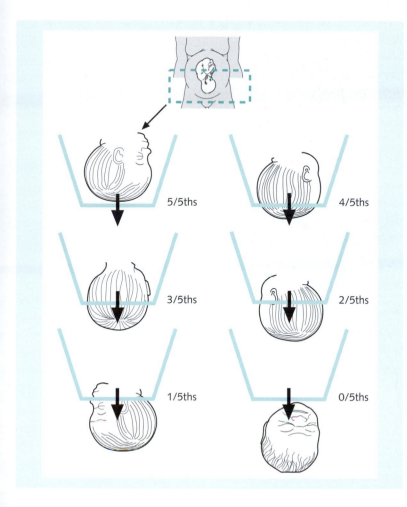

external genitalia (Fig. 46.7). Parting the labia with the left hand, the entire area should be carefully inspected for inflammation, ulceration, swellings, atrophic changes and leucoplakia (white plaques) and the clitoris and urethral orifice inspected. A deficient or scarred perineum are clues to previous trauma due to vaginal delivery. Vaginal or uterine prolapse through the introitus is assessed with and without the patient bearing down and stress incontinence might be demonstrated when the patient coughs. Assessment of prolapse can only be adequately made with the patient in the left lateral position using a Sims' speculum.

Internal inspection of the vagina and cervix

To inspect the vagina and cervix, a speculum is used. Two types of specula are used commonly, the Cusco's (bivalve) and the Sims' specula (Fig. 46.8).

The Cusco's speculum is used with the patient in the dorsal position and consists of two blades hinged outside the patient. When the blades are opened, the anterior and posterior walls of the vagina are separated allowing the vaginal fornices and cervix to be visualized. The main disadvantage of the Cusco's speculum is that the anterior and posterior walls of the vagina cannot be assessed adequately.

The Sims' speculum is used to inspect the anterior and posterior walls of the vagina and is an excellent tool for assessing uterovaginal prolapse. It was originally developed to examine vaginal fistulae. With the patient in the left lateral, or Sims', position the blade of the speculum is inserted into the vagina and used to retract either the anterior or posterior walls. Uterovaginal prolapse can then be assessed with the patient bearing down.

Bimanual examination

It is usual to perform an internal examination using the lubricated index and middle fingers of the right hand, although in nulligravid and postmenopausal

Fig. 46.5 The fetal position.

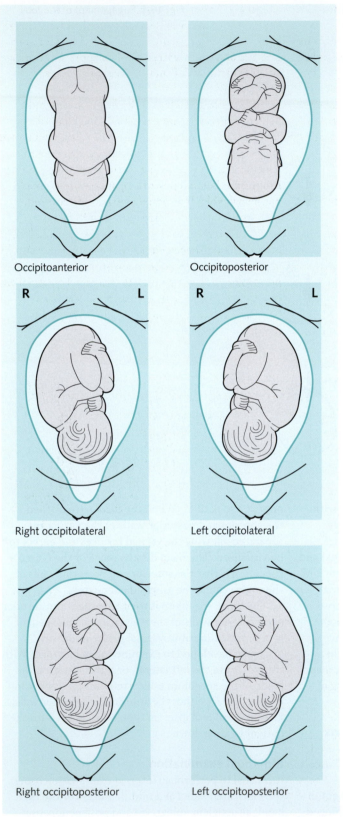

Occipitoanterior

Occipitoposterior

Right occipitolateral

Left occipitolateral

Right occipitoposterior

Left occipitoposterior

women it might be possible to use only the index finger. Palpation of the vaginal walls is important to exclude scarring, cysts and tumours that can easily be missed on inspection. The vaginal fornices should be examined for scarring, thickening and swellings that will suggest pelvic pathology. The size, shape, position, consistency, angle and mobility of the cervix should be assessed. Moving the cervix from side to side might elicit cervical excitation pain and elevating the cervix anteriorly, thereby stretching the uterosacral ligaments, might cause pain in the presence of endometriosis.

The fingers of the right hand are then used to elevate or steady the uterus while the left hand palpates abdominally. An anteverted uterus is usually palpable between the two hands. A retroverted uterus is usually felt as a swelling in the posterior fornix and is not bimanually palpable unless it is flipped forward into an anteverted position and elevated into the anterior part of the pelvis. The different combinations of version and flexion of the uterus are shown in Fig. 46.9. The size, position, consistency, outline and mobility of the uterus should all be noted. A pregnant uterus should feel soft and globular and roughly the size of an apple, large orange and grapefruit at 6, 8 and 12 weeks gestation, respectively.

To examine the adnexa, the fingers of the right hand should be positioned in one of the lateral fornices and the adnexal region palpated between the two hands. Normal premenopausal ovaries are not always palpable depending on the size of the patient. Fallopian tubes and postmenopausal ovaries should not be palpable. If an adnexal mass is discovered, then its size, shape, consistency, mobility and whether it is fixed to the uterus or not should all be noted. The presence and degree of tenderness should be noted. In the presence of a suspected ectopic, pelvic examination should not be carried out prior to inserting a large intravenous cannula as profound internal haemorrhage might occur if the ectopic pregnancy ruptures.

Situations where fetal parts might be difficult to palpate	
Types of reason	**Description**
Maternal reasons	Maternal obesity
	Muscular anterior abdominal wall
Uterine reasons	Anterior uterine wall fibroids
	Uterine contraction/Braxton Hicks contraction
Fetoplacental reasons	Anterior placenta
	Increased liquor volume

Fig. 46.6 Situations where fetal parts might be difficult to palpate.

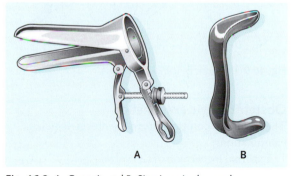

Fig. 46.8 A. Cusco's and B. Sims' vaginal specula.

Fig. 46.7 The female external genitalia.

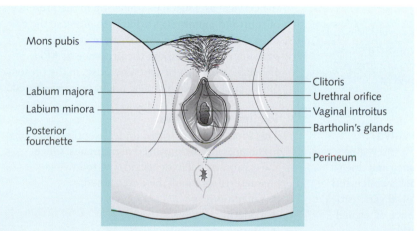

Mons pubis

Labium majora

Labium minora

Posterior fourchette

Clitoris
Urethral orifice
Vaginal introitus
Bartholin's glands

Perineum

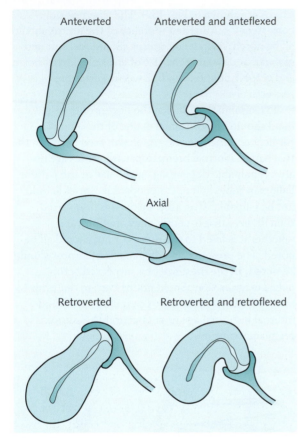

Fig. 46.9 Positions of the uterus.

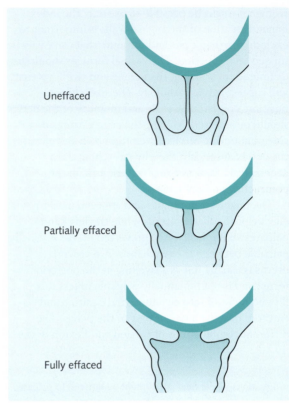

Fig. 46.10 Effacement of the cervix.

Obstetric pelvic examination

Their are four components to the obstetric pelvic examination:

1. External inspection of the vulva.
2. Internal inspection of the vagina and cervix.
3. Vaginal examination.
4. Pelvic examination.

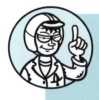

An obstetric examination is incomplete without a blood pressure check, urinanalysis and auscultation of the fetus.

External examination of the vulva

The blood flow through the vulva and vagina increases dramatically in pregnancy and due to engorgement the vulva might look swollen and oedematous. The presence of vulval varicosities should be noted. Note the presence of vaginal discharge or leaking amniotic fluid.

Internal inspection of the vagina and cervix

Examination of the vagina and cervix through a sterile Cusco's speculum should be performed using an aseptic technique. The vagina and cervix might take on a bluish tinge compared with the non-pregnant state. Increased vaginal and cervical secretions are normal in pregnancy. Inspection of the cervix might reveal amniotic fluid draining through the cervical os. Digital examination in the presence of ruptured membranes is likely to increase the risk of ascending infection. Exclusion of cervical pathology is important in the presence of APH, although care must be taken because, in the presence of placenta praevia, bleeding might be exacerbated.

Vaginal examination

This should be performed under aseptic conditions in the presence of ruptured membranes. Once the cervix has been identified, the following characteristics should be determined:

• Dilatation.
• Length.
• Station of presenting part.

- Consistency.
- Position.

Cervical dilatation

Cervical dilatation is assessed in centimetres using the examining fingers. One finger-breadth is roughly 1–1.5 cm. Full dilatation of the cervix is equivalent to 10 cm dilatation.

Cervical length

The normal length of the cervix is about 3 cm and shortening occurs as the cervix effaces due to uterine contractions (Fig. 46.10).

Station of the presenting part

The station of the presenting part is determined by how much the presenting part has descended into the pelvis. The station is defined as the number of

When taking a smear test a brush should always be used to sample the endocervix as well as a spatula.

centimetres above or below a fixed point in the maternal pelvis, the ischial spines (Fig. 46.11).

Cervical consistency

Softening of the cervix occurs as pregnancy progresses aiding cervical effacement and dilatation. The consistency of the cervix can be described as firm, mid-consistency or soft.

Cervical position

This describes where the cervix is situated in the anteroposterior plane of the pelvis. As the cervix becomes effaced and dilated it tends to be pulled from a posterior to a more anterior position.

The Bishop score

Using the above characteristics, Bishop devised a scoring system to evaluate the 'ripeness' or favourability of the cervix (Fig. 46.12). This system is often used when inducing labour to assess the likelihood of success. The higher the score, the more favourable the cervix and the more likely that induction of labour will be successful. It can also be used to assess cervical change in threatened premature labour.

Defining the position of the presenting part

With a cephalic presentation, the anterior and posterior fontanelles and the sagittal sutures should be identified. The posterior fontanelle is Y-shaped and is formed when the three sutures between the

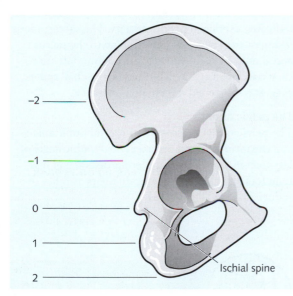

Ischial spine

Fig. 46.11 The station of the presenting part.

Fig. 46.12 The Bishop scoring system for the uterine cervix.

The Bishop scoring system for the uterine cervix				
Cervical characteristic	Score 0	1	2	3
Dilatation (cm)	0	1–2	3–4	>5
Length (cm)	3	2	1	
Station (cm)	−3	−2	−1 or 0	+1 or +2
Consistency	firm	medium	soft	
Position	posterior	mid	anterior	

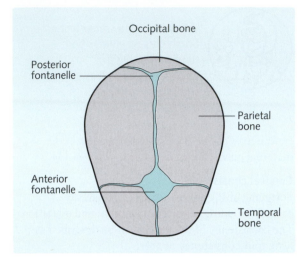

Fig. 46.13 The anterior and posterior fontanelles.

When assessing progress in labour one must always comment on engagement of head, cervical dilatation, cervical effacement, station of head in relation to ischial spines, position of head, moulding, caput and liquor colour (eg meconium staining).

occipital and parietal bones meet. The anterior fontanelle is larger, diamond-shaped and formed by the four sutures between the parietal and temporal bones meeting (Fig. 46.13). The denominator for a cephalic presentation is the occiput and for a breech presentation the sacrum. Having identified the denominator, the position of the presenting part can be defined (Fig. 46.14).

Pelvic examination

There are four basic pelvic types:
1. Gynaecoid.
2. Android.
3. Ellipsoid.
4. Platypoid.

Clinical assessment of the pelvis will reveal the characteristics of these pelvic types. Figure 46.15 summarizes the characteristics of the four basic pelvic types.

The pelvic inlet

The pelvic inlet is assessed clinically by measuring the diagonal conjugate (Fig. 46.16). This is the distance from the sacral promontory to the inferoposterior margin of the symphysis pubis (the true conjugate is measured to the anteroposterior margin of the symphysis pubis). In a normal gynaecoid pelvis the sacral promontory cannot usually be reached. If it is, the pelvic inlet is significantly reduced.

The pelvic cavity

The pelvic cavity is assessed by palpating the sacral curve, which should be concave away from the examining fingers (Fig. 46.17). A straight sacrum indicates a reduced pelvic capacity. The sacrospinous ligament runs from the ischial spine to the sacrum and should be wide enough to accommodate more than two fingers (> 3 cm). Prominent ischial spines suggest a shortened interspinous distance.

The pelvic outlet

The pelvic outlet is assessed by the subpubic angle and the intertuberous distance. A subpubic angle of less than 90° and an intertuberous distance of less than four knuckles wide indicate the possibility of a reduced outlet (Fig. 46.18).

It has become increasingly recognized that the best test of a pelvis is the dynamic process of labour itself, so formal pelvic assessment is no longer performed as a routine. However, the Bishop score is used in the assessment of cervical favourability prior to induction of labour.

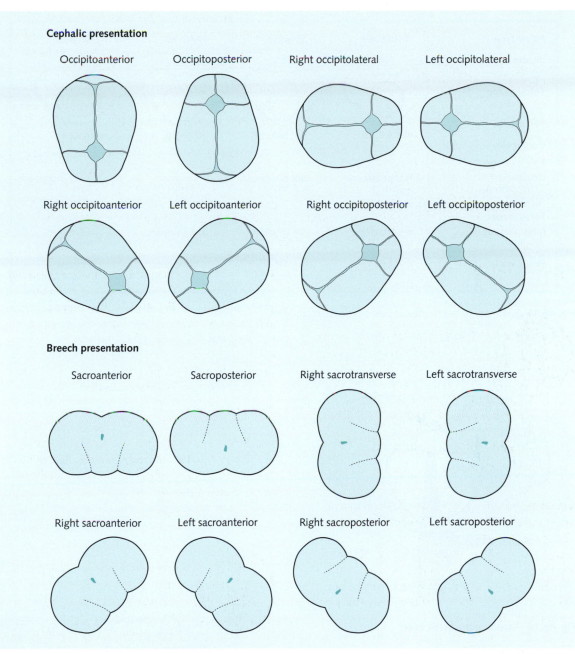

Fig. 46.14 Defining the position of the presenting part.

Pelvic type	Gynaecoid	Elllipsoid	Android	Platypoid
Incidence	50%	25%	20%	5%
Pelvic shape	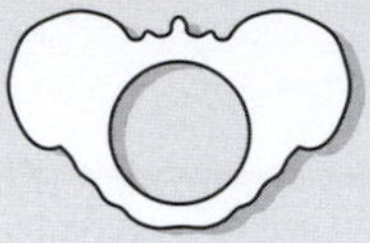	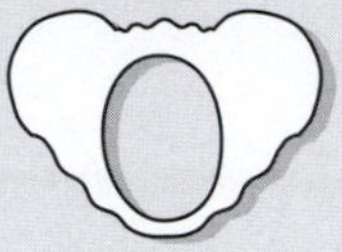	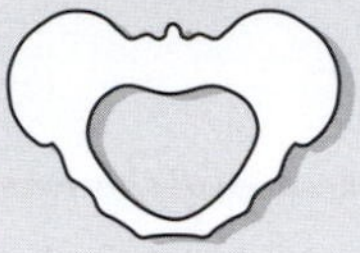	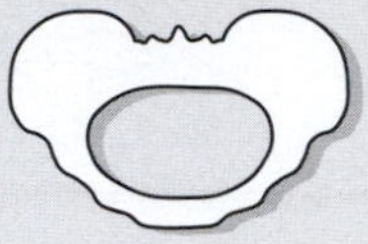
Pelvic inlet Obstetric Conjugate	Not reduced	Not reduced	Reduced	Reduced
Pelvic cavity Ischial spine Sacrospinous ligament	Not prominent > 3 cm	Not prominent > 3 cm	Prominent < 3 cm	Usually prominent > 3 cm
Pelvic outlet Intertuberous diameter	> 4 knuckles wide	< 4 knuckles wide	< 4 knuckles wide	> 4 knuckles wide
Pelvic walls	Parallel	Parallel	Convergent	Divergent

Fig. 46.15 Summary of the four basic pelvic-type characteristics.

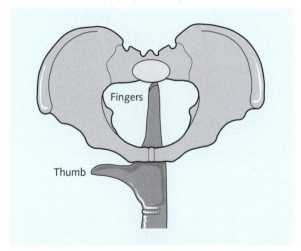

Fig. 46.16 Assessing the pelvic inlet.

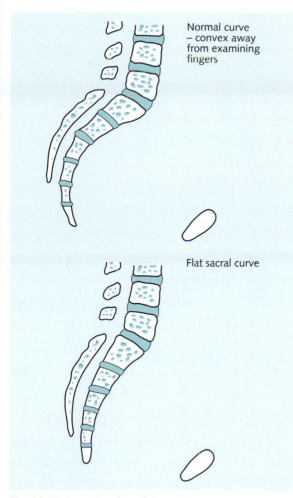

Normal curve
– convex away
from examining
fingers

Flat sacral curve

Fig. 46.17 Assessing the pelvic cavity.

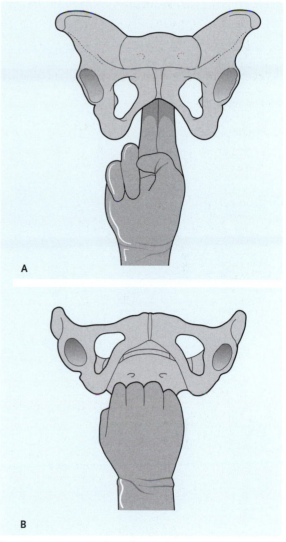

A

B

Fig. 46.18 Assessing the pelvic outlet.

47. Common Investigations

Imaging techniques

Imaging techniques are used widely in both obstetrics and gynaecology. Results of imaging tests should be interpreted carefully in the light of the history and clinical findings.

Ultrasound scanning

Ultrasound examination of the pregnant and non-pregnant pelvis is probably the most common investigation performed in obstetrics and gynaecology. Ultrasound waves passing through the pelvis are reflected in varying degrees depending on the density of the tissues present. For instance, bone is very reflective (or echogenic) and appears white on the monitor, whereas fluid is less echogenic and appears dark on the monitor. Interpretation of these echoes is the mainstay of diagnosis in ultrasound.

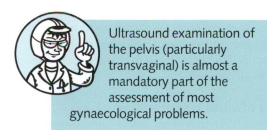

Ultrasound examination of the pelvis (particularly transvaginal) is almost a mandatory part of the assessment of most gynaecological problems.

The non-pregnant pelvis

To examine the non-pregnant pelvis a full bladder is required. This lifts the uterus from under the pubic bone, allows a 'window' through which to view the pelvic contents and helps push the bowel out of the pelvis.

The uterus

The dimensions of the uterus can be measured and the position noted. Abnormal textures in the myometrium can suggest the presence of fibroids or adenomyosis. The midline echo corresponds to the endometrial thickness and will vary depending on the menstrual cycle. Pathology of the endometrial cavity, such as endometrial hyperplasia, endometrial polyps or submucous fibroids, might be detected.

Intrauterine contraceptive devices (IUCDs) will show up as very bright echoes.

The ovaries

The size and position of the ovaries can be assessed. In polycystic ovary syndrome (PCOS, see Chapter 32), the polycystic ovary is on average twice the normal volume with thickened central stroma and 10 or more peripherally sited follicles. Follicular tracking is possible in women trying to conceive. Ovarian tumours can be identified ultrasonographically but differentiation between benign and malignant tumours cannot be made with certainty. Figure 47.1 shows some of the ultrasound characteristics of benign and malignant ovarian tumours.

The fallopian tubes

The fallopian tubes are not normally visible by ultrasound. However, when they are blocked and distended with fluid (hydrosalpinx) they will appear as cystic structures that might be mistaken for ovarian cysts.

Ultrasound and pregnancy

A gestation sac can be seen in the uterine cavity from as early as 5 weeks amenorrhoea (Fig. 47.2), especially when using a transvaginal probe. The fetal heart is detectable with ultrasound by 6 weeks amenorrhoea. Crown–rump length (CRL) is a useful measurement with which to date the fetus up to 12 weeks amenorrhoea, by which time CRL measurement becomes inaccurate due to flexion of the fetus. After the first trimester, the biparietal diameter (BPD) is a more accurate measurement with which to date the pregnancy.

Early pregnancy complications

A blighted ovum or anembryonic pregnancy occurs when the embryo fails to develop; 'missed miscarriage' is the term used when an embryo has died in utero. In the presence of an ectopic pregnancy, the usual ultrasonic finding is that of a thickened endometrium in the presence of an adnexal mass. In only about 5% of ectopic

Ultrasound characteristics of benign and malignant tumours		
	Benign	**Malignant**
Size	<5 cm	>5 cm
Laterality	Unilateral	Bilateral
Cyst walls	Thin	Thick
Septa	Absent	Thick, incomplete
Solid areas	Absent	Present
Ascites	Absent	Present

Fig. 47.1 Ultrasound characteristics of benign and malignant tumours.

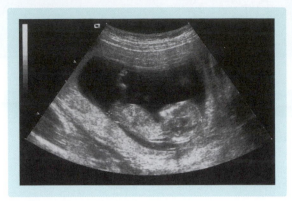

Fig. 47.2 Ultrasound in early pregnancy.

pregnancies can a viable pregnancy be seen outside the uterus with ultrasound. The most important role of ultrasound in the management of a suspected ectopic pregnancy is to confirm a viable intrauterine pregnancy.

Anomaly scans

Most obstetric units offer routine anomaly scans between 18 and 20 weeks gestation. Different fetal anomalies are best detected at different times throughout the pregnancy, but 18–20 weeks appears to be the optimum time for a screening anomaly scan. Apart from gross anatomical defects, certain 'markers', such as choroid plexus cysts, renal pelvi-caliceal dilatation and the cardiac 'golfball' sign, might be identified and can be associated with chromosomal abnormalities.

Fetal growth

Fetal growth is assessed clinically in a normal singleton pregnancy. In situations when the uterine size is not compatible with dates or clinical assessment is difficult, for instance in the presence of obesity or multiple pregnancy, objective measurements of fetal head circumference (HC), BPD and abdominal circumference (AC) can be measured using ultrasound and plotted on fetal growth charts. Scanning at regular intervals allows the growth of the fetus to be monitored.

Assessment of liquor volume

This is useful in the management of IUGR and postdates pregnancy. Reduced liquor volume can indicate the presence of placental insufficiency and might be an indication for delivery of the fetus depending on the clinical background. Reduced liquor might also be due to spontaneous rupture of the membranes.

Doppler studies

Doppler ultrasound assessment of the uteroplacental blood flow can be useful in the presence of fetal growth restriction due to placental insufficiency. Dilatation of middle cerebral vessels and absent or reversed end diastolic flow in the umbilical artery suggest a compromised fetus that is diverting its blood flow to essential organs such as the brain and kidneys and is an indication for delivery. Doppler studies need to be interpreted carefully in the light of the clinical picture.

Safety of ultrasound scanning

Experimental evidence has not shown any harmful effects of ultrasound when used as a diagnostic test.

X-ray

Two X-ray procedures that were commonly used in the past are now not used so frequently because the information gained does not always warrant the exposure to X-rays:

1. Erect lateral pelvimetry (ELP): can be used in situations where a contracted pelvis needs to be excluded, for instance in the management of a breech presentation. The inlet and outlet of the pelvis can be measured objectively as can the curve of the sacrum. This procedure can be performed using CT scanning but for reasons already discussed (see Chapter 39) is less commonly used these days.

2. Hysterosalpingography (HSG): can be used to assess the uterine cavity and the patency of the

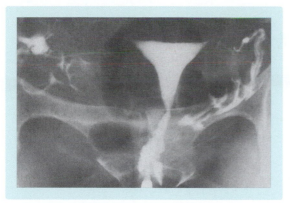

Fig. 47.3 A hysterosalpingogram.

Laparoscopy is the gold-standard investigation of pelvic pain.

fallopian tubes (Fig. 47.3). A catheter is inserted into the cervix and radiocontrast medium injected into the uterine cavity while X-rays are taken. It does not allow the exclusion of pelvic pathology as does laparoscopic assessment of the pelvic organs, but is still useful in the presence of tubal blockage to assess whether the blockage is distal or proximal; it also allows excellent delineation of the uterine cavity.

Laparoscopy

Laparoscopy is the mainstay of diagnosing pelvic disease and has effectively replaced exploratory laparotomies. The advantage of laparoscopy over imaging techniques is that the pelvic and other intra-abdominal organs can be visualized directly through endoscopes.

Technique

The vast majority of procedures are performed under general anaesthesia. Having emptied the bladder, a Veress needle is inserted into the lower abdomen through a subumbilical incision. Carbon dioxide is pumped into the peritoneal cavity to produce a pneumoperitoneum (to a pressure of approximately 18mmHg) and then a trocar and cannula are inserted through the same incision into the pneumoperitoneum. A laparoscope can then be passed down the cannula and the pelvic organs visualized (Fig. 47.4). Complications include perforation of bladder, bowel or blood vessels, and gas embolism.

Hysteroscopy

A hysteroscope is an endoscope that is inserted transcervically into the uterus to inspect the uterine cavity (Fig. 47.5). It is the best way of identifying intrauterine pathology such as endometrial polyps, submucous fibroids and endometrial carcinoma and has replaced the conventional D&C for this purpose. It can be performed under either general or local anaesthesia. A distension medium is required to separate the uterine walls, normal saline and carbon dioxide being the most commonly used. It is a relatively safe procedure but complications include perforation of the uterus, gas embolism and infection.

Hysteroscopy is now the gold-standard investigation of abnormal uterine bleeding and can be performed as an outpatient investigation.

Cervical cytology/colposcopy

Squamous carcinoma of the cervix is amenable to screening because it exhibits a pre-invasive phase. Screening is carried out by cytological examination of cervical smears using the Papanicolaou test. Using a Cusco's speculum, the visible cervix is gently scraped through 360°, first to the left and then to the right, using a cervical sampler (Fig. 47.6). A cytobrush can be used to sample the lower endocervical region. The specimens are placed on a glass slide and fixed immediately with an alcohol solution. Women with smears suggestive of CIN or women with an abnormal-looking cervix are then referred for colposcopy.

The colposcope is a binocular microscope enabling the surface epithelium of the cervix to be assessed under magnification and is usually performed in the outpatient setting. The patient is positioned in a

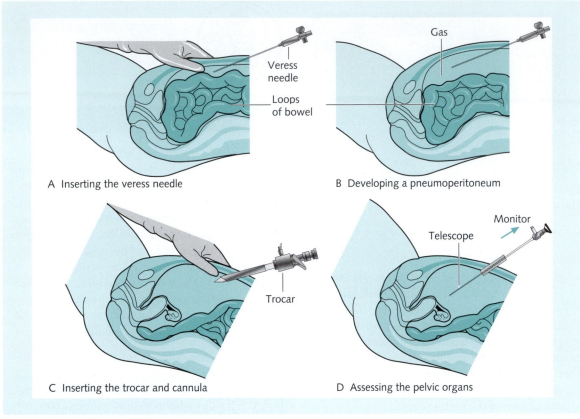

A Inserting the veress needle

Veress needle

Loops of bowel

B Developing a pneumoperitoneum

Gas

C Inserting the trocar and cannula

Trocar

D Assessing the pelvic organs

Telescope

Monitor

Fig. 47.4 Laparoscopic technique.

Fig. 47.5 Hysteroscopic technique.

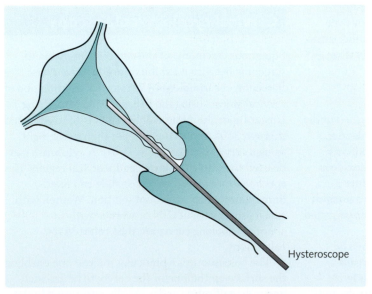

Hysteroscope

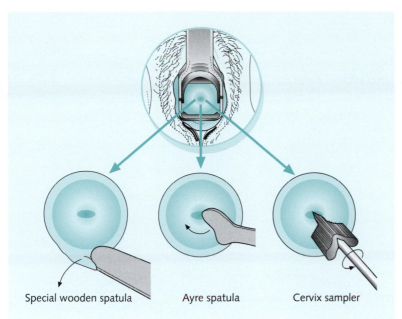

Fig. 47.6 Cervical smear technique.

Special wooden spatula   Ayre spatula   Cervix sampler

modified lithotomy position and the cervix exposed using a Cusco's or bivalve speculum. The cervix is then viewed through the colposcope to identify any lesions such as leucoplakia or frank invasion. Acetic acid solution (5%) is then gently but liberally applied to the entire surface of the cervix. Coagulation of proteins by the acetic acid in abnormal epithelial areas produces white changes, so called acetowhite changes.

Areas of CIN appear as distinct acetowhite lesions with clearly demarcated edges and the associated abnormal vessel formation produces the typical mosaic and punctate patterns. The extent of the lesion should be noted, with particular regard paid to extension into the cervical canal. All abnormal-looking areas should be biopsied for histological assessment.

Urodynamics

This term includes all the tests that assess the function of the lower urinary tract disorders, which include incontinence and voiding difficulties.

Flow studies
Using a flowmeter, the flow rate of urine can be measured. This should be above 15 mL per second and a low flow rate suggests either outflow obstruction or poor detrusor contraction.

Cystometry
The bladder is a reservoir designed to increase in volume at low pressure. Cystometry measures bladder pressure during filling or voiding. Pressure catheters are inserted into the bladder via the urethra and also the rectum. The rectal catheter represents intra-abdominal pressure and is subtracted from the intravesical pressure to give the detrusor pressure. Detrusor pressure is measured during rapid filling of the bladder to detect the presence of detrusor instability. During voiding, detrusor contractility can be measured and outflow resistance and detrusor function assessed.

Videocystourethrography
Videocystourethrography (VCU) is the most informative of urodynamic studies and involves radiologically monitoring the bladder and urethra during cystometry. Congenital anomalies, diverticulae, fistulae and ureteric reflux can all be identified during the filling phase. On coughing, bladder neck descent and genuine stress incontinence might be seen and on voiding, ureteric reflux, urethral fistulae and outflow pathology identified.

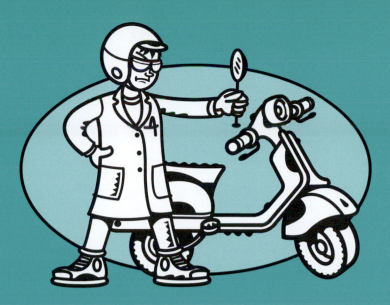

SELF-ASSESSMENT

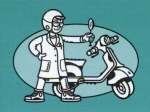

Multiple-choice Questions (MCQs)

Indicate whether each answer is true or false.

Chapter 1 Abnormal Bleeding

1. The following should be performed in the assessment of a patient with abnormal bleeding:

(a) Eliciting a menstrual history
(b) Bimanual pelvic examination
(c) Full blood count
(d) Thyroid function tests
(e) Abdominal X-ray

2. The following are associated with a history secondary dyspareunia:

(a) Pelvic inflammatory disease
(b) Endometriosis
(c) Onset at menarche
(d) Fixed retroverted uterus on bimanual examination
(e) Pelvic pain which commences at time of menstruation and lasts for 1–2 days

Chapter 2 Pelvic Pain and Dyspareunia

3. In the history from a patient complaining of pelvic pain:

(a) Secondary dysmenorrhoea suggests fibroid necrosis
(b) You must know the date of the last menstrual period and the length of the cycle to diagnose Mittelschmerz
(c) A recent change of partner predisposes the patient to pelvic inflammatory disease
(d) Recent surgical termination of pregnancy is not relevant
(e) Nausea and vomiting with acute unilateral pain is suggestive of ovarian torsion

4. When examining a patient presenting with pelvic pain:

(a) Bimanual palpation might reveal tender nodules in the anterior vaginal wall
(b) The uterus typically feels bulky with adenomyosis
(c) Hypotension and tachycardia are associated with ruptured ectopic pregnancy
(d) Ovarian torsion is the likely diagnosis in the presence of vaginal discharge
(e) The differential diagnosis of a unilateral pelvic mass includes a tubo-ovarian abscess

Chapter 3 Vaginal Discharge

5. Symptoms suggesting an infective cause of vaginal discharge include:

(a) Dysuria
(b) Anorexia
(c) Vulval irritation
(d) Constipation
(e) Fever

6. When investigating vaginal discharge:

(a) If tests are negative, the discharge may be physiological
(b) A pelvic ultrasound is mandatory
(c) Laparoscopy might be needed to confirm pelvic inflammatory disease
(d) A smear test should be performed if clinically indicated
(e) A high vaginal swab is routinely used to diagnose chlamydia infection

Chapter 4 Vulval Symptoms

7. A 45-year-old woman presents with pruritus vulvae. The following are suggestive of an infective cause:

(a) Progressively worsening symptoms over 6 months
(b) An offensive fishy odour
(c) A thick creamy white discharge
(d) Red plaques in the vulval area
(e) Fused labia

8. The following are important in the management of a woman with pruritus vulvae:

(a) A general examination of the skin in other body areas
(b) A speculum examination of the cervix and smear test
(c) Colposcopic examination of the vulva
(d) Directed biopsies of the vulva and vagina
(e) An abdominal X-ray

Chapter 5   Urinary Incontinence

9.   **A multiparous 55-year-old woman presents with a 6-month history of stress incontinence on coughing and sneezing:**

(a)   She therefore has 'genuine stress incontinence'
(b)   An obstetric history is unhelpful in making the diagnosis
(c)   A bimanual pelvic examination is important in making the diagnosis
(d)   A midstream sample of urine may help in making the diagnosis
(e)   Urodynamic studies are unnecessary

10.   **A 26-year-old woman complains of recurrent episodes of frequency, urgency and nocturia:**

(a)   A neurological history is important
(b)   The likely cause is detrusor overactivity
(c)   A pelvic examination will usually show an abnormality
(d)   A midstream urine sample is mandatory
(e)   Prolapse is usually found on examination

Chapter 6   Prolapse

11.   **In the absence of an abdominal mass, genital prolapse can present with:**

(a)   Backache
(b)   Incomplete emptying of the bladder
(c)   Vaginal discharge as the prolapse rubs on the patient's underwear
(d)   Dyspepsia
(e)   Nausea and vomiting

12.   **When examining the patient for genital prolapse:**

(a)   Abdominal palpation is essential
(b)   The lithotomy position is the best position to ask the patient to adopt
(c)   A Cusco's speculum helps to examine the vaginal wall prolapse
(d)   Bimanual palpation of the pelvis is included
(e)   A demonstration of stress incontinence might be included

Chapter 7   Bleeding and/or Pain in Early Pregnancy

13.   **Miscarriage:**

(a)   Will always present with bleeding
(b)   Is most common before 12 weeks gestation
(c)   Cannot be diagnosed by vaginal examination alone
(d)   If affecting the first pregnancy, increases the risk of miscarriage the next time
(e)   Is often provoked by intercourse, heavy lifting or a fall

14.   **When a woman with bleeding in early pregnancy presents:**

(a)   A speculum or vaginal examination could increase the risk of miscarriage
(b)   A smear test should be sent
(c)   A blood test is necessary even if her blood group is already known
(d)   An hCG level will not distinguish ectopic pregnancy from miscarriage
(e)   A history of tubal surgery should increase your suspicion of ectopic pregnancy

Chapter 8   Subfertility

15.   **Concerning male subfertility:**

(a)   A sperm count of 5 million/mL is normal
(b)   This is the sole cause of subfertility for 1 in 5 couples
(c)   If the woman is known to have tubal occlusion, investigation of the man is unnecessary
(d)   Calculation of body mass index is relevant
(e)   A viral illness 3 weeks before semenalysis is irrelevant

16.   **Concerning tubal occlusion:**

(a)   The greater the number of episodes of pelvic inflammatory disease, the more likely this is
(b)   Reversal of sterilization is more likely to result in pregnancy than tubal surgery for occlusion due to previous infection or endometriosis
(c)   It cannot be demonstrated using X-rays
(d)   Hydrosalpinx suggests a history of pelvic inflammatory disease
(e)   It is more common in women with anorexia nervosa

Chapter 9   The Menopause

17.   **Which of these are possible presenting symptoms of the menopause:**

(a)   Night sweats
(b)   Palpitations
(c)   Dyspareunia
(d)   Urgency
(e)   Fornication

18.   **Which of these are possible contributory factors towards osteoporosis:**

(a)   High body mass index
(b)   Smoking
(c)   Amenorrhoea
(d)   Oral contraceptive pill
(e)   Genetic predisposition

Chapter 10 Bleeding in the Second and Third Trimesters of Pregnancy

19. In the case of placental abruption:

(a) The uterus is typically soft on palpation
(b) Fetal parts are easily felt
(c) The uterus is usually tender
(d) Uterine contractions might be present
(e) There might not be any visible bleeding

20. When managing a major placenta praevia:

(a) Blood should be cross-matched if the patient presents with bleeding
(b) Transvaginal ultrasound scan helps with diagnosis
(c) Vaginal delivery is appropriate
(d) Inpatient admission is advised in the third trimester
(e) Consider maternal steroids in the preterm patient

Chapter 11 Large- or Small-for-Dates

21. Concerning the causes of a fetus being small-for-dates:

(a) Diabetes mellitus is a possible factor
(b) A history of cocaine use is relevant
(c) The size of the mother has no influence
(d) There is an association with pre-eclampsia
(e) Signs of fetal infection should be excluded

22. Investigations for the fetus with intrauterine growth restriction:

(a) There might be a difference on scan between the growth of the head and that of the abdomen
(b) Serial growth scans should be done weekly
(c) Doppler studies are of no benefit
(d) Abnormalites may develop in the cardiotocograph
(e) Previous obstetric history is relevant

Chapter 12 Abdominal Pain in the Second and Third Trimesters of Pregnancy

23. When diagnosing abdominal pain in a patient who is 32 weeks pregnant:

(a) Vaginal examination is contraindicated
(b) Right iliac fossa pain is diagnostic of appendicitis
(c) Placental abruption should be considered if she has vaginal bleeding
(d) Epigastric pain associated with hypertension and proteinuria suggests pre-eclampsia
(e) A previous history of gallstones might be relevant if she has right upper quadrant pain

24. Investigations of abdominal pain in pregnancy:

(a) Include urine microscopy if urinalysis shows proteinuria
(b) Liver function tests are not necessary if the patient has hypertension
(c) An ultrasound scan should be performed if gallstones are suspected
(d) A 24-h urine collection assists in the management of pre-eclampsia
(e) Hypoglycaemia is diagnostic of placental abruption

Chapter 13 Hypertension in Pregnancy

25. Regarding pre-eclampsia:

(a) A woman with high blood pressure prior to pregnancy is more prone to pre-eclampsia
(b) The presence of proteinuria makes this diagnosis
(c) If the patient's mother had pre-eclampsia in her pregnancy, the patient can be reassured that she is no more likely than anyone else to develop pre-eclampsia
(d) The priority must be to deliver the fetus
(e) Pre-eclampsia can be cured with antihypertensives

26. Concerning the investigation of high blood pressure in pregnancy:

(a) Blood tests will distinguish between underlying hypertension and pre-eclampsia
(b) A 24-h urine collection for protein showing a result of 4 g is significant
(c) Ultrasound is performed to look for evidence of the effect of blood pressure on the placenta
(d) A midstream urine sample is sent because pre-eclampsia predisposes to urinary tract infection
(e) The cuff used to take the blood pressure is not important

Chapter 14 Stillbirth

27. Regarding stillbirth:

(a) The term 'stillbirth' does not include infants who die within 1 h of delivery
(b) Multiple pregnancies are more prone to stillbirth
(c) Women who have had a stillbirth will not lactate
(d) If the fetus dies in utero, the most common presentation is in labour when no fetal heartbeat can be heard
(e) If intrauterine death is detected antenatally, caesarean section is the preferred method of delivery

Chapter 15   Failure to Progress in Labour

28.   Slow progress in labour:

(a)   Might be secondary to poor uterine contractions
(b)   Can occur with the fetus in an occipitoposterior position
(c)   Can occur with a fetal malpresentation
(d)   Does not happen if the membranes have been ruptured
(e)   Always results in instrumental delivery

29.   Regarding labour:

(a)   A multiparous patient progresses at 3 cm per hour on average
(b)   Artificial rupture of membranes should be considered if progress is slow
(c)   Caput and moulding are present with failure to progress in labour
(d)   Station is checked by abdominal palpation
(e)   Engagement is checked by vaginal examination

Chapter 16   Abnormal Cardiotocograph in Labour

30.   In a normal cardiotocograph in labour:

(a)   The baseline fetal heart rate should be more than 160 bpm
(b)   Accelerations are present
(c)   There are no decelerations
(d)   Baseline variability is <5 bpm
(e)   The strength of contractions can be monitored

31.   In the presence of a pathological cardiotocograph:

(a)   Check the liquor to exclude the presence of meconium
(b)   A fetal blood sample should be attempted at >2 cm dilatation
(c)   Expedite delivery if the pH of the fetal blood sample is greater than 7.25
(d)   The fetus might be at risk of hypoxia
(e)   A growth-restricted fetus is more at risk than one that is normally grown

Chapter 17   Bleeding After Delivery

32.   Primary postpartum haemorrhage (PPH):

(a)   Is defined as occurring within 24 h of delivery
(b)   Is defined as blood loss of more than 2000 mL
(c)   Should be anticipated in a multiple pregnancy
(d)   Might be secondary to vaginal wall lacerations
(e)   A history of antepartum haemorrhage is not associated with a risk of primary PPH

33.   Investigating secondary postpartum haemorrhage (PPH):

(a)   A high vaginal swab is indicated
(b)   An ultrasound scan of the pelvis might be appropriate
(c)   A decreased white blood cell count agrees with a diagnosis of endometritis
(d)   A persistently low serum hCG level is found in cases of molar pregnancy
(e)   A chest X-ray is essential with a confirmed diagnosis of choriocarcinoma

Chapter 18   Maternal Collapse

34.   A woman collapses on the labour ward:

(a)   Always check the condition of the fetus first
(b)   Diabetic collapse is always due to hypoglycaemia
(c)   Perform CPR, if needed, in the 'left tilt' position
(d)   Haemorrhage may result in DIC
(e)   It is wise to summon anathestic and obstetric staff

35.   Collapse associated with drug use:

(a)   Magnesium toxicity causes arrhythmias
(b)   Ecstasy use does not occur in pregnancy
(c)   Naloxone is used to reverse the effect of opiate overdose
(d)   Treat anaphylaxis with adrenaline and hydrocortisone
(e)   It is possible to overdose on Entonox

Chapter 19   Abnormal Uterine Bleeding

36.   An 18-year-old girl presents with a history of primary amenorrhoea. The following conditions usually present in this way:

(a)   Turner's syndrome
(b)   Testicular feminization
(c)   Premature ovarian failure
(d)   Polycystic ovarian syndrome (PCOS)
(e)   Imperforate hymen

37.   A 55-year-old woman presents with a 3-day vaginal bleed. Her last menstrual period was at the age of 52 years. The following would be appropriate with regards to differential diagnosis and subsequent management:

(a)   The most likely cause is atrophic vaginitis so no further action is required
(b)   An ultrasound scan would be appropriate
(c)   Ovarian carcinoma might be a cause
(d)   A cervical smear should be taken
(e)   A normal pipelle excludes endometrial carcinoma

Chapter 20   Fibroids

38.   Which of these are the possible symptoms caused by fibroids:

(a)   Pelvic pain
(b)   Subfertility
(c)   Urinary incontinence
(d)   Deep vein thrombosis
(e)   Menorrhagia

39.   What are the commonly associated complications of fibroids in pregnancy:

(a)   First trimester miscarriage
(b)   Acute severe abdominal pain
(c)   Malpresentation
(d)   Intrauterine growth restriction
(e)   Pre-eclampsia

Chapter 21   Endometriosis

40.   Which of these are possible sites for endometriotic deposits:

(a)   Ovaries
(b)   Peritoneum
(c)   Bowel
(d)   Scars
(e)   Lungs

41.   What are the possible medical treatments of endometriosis:

(a)   Danazol
(b)   Combined oral contraceptive pill
(c)   Corticosteroids
(d)   GnRH analogues
(e)   Antibiotics

Chapter 22   Benign Ovarian Tumours

42.   Clinically, the diagnosis of an ovarian cyst is suspected if:

(a)   The patient presents with unilateral iliac fossa pain
(b)   The patient is postmenopausal
(c)   Ultrasound scan shows an intrauterine pregnancy
(d)   The symptoms are of sudden onset
(e)   The patient has abdominal distension

43.   Management of an ovarian cyst:

(a)   Depends on the age of the patient
(b)   An ultrasound scan may help to differentiate between the different types of tumours
(c)   Should always include an intravenous urogram
(d)   Might include a laparotomy if the patient is symptomatic
(e)   Is not determined by the size of the cyst

Chapter 23   Gynaecological Malignancy

44.   At colposcopy:

(a)   The normal areas are stained white by acetic acid
(b)   Mosaic patterning might be seen in areas of abnormality
(c)   The cervix is investigated but not treated
(d)   Most women will have been referred following an abnormal smear
(e)   The upper extent of the transformation zone must be visualized

45.   Regarding premalignant states:

(a)   There is no known premalignant state for ovarian cancer
(b)   Complex hyperplasia is more likely than atypical hyperplasia to progress to endometrial carcinoma
(c)   Vulval intraepithelial neoplasia (VIN) is highly likely to progress to vaginal carcinoma
(d)   The progression of cervical intraepithelial neoplasia (CIN) to cervical carcinoma is more likely if the woman smokes
(e)   Human papilloma virus is an aetiological factor in CIN and VIN

Chapter 24   Vulval Disease

46.   The following are possible methods of investigation of vulval disease:

(a)   Colposcopy
(b)   Biopsy of vulva
(c)   Computed tomography (CT) scan – pelvic and abdominal
(d)   Urine testing
(e)   Vulval swabs

47.   The following are correct about lichen sclerosis:

(a)   The vulval skin can be white or red
(b)   Skin biopsy shows thinning of the epidermis
(c)   A biopsy is not necessary as the diagnosis is usually obvious
(d)   Surgical treatment is not performed because of a high incidence of symptom recurrence
(e)   A short course of medical treatment is usually required

Chapter 25   Pelvic Inflammatory Disease

48.   Typical presenting symptoms of acute pelvic inflammatory disease include:

(a)   Abnormal discharge from the vagina
(b)   Nausea and vomiting
(c)   Lower abdominal pain
(d)   Constipation
(e)   Raised temperature

49.   When managing pelvic inflammatory disease:

(a)   Always include treatment for chlamydia
(b)   Always include contact tracing
(c)   Referral to a genitourinary medicine clinic might be appropriate
(d)   Antibiotic treatment depends on the microbiology results
(e)   Consider a urine pregnancy test

Chapter 26   Urinary Incontinence

50.   Effective treatments for genuine stress incontinence include:

(a)   Pelvic floor exercises
(b)   Anticholinergics
(c)   Colposuspension
(d)   Tension free vaginal tape
(e)   Antibiotics

51.   Effective treatments for detrusor instability include:

(a)   Behavioural therapy
(b)   Antimuscarinics
(c)   Colposuspension
(d)   Antibiotic therapy for urinary tract infections
(e)   Clam cystoplasty

Chapter 27   Genital Prolapse

52.   The following factors can predispose a patient to genital prolapse:

(a)   Prolonged second stage of labour
(b)   Presence of an abdominal mass
(c)   Smoking
(d)   Constipation
(e)   Delivery of a large-for-dates infant

53.   When managing genital prolapse:

(a)   Surgery should always be included
(b)   There might be a place for hormone replacement therapy
(c)   A ring pessary should be changed every 5 years
(d)   Depending on the body mass index, advising weight loss might be appropriate
(e)   There is a risk to the pudendal nerve during sacrospinous fixation of the prolapsed vaginal vault

Chapter 28   Subfertility

54.   In vitro fertilization:

(a)   Can be used to treat couples with unexplained infertility
(b)   Requires treatment that can induce menopausal symptoms
(c)   Cannot be performed in the presence of blocked tubes
(d)   Can lead to ovarian hyperstimulation syndrome
(e)   Results in a live birth in 1 in 3 cases

55.   Intrauterine insemination:

(a)   Is a form of in vitro fertilization
(b)   Is only performed using donor sperm
(c)   Is usually preceded by drug treatment for the woman
(d)   Is usually preceded by drug treatment for the man
(e)   Is more likely to result in a live birth than intracytoplasmic sperm injection

Chapter 29   Early Pregnancy Failure

56.   Ectopic pregnancy:

(a)   Cannot occur if tubal sterilisation has been performed
(b)   Is more common in IVF pregnancies
(c)   Must be managed surgically
(d)   If viable, ie with a fetal hearbeat, can be reimplanted within the uterus
(e)   If a woman has had one ectopic pregnancy her risk of another is increased

57.   Molar pregnancy:

(a)   Never includes a fetus
(b)   If complete, contains only paternal genes
(c)   Commonly presents with bleeding in early pregnancy
(d)   hCG levels will be lower than expected in early pregnancy
(e)   May result in a need for chemotherapy

Chapter 30   The Menopause

58.   Hormone replacement therapy can be used to reduce the risk of:

(a)   Breast cancer
(b)   Osteoporosis
(c)   Venous thromboembolism
(d)   Superficial dyspareunia
(e)   Colonic cancer

59.   The following statements related to the menopause are correct:

(a)   The menopause is diagnosed retrospectively, one year after the last menstrual period
(b)   The climacteric typically lasts for 3 to 6 months
(c)   Premature ovarian failure is diagnosed if the menopause occurs before the age of 40
(d)   The average age of the menopause is 45
(e)   20% of women suffer from the short term sequelae of the menopause such as hot flushes and sweats

60.   The following are possible alternatives to HRT for treatment of hot flushes and sweats:

(a)   Clonidine
(b)   Phyto-oestrogens
(c)   Prozac
(d)   Bisphosphonates
(e)   Raloxifene

Chapter 31   Contraception, Sterilization and Unwanted Pregnancy

61.   The following are recognised advantages of the levonorgestrel intrauterine system (Mirena):

(a)   No risk of ectopic pregnancy
(b)   Reduction in menstrual flow
(c)   Efficacy equivalent to that of sterilisation
(d)   Less pain on insertion compared to traditional IUCD's
(e)   No increase in risk of pelvic inflammatory disease

62.   The following rely mainly on ovulation suppression for their contraceptive efficacy:

(a)   The levonorgestrel intrauterine system
(b)   Depo Provera
(c)   Combined oral contraceptive pill
(d)   The mini pill
(e)   Laparoscopic Sterilisation

63.   The following are recognised non contraceptive benefits of the combined oral contraceptive pill:

(a)   Reduction in incidence of breast cancer
(b)   Reduction in incidence of benign breast disease
(c)   Reduction in incidence of ovarian cancer
(d)   Improvement in endometriosis
(e)   Improvement in polycystic ovarian disease

Chapter 32   Gynaecological Endocrinology

64.   The following are possible causes of precocious puberty:

(a)   Congenital adrenal hyperplasia
(b)   Granulosa cell tumour
(c)   Hypothyroidism
(d)   Turner's syndrome
(e)   Cystic fibrosis

65.   Which of these drugs can cause hirsutism:

(a) H_2 antagonists, e.g. cimetidine
(b)   Danazol
(c)   Phenytoin
(d)   Penicillin
(e)   Progestogens

Chapter 33   Prenatal Diagnosis

66.   Concerning amniocentesis:

(a)   Culture result is available in 24 h
(b)   The procedure carries a lower risk of miscarriage than chorionic villus sampling
(c)   It is performed under general anaesthetic
(d)   It is performed after 15 weeks gestation
(e)   It cannot be used for twins

67.   Regarding prenatal diagnostic tests:

(a)   All require ultrasound
(b)   They are only performed prior to 24 weeks
(c)   Rhesus-negative women are given anti-D following chorionic villus sampling, amniocentesis and fetal blood sampling
(d)   All carry a risk of miscarriage
(e)   Fluorescent in situ hybridization and polymerase chain reaction are methods that 'speed-up' culture of fetal cells

Chapter 34   Multiple Pregnancy

68.   When diagnosing a twin pregnancy:

(a)   The uterus may palpate as small for dates
(b)   This is now usually done on the routine 12–14 week scan
(c)   The patient might present with hyperemesis gravidarum
(d)   Chorionicity should be diagnosed in the third trimester
(e)   A dichorionic pregnancy needs more surveillance than a monochorioinc pregnancy

69.   When managing delivery of a twin pregnancy:

(a)   Caesarean section is mandatory
(b)   Continuous cardiotocograph monitoring of both fetuses is advised
(c)   There is an increased risk of postpartum haemorrhage in comparison to a singleton pregnancy
(d)   If twin 1 is breech presentation, vaginal delivery is routinely advised
(e)   Regional anaesthesia is appropriate to allow assistance with delivery of the second twin

Chapter 35   Hypertension in Pregnancy

70.   Proteinuria:

(a)   Occurs in pre-eclampsia due to renal effects of the disease
(b)   Can be reversed by adequate anti-hypertensive therapy
(c)   Is not important if the woman is known to have essential hypertension
(d)   Is the reason that women with pre-eclampsia must be fluid-restricted
(e)   Is used as a screening test for pre-eclampsia

71.   Antihypertensive treatment:

(a)   Should be stopped at delivery if the woman wants to breastfeed
(b)   Can be given throughout pregnancy in tablet form
(c)   Will lead to withdrawal effects in the neonate if taken through pregnancy
(d)   Is given intravenously to reduce dangerously high blood pressure
(e)   May need to be continued for weeks post-natally

Chapter 36 Medical Disorders in Pregnancy

72. Regarding anaemia:

(a) Iron deficiency causes microcytic red blood cells
(b) Folate deficiency is treated with folate injections
(c) Women with multiple pregnancies are more at risk
(d) Drinking tea while taking tablets will aid iron absorption
(e) It is normal to have a lower haemoglobin when pregnant compared to when not pregnant

73. Regarding asthma in pregnancy:

(a) A deterioration in the peak flow is to be expected
(b) β-agonists should be continued
(c) Steroid inhalers can affect fetal growth
(d) Acute attacks in labour are common
(e) Oral steroids are not contraindicated

74. Concerning thyroid disease in pregnancy:

(a) A raised TSH level indicates hyperthyroidism
(b) Thyroid autoantibodies can cross the placenta
(c) Thyroid replacement with thyroxine has adverse fetal effects
(d) A pregnant woman with a goitre has thyroid disease of some sort
(e) Neonatal thyroid function will need to be checked if a thyrotoxic woman on treatment is breastfeeding

Chapter 37 Antepartum Haemorrhage

75. When differentiating between placenta praevia and placental abruption:

(a) An ultrasound scan is important
(b) A tender hard uterus is typical of placenta praevia
(c) There is an association between placental abruption and pre-eclampsia
(d) There may be an abnormal lie with placenta praevia
(e) The cardiotocograph may be abnormal in either condition

76. Management of a patient with an antepartum haemorrhage:

(a) Should always include checking the Rhesus status
(b) Should always include a digital vaginal examination
(c) Should always include a group and save sample in case cross-matched blood is needed
(d) Does not require a cardiotocograph
(e) Requires urinalysis if the maternal blood pressure is raised

Chapter 38 Premature Labour

77. Tocolysis:

(a) Should always be instituted when there is evidence of infection, so that antibiotics can be given to the mother
(b) With ritodrine is contraindicated in asthmatics
(c) Is always in the form of an infusion
(d) Has been proven to reduce the maternal morbidity related to preterm labour
(e) With non-steroidal anti-inflammatory drugs can result in fetal renal failure

78. The cervix in preterm labour:

(a) Should not be examined with a speculum, as this may provoke more contractions
(b) Should be swabbed for infection
(c) Might dilate relatively painlessly
(d) Can be sutured closed once it has started to open
(e) Is likely to appear shortened on transvaginal scan

Chapter 39 Malpresentation and Malpositions of the Occiput

79. A primiparous woman at 37 weeks gestation is suspected of having a breech presentation on abdominal palpation. Which of the following are appropriate in her subsequent management:

(a) If an extended breech is confirmed she should be offered external cephalic version
(b) If a footling breech is confirmed she should be advised to attempt vaginal delivery
(c) An estimated fetal weight should be requested on ultrasound scan
(d) Erect lateral pelvimetry is mandatory if vaginal delivery is to be attempted
(e) If caesarean section is chosen for delivery this should be performed as soon as possible

80. The following are malpresentations:

(a) Deep transverse arrest
(b) Breech
(c) Transverse lie
(d) Face to pubes
(e) Cord

Chapter 40 Labour

81. Labour:

(a) Is diagnosed by confirming rupture of the membranes
(b) Is diagnosed in the presence of a fully effaced cervix at least 3 cm dilated
(c) Progresses on average 2–3 cm per hour in a primiparous patient
(d) Should always be monitored with continuous fetal heart rate monitoring
(e) The third stage of labour is from delivery of the fetus until delivery of the placenta and membranes

82. When monitoring the mother and the fetus during labour:

(a) Baseline observations of maternal temperature, pulse and blood pressure should be recorded
(b) The strength of the uterine contractions can be assessed by the cadiotocograph
(c) The options for analgesia should be discussed
(d) Meconium-stained liquor is always an indication for immediate delivery
(e) Abdominal palpation is unnecessary

Chapter 41   Operative Intervention in Obstetrics

83. Regarding operative interventions in labour:

(a) An episiotomy should be sutured with a non-absorbable suture
(b) The ventouse cup can be used at any gestation
(c) The forceps can be used when the fetal head is three-fifths palpable in the maternal abdomen
(d) A fetus in the occipitotransverse position is suitable for delivery with Simpson's forceps
(e) A third-degree tear involves the anal mucosa

84. Lower segment caesarean section:

(a) Carries a reduced risk of thromboembolic disease
(b) Can be performed under regional anaesthesia
(c) After a first procedure, future deliveries should always be by caesarean section
(d) Is performed if the fetus is a breech presentation
(e) With a trial of scar, vaginal delivery can be achieved in 25% of patients

Chapter 42   Complications of the Third Stage of Labour and the Pueperium

85. Postnatal care of the mother:

(a) Up to 70% of women develop puerperal psychosis
(b) Breastfeeding is safe with tricyclic antidepressants
(c) Production of colostrum begins 2–3 days after delivery
(d) Flucloxacillin is an appropriate antibiotic for mastitis
(e) Retained products of conception must be excluded if the patient presents with postnatal pyrexia

86. Postpartum haemorrhage (PPH):

(a) Uterine atony is the most common cause of primary PPH
(b) The incidence of PPH in the developed world is about 30%
(c) An antepartum haemorrhage reduces the risk of a PPH
(d) Syntocinon should be given instead of syntometrine in the patient with hypertension
(e) Hysterectomy to treat PPH must be avoided at all costs

Chapter 43   Maternal Death

87. Concerning maternal death:

(a) The rate is 1 in 1000 in the UK
(b) IVF increases the risk of maternal death
(c) It is not related to social class
(d) It occurs more commonly in women carrying twins than in singleton pregnancies
(e) A death occurring following a medical termination would not be studied by the confidential enquiry

Chapter 44   Taking a History

88. When taking a gynaecological history it is mandatory to document the following:

(a) Date of last menstrual period
(b) Contraceptive history
(c) Social History
(d) Dyspareunia
(e) Alcohol consumption

89. When taking a routine antenatal obstetric history it is mandatory to document the following:

(a) Parity
(b) Details of previous deliveries
(c) Hx of pelvic injuries
(d) Cardiovascular history
(e) Gynaecological history

90. Typical features in the clerking of a patient with a suspected ectopic pregnancy include:

(a) Delayed menstrual period
(b) Slight pv bleeding
(c) Pyrexia
(d) Bilateral pelvic pain
(e) Shoulder tip pain

91. The following are typical features of the clerking in a woman with endometriosis:

(a) Heavy periods
(b) Pain exclusively on first two days of period
(c) Cyclical haematuria
(d) Secondary subfertility
(e) Superficial dyspareunia

92. The following are typical features of the clerking in a woman with polycystic ovarian syndrome:

(a) Hirsuitism
(b) Acne
(c) Frequent periods
(d) Obesity
(e) Hx of fractures

Chapter 45   Antenatal Booking and Ongoing Care

93.   Regarding diet and drinking in pregnancy:

(a)   Iron tablets should not be taken with tea
(b)   Eating soft cheeses can increase the risk of stillbirth
(c)   Fetal alcohol syndrome can result from a glass of wine each day in pregnancy
(d)   Dehydration is a common cause of headache in pregnancy
(e)   Women should 'eat for two' while pregnant

94.   Concerning antenatal blood tests:

(a)   Syphilis testing is no longer necessary
(b)   HIV testing requires the consent of the woman's partner
(c)   Antibody testing is unnecessary if the woman is Rhesus positive
(d)   Serum screening for Down syndrome is optional
(e)   If the woman is not immune to rubella she should be vaccinated postnatally

Chapter 46   Examination

95.   When performing a pelvic examination the following are usually palpable:

(a)   Fallopian tubes
(b)   Ovaries
(d)   Pelvic nodes
(d)   External cervical os
(e)   Internal cervical os

96.   The following can be normal findings when performing an examination in a woman with a 36 week pregnancy:

(a)   Linea Nigra
(b)   Striae Gravidarum
(c)   Symphyseal - fundal height of 34cms
(d)   2+ Proteinuria on dipstix
(e)   2+ Glycosuria on dipstix

Chapter 47   Common Investigations

97.   In order to perform a routine hysteroscopy the following are essential:

(a)   A telescope
(b)   A light source
(c)   A camera
(d)   General anaesthesia
(e)   A catheterised bladder

98.   In order to perform a routine diagnostic laparoscopy the following are essential:

(a)   A gas insufflator
(b)   A catheterised bladder
(c)   A Verress needle
(d)   A Trocar
(e)   A diathermy

99.   In order to perform a transvaginal ultrasound scan the following are essential:

(a)   A full bladder
(b)   Bowel Preparation
(c)   Ultrasound gel
(d)   A sedated patient
(e)   A light source

100.   The following can be diagnosed during a routine hysteroscopy:

(a)   Endometrial polyp
(b)   Retained IUCD
(c)   Asherman's syndrome
(d)   Meig's Syndrome
(e)   Uterine fibroids

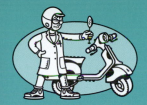

1. In a patient presenting with pelvic pain, list five symptoms that might help you to make a diagnosis. Suggest one possible diagnosis for each symptom.

2. Describe how you would examine a patient who presents with genital prolapse, and what signs you may elicit.

3. What out-patient investigations can be arranged for a couple prior to their appointment at the subfertility clinic?

4. Compare and contrast the diagnosis of placenta praevia and placental abruption.

5. List five factors in the maternal history that might be relevant when the uterus is small for dates. List five investigations that are indicated when the fetus is confirmed as small on ultrasound scan.

6. List the possible obstetric causes of abdominal pain in pregnancy and discuss how you would distinguish between them.

7. List the 4 components of a normal fetal heart rate shown by the cardiotocograph.

8. How would you investigate a patient who is suspected of having an ovarian cyst on clinical history and examination?

9. A 49 year old woman who has been taking continuous combined HRT for 4 years with no bleeding has new onset of bleeding over the last 2 months. An ultrasound scan shows a thickened endometrium. What is the differential diagnosis and what is the next step?

10. What are the potential sequelae of pelvic inflammatory disease?

11. Following a molar pregnancy, how is the patient followed up? Why is it important that she uses contraception until she is discharged from follow-up?

12. What step can women take to reduce the risk of having a baby with a neural tube defect, and what test best identifies this anomaly?

13. List the antenatal complications associated with multiple pregnancy.

14. How should the health of mother and baby be monitored in the pregnancy of a woman who is a known hypertensive, and why is monitoring necessary? She is already taking an antihypertensive medication suitable for use in pregnancy.

15. Which antenatal patients are more at risk of becoming anaemic?

16. Name two drugs commonly used to try to arrest preterm labour, and list three side-effects for each.

17. Outline a management plan for a woman diagnosed with obstetric cholestasis at 34 weeks.

18. What are the indications for ventouse delivery? How do they differ from a forceps delivery?

19. What is, currently, the commonest Direct cause of maternal death? List four risk factors.

20. A woman well known to the social services team is pregnant with her fourth baby. She has been on and off a methadone programme, and but currently admits to smoking heroin daily, and using Ecstasy 'occasionally'. She is smoking 15 cigarettes per day. What are the risks for the fetus and how should the pregnancy be monitored?

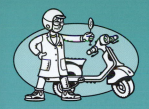

Extended-matching Questions (EMQs)

For each scenario described below, choose the *single* most likely diagnosis from the list of options.
Each option may be used once, more than once, or not at all.

1. Theme: Abnormal Bleeding

(a) Pelvic inflammatory disease
(b) Endometriosis
(c) Candida
(d) Cervical intraepithelial neoplasia
(e) Endometrial polyp
(f) Cervical carcinoma
(g) Ectopic pregnancy
(h) Hypothyroidism
(i) Fibroids
(j) Endometritis

Instruction: *For each scenario described below, choose the SINGLE most likely diagnosis from the above list of options. Each option may be used once, more than once or not at all.*

1. A 32-year-old woman complains of increasingly painful and heavy periods. The onset of pain is a few days prior to the onset of the period and lasts for 1 week after the period. ☐

2. A 55-year-old woman presents with a 6-month history of post coital bleeding. ☐

3. A 22-year-old woman presents with a 3-month history of pyrexia, lower abdominal pain and irregular vaginal discharge. On examination she is found to have lower abdominal tenderness and a purulent vaginal discharge. ☐

4. A 45-year-old woman presents with lower abdominal pain and heavy periods. On examination she is found to have a bulky uterus. ☐

5. A 47-year-old woman gives a 6-month history of increasingly heavy periods. During this time, she has gained 10 kg and is becoming increasingly lethargic. ☐

2. Theme: Pelvic Pain and Dyspareunia

(a) Endometriosis
(b) Chlamydia infection
(c) Previous ruptured appendix
(d) Ovarian torsion
(e) Urinary tract infection
(f) Fibroid degeneration
(g) Tubo-ovarian abscess

(h) Ovarian cyst rupture
(i) Acute appendicitis
(j) Pelvic tuberculosis

Instruction: *For each scenario described below, choose the SINGLE most likely diagnosis from the above list of options. Each option may be used once, more than once or not at all.*

1. A 22 year woman has had unprotected sex and is complaining of vaginal discharge. On vaginal examination she is generally tender with cervical excitation ☐

2. A 30 year old woman presents to A&E with a history of sudden onset of lower abdominal pain worse in the left iliac fossa. She has felt nauseous and vomited twice. On abdominal palpation, there is tenderness particularly in the left iliac fossa with signs of guarding and rebound. ☐

3. A 20 year old woman gives a 3 day history of increasing abdominal pain, initially generalised and now more to the right side. She has been vomiting and has lost her appetite. Her bowel movements have been loose and she feels hot. ☐

4. A 28 year old patient is referred to the out-patient clinic with a history in increasingly painful periods. She needs to take regular analgesia and occasionally needs time off work. On more direct questioning, she says that the pain actually starts 3-4 days before the period. She also complains of pain during sexual intercourse. ☐

5. A 20 year old Bangladeshi woman comes to the clinic complaining of persistent pelvic pain. She has been in the UK for 3 years and gives a long history of lower abdominal pain, as well as painful sexual intercourse. ☐

3. Theme: Vaginal Discharge

(a) *Candida albicans*
(b) Retained tampon
(c) Granulation tissue
(d) Cervical carcinoma
(e) Vesicovaginal fistula
(f) Bacterial vaginosis
(g) Uterine carcinoma

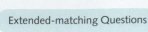

(h) Ring pessary
(i) *Chlamydia trachomatis*
(j) Postmenopausal atrophic changes

Instruction: *For each scenario described below, choose the SINGLE most likely diagnosis from the above list of options. Each option may be used once, more than once or not at all.*

1. A 75-year-old non-insulin-dependent diabetic woman has recently been on a course of antibiotics for a chest infection. She has been to see her GP complaining of a thick white itchy vaginal discharge. ☐

2. A 45-year-old woman has been referred to the hospital with a history of intermittent offensive brown vaginal discharge and postcoital bleeding. She has not attended for cervical smear tests for the past 10 years. ☐

3. A 55-year-old woman had an abdominal hysterectomy 2 months previously. She has started to notice the constant presence of a clear watery vaginal discharge. ☐

4. A 22-year-old woman presents to her GP with a 5-day history of generalized lower abdominal pain and a watery vaginal discharge. She is using the oral contraceptive pill for contraception. ☐

5. A 32-year-old woman gives a history of a grey-coloured watery vaginal discharge, which smells unpleasantly strong but does not itch. It seems to be associated with the use of barrier contraception. ☐

4. Theme: Subfertility

(a) Polycystic ovarian syndrome
(b) Klinefelter's syndrome
(c) Obstructive azoospermia
(d) Anorexia nervosa
(e) Turners syndrome
(f) Pelvic inflammatory disease
(g) Submucous fibroids
(h) Poorly controlled hyperthyroidism

The following are the results of investigations performed for couples seen in the subfertility clinic. Only abnormal results are listed. *Please choose the diagnosis that best explains the result found.*

1. Laparoscopy and dye test showed bilateral hydrosalpinges and lack of spill. ☐

2. LH : FSH ratio is raised, Day 21 progesterone level is 5 ☐

3. LH:FSH ratio is normal, Day 21 progesterone is 2 ☐

4. Semenalysis shows azoospermia, testicular biopsy shows spermatazooa ☐

5. Semenalysis shows azoospermia, testicular biopsy shows no spermatogenesis ☐

5. Theme: Bleeding in the Second and Third Trimesters of Pregnancy

(a) Molar pregnancy
(b) Ectopic pregnancy
(c) Early miscarriage
(d) Placenta praevia
(e) Placental abruption
(f) Cervical ectropion
(g) Retained placenta
(h) Vaginal tear
(i) Uterine atony
(j) Cervical tear

Instruction: *For each scenario described below, choose the SINGLE most likely diagnosis from the above list of options. Each option may be used once, more than once or not at all.*

1. A 20 year old woman has a history of 8 weeks amenorrhoea. She has light fresh vaginal bleeding associated with lower abdominal pain. On examination she is tender in the left adnexa with cervical excitation. Ultrasound scan shows an empty uterus. ☐

2. A 34 year old woman in her second pregnancy had just had a normal vaginal delivery of a twin pregnancy. She is now bleeding heavily. On abdominal examination the uterine fundus is above the umbilicus and is poorly contracted. ☐

3. A 28 year old woman has a history of 12 weeks amenorrhoea. She has severe nausea and vomiting, as well as light vaginal bleeding. On abdominal palpation the uterus is 18 weeks size. Ultrasound scan shows a vesicular pattern with no intrauterine sac. ☐

4. A 32 year old woman is 28 weeks pregnant. She has a 2 hour history of vaginal bleeding. She is also complaining of a headache, nausea and constant abdominal pain. On examination, she is hypertensive and the uterus is firm and tender. There is proteinuria on urinalysis. ☐

5. A 24 year old woman in her first pregnancy has laboured spontaneously. After a normal first stage of labour, the second stage is long and she requires a rotational ventouse delivery for a fetal malposition. ☐

6. Theme: Abdominal Pain in the Second and Third Trimesters of Pregnancy

(a) Fibroid degeneration
(b) Gastroenteritis
(c) Symphysis pubis dysfunction
(d) Placental abruption
(e) Acute appendicitis
(f) Ovarian torsion
(g) Pre-eclampsia
(h) Urinary tract infection
(i) Gallstones
(j) Preterm labour

For each of the clinical findings below, select the pathological process most likely to account for them from the above list.

1. On abdominal palpation, hard tender uterus, difficulty defining the fetal parts ☐

2. Leucocytosis on urinalysis ☐

3. Regular contractions palpated on abdominal examination, cervical change on vaginal examination ☐

4. The uterus palpates large-for-dates, with tenderness elicited over a specific site ☐

5. The patient is hypertensive and hyperreflexic, with tenderness over the right hypochondrium ☐

7. Theme: Stillbirth

(a) Maternal ALT = 60 iu/l
(b) Maternal HbA1c = 15%
(c) Fetal Hb = 3g/dl, positive Coombs test
(d) Parvovirus IgM positive, IgG negative
(e) Maternal Rubella IgG positive
(f) 24 hour urinary protein 5.1g/l
(g) Fetal karyotype 47XY
(h) Fetal karyotype 45XO
(i) 24 hour urinary protein 0.2g/l

The conditions below are the underlying diagnoses of causes of stillbirth, made on the basis of investigations performed soon after delivery. *Please match the diagnosis to the test result from the list above.*

1. Fetus with Down's syndrome ☐

2. Pre-eclampsia ☐

3. Intrauterine fetal infection ☐

4. Obstetric cholestasis ☐

5. Rhesus isoimmunisation ☐

6. Maternal diabetes ☐

8. Theme: Failure to Progress in Labour

(a) Cervical fibroid
(b) Persistent OP position
(c) Previous pelvic fracture
(d) Fetal macrosomia
(e) Irregular contractions
(f) Breech presentation
(g) OT position
(h) Rickets
(i) Transverse lie
(j) Face presentation

Instruction: *For each scenario described below, choose the SINGLE most likely diagnosis from the above list of options. Each option may be used once, more than once or not at all.*

1. A 26 year old woman who has been an insulin-dependent diabetic since the age of 10 ☐

2. A primiparous patient with a term pregnancy and a cephalic presentation. Over the past 4 hours, she has remained at 4cm dilatation on vaginal examination. She is not yet requiring analgesia. ☐

3. A 35 year old Nigerian woman who is in spontaneous labour. She has a history of having had a previous myomectomy for menorrhagia ☐

4. A 40 year old grand multiparous woman who has attended labour ward at term with a 3 hour history of regular contractions and no PV loss. On abdominal palpation, there is nothing in the maternal pelvis. ☐

5. A 28 year old multiparous patient has had a long latent phase of labour and is now progressing at less than 1 cm per hour ☐

9. Theme: Maternal Collapse

(a) Uterine atony
(b) Amniotic fluid embolism
(c) Postural hypotension
(d) Opiate use
(e) Pulmonary embolism
(f) Epileptic seizure
(g) Eclampsia
(h) Sepsis
(i) Myocardial infarction
(j) Uterine rupture

Instruction: *For each scenario described below, choose the SINGLE most likely diagnosis from the above list of options. Each option may be used once, more than once or not at all.*

1. This 18 year old had a forceps delivery of a 4.3kg baby about 1 hour ago after a long labour that was

augmented with syntocinon. She had syntometrine for the third stage. Her pulse is 100bpm, her blood pressure is 90/45 mmHg. Her uterus is palpable above the umbilicus and feels 'boggy'. She is lying in a pool of blood. ☐

2. This woman had her fourth Caesarean section yesterday. She was kept on the labour ward overnight as the estimated blood loss at delivery was 800mls. Her husband helped her get up to go to the shower, but then she collapsed by the side of her bed. Her pulse is 94bpm, her blood pressure is 110/55 and her lochia is normal. There is no respiratory distress. ☐

3. This 35 year old, whose BMI is 28, has had frequent admissions in her pregnancy, early on with hyperemesis, now, in the third trimester, with symphysis pubis pain. When found she is tachycardic but normotensive, with cyanosis and dyspnoea. ☐

4. This primigravid woman was aiming for home delivery, and wanted to avoid contact with the hospital if at all possible. Her membranes ruptured 3 days ago, at term, and she has had irregular contractions ever since but labour has not established. She came in because she started to feel unwell, and because fetal movements had reduced over the previous 12 hours. On examination she is tachycardic and pyrexial, and the liquor is yellowish in colour. ☐

5. At 32 weeks, this woman had been referred in by her community midwife who found her blood pressure to be elevated and some proteinuria at a routine antenatal check. She is generally fit and well with no medical history. On arrival she is asked to provide another urine specimen. When she fails to emerge from the toilet the midwife goes in and finds her having a generalized tonic-clonic seizure. ☐

10. Theme: Urinary Incontinence

(a) Multiple sclerosis
(b) Urinary tract infection
(c) Genuine stress incontinence
(d) Idiopathic detrusor overactivity
(e) Sensory urgency
(f) Fibroids
(g) Fistula
(h) Bladder tumour
(i) Prolapsed disc
(j) Detrusor overactivity due to menopause

Instruction: *For each scenario described below, choose the SINGLE most likely diagnosis from the above list of options. Each option may be used once, more than once or not at all.*

1. A 55-year-old multiparous woman presents with a 6-month history of loss of urine on coughing and bending. Urodynamic investigations show no evidence of detrusor instability. ☐

2. A 26-year-old woman presents with a 5-day history of worsening urinary frequency, nocturia and dysuria. Urinary testing indicates proteinuria. ☐

3. A 60-year-old woman presents with a 6-week history of urgency nocturia and urge incontinence. ☐

4. A 30-year-old woman, 6 weeks postpartum and recently arrived from Somalia, gives a history of continually feeling damp 'down below'. ☐

5. A 52-year-old woman presents with a 6-week history of hot flushes, sweats and vaginal dryness and urinary frequency. ☐

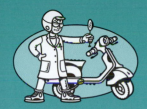
1. A 24-year-old woman presents to the gynaecology outpatient clinic with a 12-month history of increasing pelvic discomfort and deep dyspareunia. Discuss the relevant factors in the history and examination that would help you to reach a diagnosis. How would you investigate the patient?

2. A 45-year-old woman presents with a 1-year history of progressively worsening urinary incontinence. Discuss the management – including those salient aspects of the history that should be elicited – examination and investigation.

3. A 47-year-old woman presents with a 6-month history of irregular periods and progressively worsening hot flushes and sweats. Discuss other symptoms that might be elicited in the history, possible examination findings and relevant investigations that could be used to reach a diagnosis.

4. A multiparous woman presents to the labour ward at 28 weeks gestation with a 3-day history of increasing right upper quadrant pain. List the points that you would elicit from the history and examination, and the investigations you would plan to perform to establish the cause of the pain.

5. A 26-year-old woman is in established labour. The cervical dilatation has been unchanged for the last 6 h at 7 cm; she has been receiving intravenous oxytocin for the last 2 h and has a temperature of 38.2°C. The cardiotocograph shows a baseline of 175 bpm with a variability of 5–10 bpm. There have been late decelerations for the last 20 min. Discuss any further points in the patient's history that might be relevant. What would be your plan for this patient's future management.

6. A 38-year-old nulliparous woman presents with menorrhagia and pelvic discomfort. Examination reveals a 12-week-sized uterus consistent with fibroid enlargement. Discuss the subsequent management of this patient including her further investigation and treatment.

7. A 22-year-old woman presents to A&E with a 6-day history of increasing lower abdominal pain. List the possible differential diagnoses. Consider what are the relevant points in the history, examination and investigations to enable you to make a diagnosis.

8. A 26-year-old woman presents with a 4-week history of increasing facial and body hair, greasy skin and deepening of her voice. What is the differential diagnosis and management.

9. A 30-year-old woman attends the antenatal clinic at 18 weeks gestation, having been diagnosed with a twin pregnancy at the 12-week scan. As her consultant, discuss the plan for her antenatal care.

10. A 32-year-old woman presents to the labour ward with a 6-hour history of contractions. List the points in the history and examination that would be made at the time of her initial assessment. How would you proceed to monitor her labour?

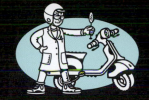

1. (a) T—A menstrual history is essential in a patient with abnormal bleeding
    (b) T—A bimanual examination is an important part of the examination
    (c) T—A full blood count is necessary to exclude anaemia due to abnormal bleeding
    (d) F—Thyroid function tests are not an essential part of the routine work up for the investigation of abnormal periods unless other symptoms suggest a thyroid disorder
    (e) F—An abdominal X-ray is not usually required for investigation of abnormal genital tract bleeding. Caution should be exercised if one is ordered as the patient could be pregnant

2. (a) T—Occasionally associated with chronic pelvic inflammatory disease
    (b) T—Typically associated with endometriosis
    (c) F—This is typical of primary dysmenorrhoea
    (d) T—Uterus can be fixed and retroverted due to adhesions caused endometriosis and pelvic inflammatory disease
    (e) T—This is typical of primary dysmenorrhoea

3. (a) F—Secondary dysmenorrhoea suggests endometriosis
    (b) T—You must know the date of the last menstrual period and the length of the cycle to diagnose Mittelschmerz, which is the name for pain associated with ovulation
    (c) T—A recent change of partner does predispose the patient to pelvic inflammatory disease due to exposure to new pathogens
    (d) F—Recent surgical termination of pregnancy is relevant since instrumenting the uterus increases the risk of pelvic inflammatory disease
    (e) T—Nausea and vomiting with acute unilateral pain is suggestive of ovarian torsion

4. (a) F—Bimanual palpation may reveal tender nodules in the posterior fornix if the patient has endometriosis
    (b) T—The uterus does typically feel bulky with adenomyosis
    (c) T—Hypotension and tachycardia are associated with ruptured ectopic pregnancy due to bleeding
    (d) F—Pelvic inflammatory disease is the likely diagnosis in the presence of vaginal discharge
    (e) T—The differential diagnosis of a unilateral pelvic mass includes a tubo-ovarian abscess, particularly in the presence of fever

5. (a) T—Urinary symptoms can be present with a sexually transmitted infection
    (b) F—Anorexia is more likely to be a symptom of malignancy
    (c) T—Vulval irritation can suggest infection such as candida, but might also be present with other pathology
    (d) F—Bowel symptoms are not typical of infection
    (e) T—Fever is a typical symptom of infection

6. (a) T—If tests are negative, the discharge may be physiological
    (b) F—A pelvic ultrasound is indicated if history and examination suggests malignancy or a pelvic mass
    (c) T—Laparoscopy may be needed to confirm pelvic inflammatory disease to visualise pus and inflammations
    (d) T—A smear test should be performed if clinically indicated—this may also indicate infection
    (e) F—An endocervical swab is necessary to exclude chlamydial infection

7. (a) F—An acute onset suggests infection
    (b) T—This suggests bacterial vaginosis
    (c) T—This supports a diagnosis of infection, possibly candidal
    (d) F—This suggests psoriasis or eczema
    (e) F—This suggests lichen sclerosis

8. (a) T—To exclude generalized dermatoses affecting the vulval area
    (b) T—CIN is often associated with VIN
    (c) T—Colposcopy allows closer inspection of the vulva
    (d) T—Biopsies give a histological diagnosis
    (e) F—Abdominal X-ray is not a usual part of the routine work-up for pruritus vulvae

9. (a) F—Not necessarily; the diagnosis of genuine stress incontinence can be made only in the absence of detrusor overactivity on urodynamic investigation
    (b) F—An obstetric history indicating traumatic deliveries of large infants would support a diagnosis of genuine stress incontinence
    (c) T—Occasionally, stress incontinence can be due to pressure from a large pelvic tumour, e.g. fibroid, ovarian cyst
    (d) T—A midstream urine sample will exclude a urinary tract infection as the cause of the urinary symptoms
    (e) F—Urodynamic studies are essential to exclude detrusor overactivity as a cause for the symptoms

10. (a) T—A neurological examination is important to exclude causes such as multiple sclerosis.
(b) F—In this age group the likely diagnosis is sensory urgency where DO is absent
(c) F—It is unlikely that a pelvic abnormality will be found
(d) T—A midstream urine will exclude a urinary tract infection as the cause of the symptoms
(e) F—Genital prolapse is unlikely to be found in this scenario

11. (a) T—This is one of the more common symptoms a patient presents with
(b) T—A cystocoele may present with this symptom
(c) T—A procidentia can cause discharge as it is irritated by clothing
(d) F—This symptom suggests upper abdominal pathology
(e) F—These symptoms suggest an acute condition rather than a more longstanding one such as a genital prolapse

12. (a) T—Abdominal palpation is essential to exclude a mass which may be causing a prolapse as a pressure effect
(b) F—It is generally agreed that the left lateral position allows better assessment
(c) F—A Sims speculum is preferable
(d) T—This will help to exclude a pelvic mass responsible for the prolapse
(e) T—This may be appropriate if the patient presents with urinary symptoms

13. (a) F—Miscarriage can be found on ultrasound scan before any bleeding is seen
(b) T—This is the most common time for miscarriage
(c) F—If the cervical os is open, miscarriage is inevitable
(d) T—After one miscarriage the risk increases from 15% to 20%, but it should be stressed to the patient that this means there is still an 80% chance that her next pregnancy will be successful
(e) F—Most miscarriages are unprovoked and any recent events to which the patient might attribute her loss are purely coincidental

14. (a) F—Examination will not affect the pregnancy, but may result in more bleeding being revealed as it had previously collected in the vagina
(b) F—A smear taken while the woman is bleeding will not be helpful, as the cells will be obscured by blood, but can be arranged for a future date
(c) T—Antibody levels must also be checked following an episode of bleeding
(d) T—A single level will not be helpful; if the scan is equivocal two levels must be checked, 48h apart
(e) T—Tubal scarring following surgery makes tubal implantation and therefore tubal ectopic pregnancy more likely

15. (a) F—A count of >20 million/mL is normal
(b) T—Male factor contributes to a further 20% when both members of the couple are considered
(c) F—If assisted fertility is being proposed, it is important to assess the quality of the sperm
(d) T—Obesity reduces testosterone levels and therefore affects spermatogenesis
(e) F—Spermatogenesis takes 72 days and is adversely affected by viraemia

16. (a) T—One episode of pelvic inflammatory disease gives a 10% chance, three episodes increase the risk to 50%
(b) T—Underlying pathology makes it less likely that tubal surgery will result in pregnancy
(c) F—Hysterosalpingography involves the introduction of dye through the cervix while taking X-rays of the pelvis to look for fill and spill from the tubes
(d) T—Hydrosalpinx means 'fluid-filled tube', and suggests tubal infection has occurred in the past
(e) F—Women with anorexia are more likely to experience fertility problems due to infrequent ovulation rather than tubal occlusion

17. (a) T—Classic vasomotor symptom
(b) T—Classic vasomotor symptom
(c) T—Hypoestrogenic symptom due to atrophic vaginitis
(d) T—Hypoestrogenic symptom due to atrophic changes in the urinary tract
(e) T—Less common symptom – feeling of ants crawling all over body

18. (a) F—A low body mass index contributes to osteoporosis due to less peripheral conversion to oestrogen of androgenic precursors
(b) T—Possibly due to earlier ovarian failure
(c) T—Due to hypoestrogenic state (except in polycystic ovary syndrome, when the oestrogen level is usually normal)
(d) F—Although the pill inhibits ovulation, ethinyloestradiol acts as add-back therapy
(e) T—One-third of women with osteoporosis have a significant family history

19. (a) F—The uterus is typically hard
(b) F—Fetal parts are difficult to palpate because the uterus is hard
(c) T—The uterus is usually tender
(d) T—Uterine contractions might be present
(e) T—Placental abruption can be either concealed or revealed

20. (a) T—Blood should be cross-matched if the patient presents with bleeding
(b) T—Transvaginal ultrasound scan helps with diagnosing the position of the placental edge from the internal cervical os
(c) F—Delivery by caesarean section is advised
(d) T—Inpatient admission is advised in the third trimester
(e) T—Consider maternal steroids in the preterm patient in case delivery is needed

21. (a) F—Diabetes mellitus is a cause of a large-for-dates abdomen
(b) T—Illegal drug use is associated with the small-for-gestational age fetus
(c) F—A fetus that is small may be constitutionally small
(d) T—Pre-eclampsia is associated with intrauterine growth restriction
(e) T—Fetal infection is associated with being small-for-gestational age

22. (a) T—In asymmetrical growth restriction, there is a discrepancy between the growth of the fetal head and the abdomen
(b) F—Serial growth scans should be performed every 2 weeks to see a significant difference in the pattern
(c) F—Doppler studies can be useful to determine if there are signs of increased placental resistance and re-distribution of blood flow within the fetus
(d) T—Abnormalities might appear in the cardiotocograph
(e) T—A previous pregnancy affected by intrauterine growth restriction increases the risk of the current pregnancy being affected

23. (a) F—Vaginal examination is necessary if the history and the findings of abdominal palpation suggest pre-term labour
(b) F—Appendicitis in pregnancy may not present with typical symptoms and signs present outside pregnancy
(c) T—Placental abruption is a possible diagnosis if the patient has vaginal bleeding
(d) T—Epigastric pain associated with hypertension and proteinuria does suggest pre-eclampsia due to streching of the liver capsule
(e) T—A previous history of gallstones may be relevant (cholecystitis biliary colic) if she has right upper quadrant pain

24. (a) T—Urine microscopy should be performed to exclude a urinary tract infection
(b) F—Liver function tests are important if the patient has hypertension to exclude pre-eclampsia
(c) T—An ultrasound scan is a good way to pick up suspected gallstones
(d) T—A 24-h urine collection assists in the management of pre-eclampsia
(e) F—Hypoglycaemia is diagnostic of acute fatty liver of pregnancy

25. (a) T—Pre-existing hypertension makes pre-eclampsia more likely in pregnancy
(b) F—Infection must be excluded
(c) F—A family history increases the risk
(d) F—The mother's condition must be stabilized first
(e) F—Delivery is the only cure for pre-eclampsia, although anti-hypertensives are used to control the blood pressure while it is high

26. (a) F—Pre-eclampsia may occur in the presence of normal blood results
(b) T—Any level greater than 0.3 g is significant
(c) T—Ultrasound signs of placental insufficiency are growth restriction and oligohydramnios
(d) F—A midstream urine sample is sent to exclude urinary tract infection, which can also cause proteinuria
(e) F—The size of cuff is important to obtain an accurate blood pressure

27. (a) T—Only deaths prior to delivery are included i.e. the baby is born with no signs of life
(b) T—Twin, triplet and other multiple pregnancies are more prone to stillbirth and pose a particularly difficult management problem for the clinician if only one fetus has died
(c) F—Lactation occurs as usual and, although it might not become established (because of the lack of the suckling stimus), it can be distressing and painful
(d) F—Most stillbirths occur before labour, with the mother presenting due to reduced fetal movements
(e) F—Labour is induced in almost all cases

28. (a) T—Slow progress may be secondary to poor uterine contractions
(b) T—Slow progress is more likely to occur with the fetus in an occipito-posterior position
(c) T—Slow progress commonly occurs with a fetal malpresentation
(d) F—Slow progress may happen if the membranes have been ruptured
(e) F—Slow progress does not always result in instrumental delivery but it is more likely

29. (a) F—A multiparous patient progresses at 2cm per hour on average
(b) T—Artificial rupture of membranes should be considered if progress is slow
(c) T—Caput and moulding are present with failure to progress
(d) F—Station is the relation of the fetal head to the ischial spines and is checked by vaginal examination
(e) F—Engagement is the amount of head palpable above the pelvic brim and is checked by abdominal palpation

30.
(a) F—Normal baseline fetal heart rate is 110–160 bpm
(b) T—Accelerations are a normal feature
(c) T—Decelerations are an abnormal feature
(d) F—Normal baseline variability is ≥5 bpm
(e) F—Frequency of contractions can be monitored

31.
(a) T—Meconium-stained liquor is associated with fetal hypoxia
(b) T—Fetal blood sampling should be attempted at > 2cm dilatation
(c) F—Expedite delivery if the fetal blood sample pH is ≤7.20
(d) T—A pathological cardiotocograph indicates that the fetus may be at risk of hypoxia
(e) T—A growth-restricted fetus might already be compromised in utero and so less able to withstand uterine contractions

32.
(a) T—Primary postpartum haemorrhage is defined as occurring within 24h of delivery
(b) F—Primary postpartum haemorrhage is defined as blood loss of more than 500mL
(c) T—Should be anticipated in a multiple pregnancy since there is a risk of uterine atony
(d) T—Vaginal and cervical lacerations can cause primary postpartum haemorrhage
(e) F—A history of antepartum haemorrhage is associated with a risk of primary postpartum haemorrhage

33.
(a) T—A high vaginal swab is indicated to exclude endometritis
(b) T—An ultrasound scan can help in the diagnosis of retained products of conception or molar pregnancy
(c) F—An increased white blood cell count agrees with a diagnosis of endometritis
(d) F—A persistently raised serum hCG level is found in cases of molar pregnancy
(e) T—A chest X-ray is essential with a confirmed diagnosis of choriocarcinoma to exclude lung metastases

34.
(a) F—Follow the ABC of resuscitation
(b) F—Never assume the cause
(c) T—This posture displaces the pregnant uterus, preventing caval compression
(d) T—Due to exhaustion of clotting factors
(e) T—Anathestic input is extremely helpful in this situation

35.
(a) T—Due to cardiac effects
(b) F—A drug history should always be taken from a patient at booking
(c) T—But the effect may be short-lived
(d) T—This is a standard medical emergency
(e) F—This is one of the advantages of this form of analgesia

36.
(a) T—Turner's syndrome typically presents with primary amenorrhoea
(b) T—The genotype is XY therefore by definition there is primary amenorrhoea
(c) F—Premature ovarian failure can occur at this age but it usually present as secondary amenorrhoea
(d) F—Polycystic ovary syndrome usually presents as secondary amenorrhoea
(e) T—There is a physical obstruction to menstrual flow

37.
(a) F—Action is always required for postmenopausal bleeding
(b) T—Standard investigation for postmenopausal bleeding for endometrial thickness
(c) T—Ovarian carcinoma can cause bleeding by direct invasion or release of oestrogen leading to endometrial hyperplasia
(d) T—To exclude cervical carcinoma
(e) F—A pipelle sample of the endometrium is reassuring but does not absolutely exclude malignancy

38.
(a) T—Pressure symptoms or degeneration
(b) T—Due interference with implantation mechanism
(c) T—Pressure on the bladder
(d) T—Reduction in blood flow of blood in pelvic veins due to occlusion
(e) T—Usually due to submucous fibroids leading to increased endometrial surface area

39.
(a) T—Due to interference with implantation mechanism
(b) T—Due to red degeneration of rapidly growing fibroid
(c) T—Due to obstruction by fibroid in the lower segment/cervix
(d) F—Not a recognized complication of fibroids
(e) F—Not a recognized complication of fibroids

40.
(a) T—Common
(b) T—Common
(c) T—Common but underdiagnosed (up to 30% of women with endometriosis)
(d) T—Rare
(e) T—Rare

41.
(a) T—Androgenic steroid with ovulation suppression capabilities
(b) T—Ovulation suppression plus continuous progestogenic activity
(c) F—No known benefits for endometriosis
(d) T—Profound ovulation suppression by down regulation of pituitary gonadotrophins
(e) F—No known benefits for antibiotics

42. (a) T—Unilateral iliac fossa pain is the typical presentation of torsion, rupture or haemorrhage into an ovarian cyst
(b) F—Ovarian cysts present at any age but malignancy should be suspected in the postmenopausal woman
(c) T—An ovarian cyst can become symptomatic during pregnancy
(d) T—Typically the symptoms from an ovarian cyst are of sudden onset
(e) T—A large ovarian cyst can present with abdominal distension or symptoms of pressure

43. (a) T—Over the age of 40, operative management should be considered depending on the clinical features
(b) T—An ultrasound scan may help to differentiate between the different types of tumours
(c) F—An intravenous urogram is only warranted if malignancy is suspected or confirmed, or if the patient has urological symptoms ; it is not part of routine investigations
(d) T—A laparotomy or laparoscopy is necessary if the patient is symptomatic
(e) F—If the cyst is ≥5cm surgery is more likely

44. (a) F—Areas of abnormality stain white with acetic acid
(b) T—The abnormal vasculature in areas of cervical intraepithelial neoplasia produces the mosaic patterning
(c) F—Initially the cervix is inspected, and biopsy is a form of investigation, but treatment in the form of LLETZ is also performed
(d) T—Other reasons for referral are abnormal bleeding (e.g. intermenstrual or postcoital) or a cervix that looks abnormal
(e) T—If the upper limit of the transformation zone is high in the endocervical canal, the colposcopy is said to be 'inadequate'

45. (a) T—The lack of a premalignant state is one of the obstacles to screening
(b) F—Complex hyperplasia is unlikely to result in malignancy, whereas atypical hyperplasia is very likely to progress and might point to the fact that carcinoma is already present
(c) F—The risk is small
(d) T—Smoking makes it more difficult for the body to 'cure itself' of cervical intraepithelial neoplasia
(e) T—Human papilloma virus is implicated in both of these premalignancies

46. (a) T—Allows closer inspection of vulval skin
(b) T—For histological examination
(c) T—If vulval malignancy is suspected to look for possibility of spread
(d) T—To look for urinary tract infection and/or diabetes
(e) T—To exclude infective causes

47. (a) T—Lichen sclerosis can appear as white or reddish plaques
(b) T—The epidermis is usually thin and hyalinized
(c) F—A skin biopsy is mandatory to exclude malignant change
(d) T—50% of symptoms of pruritus vulvae can recur
(e) F—A long course of medical therapy is often required

48. (a) T—Abnormal vaginal discharge is a typical presenting symptom of acute PID
(b) F—Nausea and vomiting is not a typical presenting symptom of acute PID
(c) T—Lower abdominal pain is a typical presenting symptom of acute PID
(d) F—Constipation is not a typical presenting symptom of acute PID
(e) T—Raised temperature is a typical presenting symptom of acute PID

49. (a) T—Treating PID must include treatment for chlamydia
(b) T—Contact tracing is important to prevent reinfection
(c) T—Screening for all sexually transmitted infections and contact tracing can be best managed by a genitourinary medicine clinic, depending on local arrangements
(d) F—With a reasonable clinical diagnosis of PID, antibiotic treatment should be initiated prior to obtaining microbiology results
(e) T—A pregnancy test might be appropriate, depending on the date of last menstrual period

50. (a) T—Improves tone of pelvic floor muscles to prevent loss of urine
(b) F—Indicated for detrusor instability to prevent involuntary muscle contraction
(c) T—To raise urinary sphincter above pelvic floor
(d) T—Same principle as (c)
(e) F—Only helpful for detrusor instability caused by a urinary tract infection

51. (a) T—To train the CNS to resist the urge to micturate
(b) T—To relax the detrusor muscle
(c) F—Indicated for GSI
(d) T—A typical cause of detrusor instability
(e) T—A rare operation carried out to increase bladder capacity by adding a piece of small bowel to the bladder

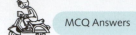

52. (a) T—Prolonged second stage can result in denervation of the pelvic floor muscles
(b) T—The pressure of an abdominal mass may cause genital prolapse
(c) T—A chronic cough resulting from smoking causes increased intra-abdominal pressure and therefore the risk of the patient developing prolapse
(d) T—Straining with constipation also increases intra-abdominal pressure
(e) T—Delivering a large infant can cause trauma to pelvic tissues resulting in prolapse

53. (a) F—In certain situations, such as in the frail elderly patient, conservative options might be more appropriate
(b) T—Hormone replacement therapy may be beneficial in patients with minor degrees of prolapse
(c) F—A ring pessary should be changed every 6–12 months
(d) T—Weight loss should be advised if necessary
(e) T—There is a risk to the pudendal nerve during sacrospinous fixation as it curves around the ischial spine, into which the sacrospinous ligament inserts

54. (a) T—IVF might help these patients, but IUI can be tried first
(b) T—GnRH agonists are given to down-regulate the woman's own hormones
(c) F—IVF is often used in cases of tubal blockage
(d) T—OHSS is a recognized complication of IVF
(e) F—The livebirth rate is 15–20%

55. (a) F—Fertilization occurs 'in vivo'
(b) F—Sperm from the man can be used, but donor sperm is an option
(c) T—Success rates are higher when the woman has had ovulation-inducing drugs
(d) F—No treatment is given to the man prior to collection of the semen sample
(e) F—ICSI success rates are more than double those of IUI, but the complication rate is higher

56. (a) F—A pregnancy occurring after tubal sterilisation is at higher risk of tubal implantation
(b) T
(c) F—Some ectopic pregnancies can be treated with methotrexate
(d) F—This is impossible
(e) T—The background population risk is 1 in 100, after an ectopic the risk is around 1 in 10

57. (a) F—A partial molar pregnancy may contain a fetus (usually non-viable)
(a) T
(a) T—An early scan will lead to diagnosis
(a) F—hCG levels are very high, leading to exaggerated symptoms of pregnancy eg hyperemesis
(a) T—in the instance of the trophoblast behaving in a malignant fashion eg proliferation

58. (a) F—Risk is slightly increased
(b) T—A recognised benefit
(c) F—Risk is trebled
(d) T—A recognised benefit due to relef of atrophic vaginitis
(e) T—Risk is reduced by one third

59. (a) T
(b) F—The climacteric typically lasts for 1 to 5 years
(c) T
(d) F—The average age is 51
(e) F—75-80% suffer from vasomotor symptoms

60. (a) T—Mild symptom relief through alpha receptor blockade
(b) T—Mild symptom relief through the action of isoflavones (compounds with a mild oestrogen like effect)
(c) T—Mild effect by increasing serotonin levels
(d) F—No effect on vasomotor symptoms
(e) F—Makes hot flushes worse

61. (a) F—Even with Mirena there is a very small risk ectopic pregnancy
(b) T—Due to endometrial atrophy
(c) T
(d) F—The Mirena is slightly wider than traditional coils due to its hormone releasing stem
(e) T—Due to the cervical mucus thickening effect of the levonorgestrel preventing ascending infection

62. (a) F—The main mechanism of action is through endometrial suppression
(b) T—There is significant ovulation suppression effect as well as endometrial suppression
(c) T—Profound ovulation suppression
(d) F—Endometrial, cervical mucus and tubal motility effects
(e) F—Obstruction of tubal ostia

63. (a) F—Risk neutral or increased
(b) T—A recognised benefit
(c) T—Through ovulation suppression
(d) T—Effective when taken continuously for mild endometrisis
(e) T—Through suppression of androgen release by ovary

64. (a) T—Due to adrenal hyperandrogenism
    (b) T—Due to oestrogen secreting tumour
    (c) F—Delayed puberty
    (d) F—Delayed puberty
    (e) F—Delayed puberty

65. (a) F—These drugs can cause gynaecomastia in men
    (b) T—Profound virilizing effect as androgenic steroid
    (c) T—Displaces androgens from sex hormone binding globulin and affects hepatic catabolism
    (d) F—No link at all!
    (e) T—Most synthetic progestogens can have androgenic side effects due to stimulation of androgen receptors

66. (a) F—A culture result takes at least 6 days
    (b) T—The miscarriage rate for chorionic villus sampling is 2% compared to 1% for amniocentesis
    (c) F—Some local anaesthetic can be used at the needle site
    (d) T—Prior to this there are insufficient fetal cells in the amniotic fluid
    (e) F—If the twins are in separate sacs, amniocentesis can be performed

67. (a) T
    (b) F—Amniocentesis, fetal blood sampling, and ultrasound for anomaly can be performed into the third trimester
    (c) T—Any procedure that involves a needle passing into the uterus gives a risk of fetomaternal haemorrhage
    (d) F—Ultrasound alone is used for prenatal diagnosis, and does not carry a risk of miscarriage
    (e) F—These techniques allow the genetic material of fetal cells to be examined without culture

68. (a) F—The uterus usually feels large for dates
    (b) T—Diagnosing multiple pregnancy and determining chorionicity is a good indication for a routine 12–14-week scan
    (c) T—The patient may present with hyperemesis gravidarum
    (d) F—Chorionicity should be diagnosed at the end of the first or start of the second trimester
    (e) F—A monochorionic pregnancy needs more surveillance due to the risk of discordant fetal growth caused by shared placentation

69. (a) F—Vaginal delivery is appropriate if twin one is cephalic and the pregnancy is uncomplicated
    (b) T—Continuous CTG is advised as this is a high risk pregnancy
    (c) T—There is an increased risk of postpartum haemorrhage because of the increased size of the placental bed
    (d) F—If twin one is breech presentation, caesarean section is routinely advised
    (e) T—Regional anaesthesia is appropriate to allow assistance with delivery of the second twin, for example, external cephalic version

70. (a) T—The renal capillaries become 'leaky', allowing protein into the urine
    (b) F—Antihypertensive treatment is important to reduce the risk of maternal intracerebral haemorrhage, but it will not reverse the pre-eclampsia disease process
    (c) F—Women with essential hypertension are also prone to pre-eclampsia
    (d) F—Women with pre-eclampsia are at risk of pulmonary oedema secondary to fluid overload, not related to proteinuria
    (e) T—Urinalysis should be performed at every antenatal check

71. (a) F—Breastfeeding is not a contraindication to antihypertensive treatment
    (b) T—Women already on antihypertensives might need to have their medication changed
    (c) F—The neonate does not suffer ill-effects
    (d) T—Hydralazine and labetalol can be given as intravenous bolus or infusion
    (e) T—Blood pressure might not settle with delivery

72. (a) T—The mean cell volume is low
    (b) F—Folate tablets are prescribed
    (c) T—Some doctors give iron and folate tablets routinely throughout multiple pregnancies
    (d) F—Tea contains caffeine, which reduces iron absorption
    (e) T—Plasma expansion means that haemoglobin concentration drops

73. (a) F—The peak flow is unaffected by pregnancy
    (b) T—Salbutamol (Ventolin™) is the most commonly used for acute attacks
    (c) F—Steroids have no effect on fetal growth
    (d) F—Acute attacks in labour are uncommon
    (e) T—Asthma can be treated in the same ways as when not pregnant

74. (a) F—If the TSH is high, hypothyroidism is more likely
    (b) T—Thyroid autoantibodies can result in fetal thyrotoxicosis (in Graves' disease) or fetal hypothyroidism (with maternal autoimmune hypothyroidism)
    (c) F—Thyroxine is safe in pregnancy
    (d) F—Some women develop a goitre as a result of pregnancy, but there is no thyroid disease
    (e) T—Antithyroid drugs are transmitted in breast milk

75. (a) T—An ultrasound scan is used to diagnose placenta praevia
    (b) F—A tender hard uterus is typical of placental abruption
    (c) T—There is an association between placental abruption and pre-eclampsia
    (d) T—Placenta praevia is associated with an abnormal lie
    (e) T—The cardiotocograph may be abnormal in either condition

76. (a) T—Management should always include checking the Rhesus status and giving anti-D if the patient is Rhesus negative
(b) F—A digital vaginal examination is contraindicated in placenta praevia
(c) T—Management should always include a group-and-save sample in case cross-matched blood is needed
(d) F—A cardiotocograph is always advised
(e) T—Urinalysis is indicated if the maternal blood pressure is raised to exclude pre-eclampsia in a patient with a history suggesting placental abruption

77. (a) F—If infection is present it is important to expedite delivery, so tocolysis should not be given.
(b) F—Ritodrine is a β-agonist; β-antagonists are dangerous for asthmatics
(c) F—Some tocolytics are given orally
(d) F—Tocolysis is more likely to increase maternal morbidity, due to side-effects
(e) T—This will be shown on scans as oligohydramnios

78. (a) F—speculum examination is an important part of the clerking
(b) T—infection may precipitate preterm labour
(c) T
(d) T—in the case of cervical incompetence
(e) T

79. (a) T—Most obstetricians would offer external cephalic version as an option in primiparae with no other complicating factors
(b) F—Footling breech is an indication for casarean section because of the high risk of cord prolapse
(c) T—An estimated fetal weight is one of the factors used to decide whether vaginal breech delivery is advisable
(d) F—Erect lateral pelvimetry has been discredited as a useful investigation for assessing pelvic capacity. The pelvic bones are not fixed and allow some expansion to occur (up to 1 cm) and the pelvis is 3-dimensional, which makes 2-dimensional measurements of the pelvic inlet and outlet very limited in the information they give
(e) F—Elective caesarean for breech presentation should not be carried out before 39 weeks to minimize the risk of respiratory distress syndrome occurring

80. (a) F—This is a malposition of the occiput
(b) T
(c) T
(d) F—This is a malposition of the occiput
(e) T

81. (a) F—Rupture of the membranes is not necessary to confirm the onset of labour
(b) T—Labour is diagnosed in the presence of a fully effaced cervix at least 3 cm dilated
(c) F—Progresses on average 1 cm per hour in a primiparous patient
(d) F—Intermittent fetal heart rate monitoring might be sufficient in a low-risk patient
(e) T—The third stage of labour is from delivery of the fetus until delivery of the placenta and membranes

82. (a) T—Baseline observations of maternal temperature, pulse and blood pressure should be recorded
(b) F—The strength of the uterine contractions is assessed by uterine palpation or intrauterine pressure catheter
(c) T—The options for analgesia should be discussed
(d) F—Meconium-stained liquor is an indication for continuous fetal heart rate monitoring since it may be a sign of fetal distress, but it does not necessarily warrant immediate delivery if the fetal monitoring is normal
(e) F—Abdominal palpation is necessary to ensure descent of the head into the maternal pelvis

83. (a) F—An episiotomy should be sutured with an absorbable suture
(b) F—The ventouse cup can be used after 34 weeks gestation
(c) F—The forceps must only be used when the fetal head is 1/5 or 0/5 palpable in the maternal abdomen; if the head is higher than this, then caesarean section is indicated
(d) F—A fetus in the occipitotransverse position is suitable for delivery with the ventouse cup or with Keilland's forceps if the operator is suitably trained
(e) F—A third-degree tear involves the anal sphincter only and not the mucosa

84. (a) F—Carries an increased risk of thromboembolic disease
(b) T—Can be performed under regional anaesthesia
(c) F—Future delivery depends on the indication for the procedure
(d) T—Is performed if the fetus is a breech presentation; this is one of the indications
(e) F—With a trial of scar, vaginal delivery can be achieved in 75% of patients

85. (a) F—0.2% of women develop puerperal psychosis
(b) T—Breastfeeding is safe with tricyclic antidepressants
(c) F—Production of colostrum begins late in pregnancy
(d) T—Flucloxacillin is an appropriate antibiotic for mastitis
(e) T—Retained products of conception must be excluded if the patient presents with postnatal pyrexia

86. (a) T—Uterine atony is the most common cause of primary postpartum haemorrhage
    (b) F—The incidence of postpartum haemorrhage in the developed world is about 5%
    (c) F—An antepartum haemorrhage increases the risk of a postpartum haemorrhage
    (d) T—Syntocinon should be given instead of syntometrine in the patient with hypertension because the hypertension can be exacerbated by the ergometrine component
    (e) F—In some cases, hysterectomy is vital and reduces both maternal mortality and morbidity

87. (a) F—The rate is 1 per 10 000 maternities
    (b) T
    (c) F—Women in the lowest social class are 20 times more likely to die than those in the highest
    (d) T—Multiple pregnancy is a risk factor
    (e) F—Any death following a pregnancy is studied

88. (a) T—Essential in any gynaecological history
    (b) T—Especially when considering the possibility of ectopic pregnancy
    (c) F—Not part of core gynaecological history
    (d) T—Important in conditions such as atrophic vaginitis and endometriosis
    (e) F—Not part of core gynaecology history

89. (a) T—Essential in any obstetric history
    (b) T—Pertains to potential complications in current pregnancy
    (c) T—Serious pelvic injuries can prevent vaginal delivery
    (d) T—It is imperative to establish cardiovascular health in pregnancy
    (e) T—May have great relevance to current pregnancy e.g. History of cervical cone biopsy might predispose to pre term labour

90. (a) T—Suggesting pregnancy
    (b) T—Typically slight dark pv loss although may not be any bleeding
    (c) F—Not an associated symptom
    (d) F—Pain is usually unilateral
    (e) T—Due to diaphragmatic irritation from intra-peritoneal bleeding

91. (a) T—Typical symptom of endometriosis
    (b) F—Pain typically starts before period and lasts beyond period (secondary dysmenorrhoea)
    (c) T—Due to endometriosis in the bladder
    (d) T—The cause of subfertility in 5% of cases
    (e) F—Endometriosis typically causes deep dyspareunia

92. (a) T—Due to hyperandrogenism
    (b) T—As above
    (c) F—Typically causes oligomenorrhoea
    (d) T—Due to insulin resistance
    (e) F—Oestrogen levels are usually normal therefore patients are not predisposed to osteoporosis

93. (a) F—Tea reduces iron absorption
    (b) T—Listeria can be carried by the rind of soft cheese
    (c) F—Fetal alcohol syndrome is a risk when alcohol consumption exceeds 8 units/day
    (d) T—Fluid requirements are higher in pregnancy
    (e) F—A healthy diet should be maintained, and women who are obese should be counselled and referred to the dietitian as obesity increases the risk of complications

94. (a) F—Syphilis cases still occur in the twenty-first century
    (b) F—HIV testing is a confidential, individual decision
    (c) F—Antibodies other than anti-D can develop in pregnancy
    (d) T—Careful counselling is necessary, emphasizing that the test is not diagnostic
    (e) T—Vaccine cannot be given during pregnancy because it is live

95. (a) F—Unless there is a big hydrosalpinx the tubes are not usually palpable
    (b) T—Usually palpable except in very obese women
    (c) F—Not usually palpable
    (d) T—Usually palpable in upper vagina
    (e) F—Not usually palpable unless cervix very patulous

96. (a) T
    (b) T
    (c) T—Symphyseal fundal height +/− 2cms = number of weeks gestation in normally progressing pregnancy
    (d) F—This degree of proteinuria is abnormal and should be investigated for such problems as urinary tract infection and pre eclampsia
    (e) T—Glycosuria may be normal in pregnancy after a heavy glucose load due to a reduced renal threshold due to an increased glomerular filtration rate

97. (a) T—Essential
    (b) T—Essential
    (c) F—The surgeon can look directly down the telescope
    (d) F—Outpatient hysteroscopy under local anaesthesia is possible
    (e) F—No need to catheterise—does not facilitate insertion of telescope

98. (a) T—To introduce CO2 into the peritoneal cavity to avoid injury to organs and facilitate view
    (b) T—To avoid injury to the bladder
    (c) F—Direct insertion of the trocar is possible by dissection under direct vision
    (d) T—Essential port to allow insertion of telescope and instruments
    (e) F—A diathermy is not usually required for diagnostic laparoscopy

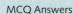

99. (a) F—A full bladder is only required for trans abdominal ultrasound
 (b) F—Not a usual requirement
 (c) T—To allow transmission of sound waves
 (d) F—Procedure does not usually cause discomfort
 (e) F—The procedure relies on sound, not light

100. (a) T—Has typical polypoid appearance
 (b) T—A good way to diagnose and remove a retained IUCD where the threads have disappeared
 (c) T—Typical appearance of multiple synechiae obliterating the uterine cavity
 (d) F—Peritoneal fluid / pleural effusions associated with ovarian cancer
 (e) T—If in sub-mucous position

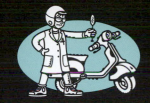

1. (a) Timing in the menstrual cycle. If the patient is midcycle, then sudden onset of unilateral lower abdominal pain might be Mittelschmerz.

(b) Presence of vaginal discharge. A patient who has pelvic inflammatory disease usually presents with generalized lower abdominal pain and vaginal discharge.

(c) Associated nausea and vomiting. A patient with an ovarian torsion commonly presents with a sudden onset of unilateral lower abdominal pain, radiating down the legs, and nausea and vomiting.

(d) Date of the last menstrual period. An ectopic pregnancy must be excluded in the patient who presents with lower abdominal pain.

(e) Presence of deep dyspareunia. A patient who has endometriosis typically presents with chronic pelvic pain, which begins up to 2 weeks before her period starts, and also deep pelvic pain during sexual intercourse.

2. General examination
Cardiovascular and respiratory systems to check fitness for anaesthesia if an operation is considered or if relevant to the patient's medical history

Abdominal palpation
Exclude an abdominal mass which may be the cause of the prolapse. If present, check for organomegaly and ascites

Sims speculum examination
- Left lateral position
- Examine for prolapse of the vaginal walls
- Assess the descent of the cervix

Bimanual palpation
- Assess uterine size and mobility
- Exclude adnexal masses

3. For the woman:
- Serum progesterone, sent 7 days before the next period is due.
- Rubella antibodies—so that vaccination can be given if necessary.
- Ultrasound scan—to look at the structure of uterus and ovaries.
- Chlamydia testing—in the form of serum or urine ELISA or swabs.

For the man:
- Semen analysis on at least two occasions.

Other investigations would only be arranged if the history or examination in the clinic suggested a particular underlying diagnosis.

4. Placenta praevia
History: bleeding.
Examination: soft uterus, presenting part of the fetus high, fetal lie might be abnormal, fetal heart beat present.
Investigation: full blood count, group-and-save and possibly cross-match blood, cardiotocograph, ultrasound scan.

Placental abruption
History: might or might not be bleeding, constant abdominal pain, uterine contractions, loss of fetal movements.
Examination: hard tender uterus, uterine contractions, unable to distinguish fetal parts, absent fetal heart.
Investigation: full blood count, group-and-save and possibly cross-match, cardiotocograph.

5. Relevant factors in the maternal history
(a) Previous history of intrauterine growth restriction.
(b) Maternal disease prior to pregnancy.
(c) Smoking.
(d) Ethnicity.
(e) Illicit drug use.

Investigations indicated for a small-for-dates fetus
(a) Ultrasound assessment of liquor volume.
(b) Doppler studies of the umbilical artery.
(c) Cardiotocography.
(d) Fetal chromosome analysis.
(e) Maternal serum testing for intrauterine infection.

6. Possible causes of pain are:
- Labour.
- Placental abruption.
- Symphysis pubis dysfunction.
- Ligament pain.
- Pre-eclampsia/HELLP syndrome.
- Acute fatty liver of pregnancy.

The following information needs to be obtained to distinguish between these:

- History of the pain: intermittent suggests labour; constant occurs with placental abruption; right upper quadrant or epigastric occurs with pre-eclampsia or acute fatty liver; suprapubic pain suggests symphysis pubis dysfunction
- Associated symptoms: PV bleeding is seen with abruption; nausea and vomiting associated with acute fatty liver, as well as pre-eclampsia, when there may also be cerebral symptoms such as headache or blurred vision
- Examination: general observations; abdominal palpation for site of tenderness, to exclude uterine contractions and to check fetal presentation and lie; speculum examination if there is bleeding and vaginal examination to exclude cervical change
- Investigations: blood tests if there is bleeding or if there is hypertension to exclude pre-eclampsia; urinalysis with hypertension; ultrasound scan

7. (a) Baseline rate 110-160 beats per minute
   (b) Baseline variability ≥5 beats per minute
   (c) Presence of accelerations
   (d) Absence of decelerations

8. Haemoglobin to exclude intraperitoneal bleeding, for example, from a ruptured corpus luteal cyst or a ruptured ectopic pregnancy, or to give a baseline level.

White blood cell count if infection is suspected in the differential diagnoses, for example, pelvic inflammatory disease or appendicitis.

Urine pregnancy test and/or serum β-hCG level to exclude miscarriage or ectopic pregnancy.

Pelvic ultrasound scan to diagnose an ovarian cyst and examine the nature, size and echogenicity of the cyst. Scan will also exclude fibroids and examine for a pregnancy if suspected.

Serum CA 125 level, chest X ray, intravenous urogram if malignancy is suspected.

9. She may have an endometrial polyp, or an endometrial carcinoma. The next step is to visualize the uterine cavity and obtain a histology sample. Hysteroscopy may be performed under local, regional or general anaesthetic and a biopsy could be taken either under direct vision or with a pipelle sample in combination with saline hysterography.

10. Short term
- pelvic abscess formation
- septicaemia
- septic shock

Long term
- infertility
- ectopic pregnancy
- chronic pelvic pain
- dyspareunia
- menstrual disturbances
- psychological effects

11. Follow-up is co-ordinated by the nearest specialist centre and consists of monitoring hCG levels by testing blood or urine. Initially blood samples are sent every 2 weeks. Once the hcg levels are back to normal, monthly urine samples are sent. If the levels normalized within 8 weeks after the end of the pregnancy, follow-up is for 6 months. If it took longer than 8 weeks, follow-up is for 2 years. Chemotherapy is advised if levels do not fall, or if hCG starts to rise again within the follow-up period.

Women are advised not to conceive again until levels have been normal for 6 months because there is a worry that a pregnancy soon after the mole will heighten the risk of malignant change. Hormonal contraceptives are not advisable.

Possible answers:
- Previous ectopic pregnancy
- Past history of PID, peritonitis, abdominal surgery, tubal surgery (including sterilization and it's reversal), endometriosis
- Conception with IUCD in situ

- IVF pregnancy
- Conceived whilst on the progestogen-only pill

12. 400 microgrammes of folic acid daily taken prior to conception and for the first 12 weeks of pregnancy reduces the risk of the fetus having a neural tube defect. Women who have had a previous child with a neural tube defect and those who suffer from epilepsy should take a higher dose of folic acid (5mg daily) due to the higher risk. Ultrasound is the best test for identifying neural tube defects.

13. • Congenital fetal malformations.
- Preterm labour.
- Pregnancy induced hypertension or pre-eclampsia.
- Antepartum haemorrhage.
- Intrauterine growth restriction.
- Twin-to twin transfusion syndrome.

14. She must be seen regularly for blood pressure checks, urinalysis and palpation to check for fetal growth, which should also be monitored by ultrasound after 28 weeks. Her pre-existing hypertension means that there is an increased risk of intrauterine growth retardation, which will be detected with serial scans, and of pre-eclampsia, which may cause raised blood pressure and proteinuria.

15. • High number of pregnancies
- Short gaps between pregnancies, especially if breastfeeding
- History of menorrhagia
- Poor diet
- High tea intake
- Anaemia prior to pregnancy
- Multiple pregnancy

16. Possible answers:

Ritodrine
Side-effects: Nausea and vomiting
Flushing and sweating
Tremor and tachycardia
Palpitations
Hypotension
Pulmonary oedema

Nifedipine
Side-effects: Headache
Flushing
Dizziness
Tachycardia
Palpitations

Indomethacin
Side-effects: Gastrointestinal disturbance eg diarrhoea and nausea
Headache
Dizziness
Gastrointestinal bleeding
Rash
Renal failure with pre-existing renal impairment

Atosiban
Side-effects: Flushing
Headache
Nausea
Palpitations

17. Prescribe treatment for itching eg piriton, UDCA. See for regular monitoring of fetal condition eg scans and CTGs. Start oral Vitamin K supplements at 36 weeks and recommend that the baby has IM Vitamin K at delivery. Advise her to watch fetal movements very carefully and consider induction of labour at term, as there is an increased risk of stillbirth. Counsel her that she is at risk of the same condition in her next pregnancy.

18. Maternal
Delay in 2nd stage due to maternal exhaustion.

Fetal
Delay in 2nd stage due to fetal malposition (occipito-posterior or occipito-transverse position).
Abnormal CTG.

Forceps can be performed without maternal effort or adequate contractions, for example if the mother is unconscious, or if a medical condition such as a cardiovascular disorder prevents her from pushing. It is also appropriate if the fetus is at risk of having an undiagnosed bleeding disorder such that the ventouse may precipitate bleeding. Other uses include:

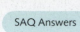

- Gestation less than 34 weeks.
- Face presentation.
- After-coming head of a breech.
- At caesarean section.

19. Thromboembolic disease. Risk factors include: previous thromboembolism, grandparity, age >35 years, immobility, significant concurrent illness, emergency caesarean section, obesity >90 kg, multiple pregnancy.

20. Miscarriage and intrauterine death are more common with opiate use, and intrauterine growth retardation is part of the spectrum. Smoking is another risk factor for IUGR. Hepatitis B, C and HIV are prevalent in the drug using population (although she is smoking heroin, she may have injected in the past, or had unprotected intercourse with an infected man). Ecstasy is associated with congenital anomalies.

Initially she should be fully counseled and offered screening for hepatitis and HIV. A careful anomaly scan will be performed at 20 weeks. Fetal growth should be monitored regularly from 24 weeks. Liaison with the paediatricians is important as the baby will go through withdrawal after delivery.

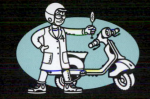

EMQ Answers

1. Theme: Abnormal Bleeding

1. Endometriosis (b)
   One of the classic ways in which endometriosis presents is with increasingly heavy and painful periods. The pain typically commences before the period and/or lasts for a few days after the period (secondary dysmenorrhoea).
2. Cervical Carcinoma (f)
   Cervical carcinoma typically presents with painless post-coital bleeding and is particularly likely in this age group.
3. Pelvic Inflammatory Disease (PID) (a)
   Lower abdominal pain and tenderness (typically bilateral) associated with a temperature and vaginal discharge are commonly due to PID.
4. Fibroids (i)
   A bulky uterus in this age group associated with heavy periods is often due to uterine enlargement secondary to fibroids.
5. Hypothyroidism (h)
   This must not be forgotten as a possible medical cause of menorrhagia, particularly in the perimenopausal era. Two of the commonest symptoms are increasing tiredness and weight gain.

2. Theme: Pelvic Pain and Dyspareunia

1. Chlamydia infection (b)
2. Ovarian torsion (d)
3. Acute appendicitis (i)
4. Endometriosis (a)
5. Pelvic tuberculosis (j)

3. Theme: Vaginal Discharge

1. *Candida albicans* (a)
2. *Cervical carcinoma* (d)
3. *Vesicovaginal fistula* (e)
4. *Chlamydia trachomatis* (i)
5. *Bacterial vaginosis* (f)

4. Theme: Subfertility

1. Pelvic inflammatory disease (f)
   PID has caused hydrosalpinges and bilateral tubal occlusion
2. Polycystic ovary syndrome (a)
   The progesterone level indicates anovulation, and the raised LH:FSH ratio points to PCOS as the cause of anovulation.
3. Anorexia nervosa (d)
   The progesterone level indicates anovulation
4. Obstructive azoospermia (c)
   The testes are producing sperm but they are not passing into the seminal fluid, due to obstruction or absence of the vas, or obstruction of the epididymis.
5. Klinefelter's syndrome (b)
   Men who are XXY have small soft testes which do not produce sperm.

5. Theme: Bleeding in the Second and Third Trimesters of Pregnancy

1. Ectopic pregnancy (b)
2. Uterine atony (i)
3. Molar pregnancy (a)
4. Placental abruption (e)
5. Vaginal tear (h)

6. Theme: Abdominal Pain in the Second and Third Trimesters of Pregnancy

1. Placental abruption (d)
2. Urinary tract infection (h)
3. Preterm labour (j)
4. Fibroid degeneration (a)
5. Pre-eclampsia (g)

7. Theme: Stillbirth

1. 47XY (g)
   A normal karyotype is 46XX or 46XY. This analysis shows 47XY, indicating that the fetus is male and has an extra chromosome—trisomy 21 is seen in Down's syndrome.

2. Protein = 5.1g/l (f)
   Proteinuria of greater than 0.3g/l is significant and can point to a diagnosis of pre-eclampsia.
3. Parvovirus IgM positive, IgG negative
   Parvovirus infection can pass across the placenta and cause fetal cardiac failure (leading to hydrops) and fetal death. Positive IgM and negative IgG confirms recent infection. (d)
4. ALT= 60iu/l (a)
   Transaminases are often raised in cholestasis, as are bile acids. However, the levels of liver function tests alone do not make the diagnosis, which must also be based on the clinical picture and the absence of hepatitis.
5. Fetal anaemia and positive Coombs test
   Rhesus disease causes fetal haemolysis, and therefore anaemia. Coombs test proves the presence of antibodies. (c)
6. HbA1c = 15% (b)
   This level of glycosylated haemoglobin indicates poor control, which predisposes to congenital anomalies and intrauterine death.

8. Theme: Failure to Progress in Labour

1. Fetal macrosomia (d)
2. Irregular contractions (e)
3. Cervical fibroid (a)
4. Transverse lie (i)
5. Persistent OP position (b)

9. Theme: Maternal Collapse

1. Uterine atony (a)
   A long labour, the need for syntocinon augmentation and a big baby all predispose to poor uterine contraction after delivery leading to post-partum haemorrhage.
2. Postural hypotension (c)
   This multipara is predisposed to anaemia, which will have been exacerbated by her blood loss at caesarean section. The standing up has led to her fainting.
3. Pulmonary embolism (e)
   Pregnancy, obesity and immobility are all risk factors for thromboembolic disease.

4. Sepsis (h)
   This woman has developed chorioamnionitis, with infection ascending up and around the baby, producing a systemic illness. She needs antibiotic treatment and delivery.
5. Eclampsia (g)
   Hypertension and proteinuria raise suspicion of pre-eclampsia, which can rapidly deteriorate into an eclamptic episode. Fits in pregnancy, even in those previously labeled epileptic, should always be suspected of being related to pre-eclampsia.

10. Theme: Urinary Incontinence

1. Genuine Stress Incontinence (c)
   It is essential that urodynamic investigations have been performed to exclude detrusor overactivity as a cause of incontinence during laughing, sneezing etc.
2. Urinary tract infection (b)
   Symptoms of frequency, dysuria and nocturia are often due to a urinary tract infection and this diagnosis is supported by presence of protein in the urine.
3. Idiopathic detrusor overactivity (d)
   Symptoms of urgency, nocturia and urge incontinence in this age group are often due to detrusor overactivity – the diagnosis should be confirmed with urodynamics.
4. Fistula (g)
   This is a recognised complication of prolonged obstructed labour and leads to continuous incontinence due to the presence of a urinary fistula, often connecting to the vagina. It is a particular problem in Somalia where women often have to walk miles to reach the nearest hospital.
5. Detrusor Overactivity (DO) due to menopause (j)
   DO symptoms are common in the menopause due to deterioration the collagen in the urethra and bladder from oestrogen deficiency.

Glossary

ABC	airways, breathing, circulation		GnRH	gonadotrophin-releasing hormone
AC	abdominal circumference		GSI	genuine stress incontinence
AFE	amniotic fluid embolism		HbA1c	glycosylated haemoglobin
AFI	amniotic fluid index		HC	head circumference
ALT	alanine transaminase		hCG	human chorionic gonadotrophin
APH	antepartum haemorrhage		HELLP	hypertension, elevated liver enzymes, low platelets
APTT	activated partial thromboplastin time		HFEA	Human Fertilization and Embryology Authority
ARDS	adult respiratory distress syndrome			
ARM	artificial rupture of the membranes		hMG	human menopausal gonadotrophin
AST	aspartate transaminase		HPV	human papilloma virus
AZT	zidovudine		HRT	hormone replacement therapy
BMI	body mass index		HSG	hysterosalpingogram
BPD	biparietal diameter		HyCoSy	hysterosalpingo contrast sonography
bpm	beats per minute		ICSI	intracytoplasmic sperm injection
BSO	bilateral salpingo-oophrectomy		Ig	immunoglobulin
CAH	congenital adrenal hyperplasia		IMB	intermenstrual bleeding
CEMD	Confidential Enquiries into Maternal Deaths		IUGR	intrauterine growth restriction
			IUI	intrauterine insemination
CIN	cervical intraepithelial neoplasia		IVF	in vitro fertilization
CNS	central nervous system		IVU	intravenous urogram
COCP	combined oral contraceptive pill		JVP	jugular venous pressure
CPD	cephalopelvic disproportion		LFD	large for dates
CRL	crown–rump length		LH	luteinizing hormone
CT	computed tomography		LLETZ	large loop excision of the transformation zone
CTG	cardiotocograph			
CVS	chorionic villus sampling		LMP	last menstrual period
CXR	chest X-ray		LMWH	low molecular weight heparin
D&C	dilatation and curettage		LSCS	lower segment caesarean section
DEXA	dual energy X-ray absorptiometry		MAP	mean arterial pressure
DHEAS	dehydroepiandrosterone sulphate		MBL	menstrual blood loss
DI	donor insemination		MI	myocardial infarction
DO	detrusor overactivity		MRI	magnetic resonance imaging
DIC	disseminated intravascular coagulation		MS	multiple sclerosis
DUB	dysfunctional uterine bleeding		MSU	midstream urine
DVT	deep vein thrombosis		NSAID	non-steroidal anti-inflammatory drug
ECG	electrocardiogram		NSU	non-specific urethritis
ECT	electroconvulsive therapy		OHSS	ovarian hyperstimulation syndrome
ECV	external cephalic version		OP	occipitoposterior
EFW	estimated fetal weight		OT	occipitotransverse
ERPC	evacuation of the retained products of conception		PCB	postcoital bleeding
			PCOS	polycystic ovary syndrome
FBC	full blood count		PCR	polymerase chain reaction
FBS	fetal blood sampling		PE	pulmonary embolism
FHR	fetal heart rate		PGD	pre-implantation genetic diagnosis
FISH	fluorescent in situ hybridization		PID	pelvic inflammatory disease
FSH	follicle stimulating hormone			

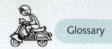

PIH	pregnancy-induced hypertension	TENS	transcutaneous electrical nerve stimulation
PMB	postmenopausal bleeding		
PMS	premenstrual syndrome	TOP	termination of pregnancy
PPH	postpartum haemorrhage	TSH	thyroid stimulating hormone
PV	per vagina	TTTS	twin-to-twin transfusion syndrome
SERM	selective oestrogen receptor modulator	TURP	transurethral resection of the prostate
SFD	small for dates	TVT	tension-free vaginal tape
SGA	small for gestational age	UDCA	ursodeoxycholic acid
SHBG	sex hormone binding globulin	USS	ultrasound scan
SLE	systemic lupus erythematosus	UTI	urinary tract infection
SSRI	selective serotonin reuptake inhibitor	VCU	videocystourethrography
STD	sexually transmitted disease	VIN	vulval intraepithelial neoplasia
TAH	total abdominal hysterectomy	V/Q	ventilation perfusion isotope (scan)
TCRE	transcervical resection of endometrium	WBC	white blood cell count
TED	thromboembolic disease		

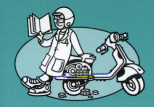

Index

Page numbers in **bold** refer to figures or tables.